Teaching Students

with Mild Disabilities

Teaching Students

with Mild Disabilities

Tom E. C. Smith

David M. Finn

Carol A. Dowdy

Harcourt Brace Jovanovich College Publishers

Fort Worth   Philadelphia   San Diego   New York   Orlando   Austin   San Antonio
Toronto   Montreal   London   Sydney   Tokyo

Publisher:	*Ted Buchholz*
Acquisitions Editor:	*Jo-Anne Weaver*
Project Editor:	*Nancy Lombardi*
Book Designer:	*Nick Welch*
Production Manager:	*Cynthia Young*
Cover:	*photograph by Skeeter Hagler*

Address for Editorial Correspondence:
Harcourt Brace Jovanovich, Inc., 301 Commerce Street, Suite 3700, Fort Worth, TX 76102.

Address for Orders:
Harcourt Brace Jovanovich, Inc., 6277 Sea Harbor Drive, Orlando, FL 32887.
1-800-782-4479, or 1-800-433-0001 (in Florida).

Table and figure credits appear on pages 499–500 which constitute a continuation of the copyright page

ISBN: 0-03-047519-8

Library of Congress Card Catalog Number 92-70786

Printed in the United States of America

2 3 4 5 6 7 8 9 0 1   0 3 9   9 8 7 6 5 4 3 2 1

To
Bonnie, Jake, Alex
Jim, Cameron, Meredith
Edward, and Elizabeth Finn

PREFACE

Students with mild disabilities are currently being served in public schools more effectively than ever before. Thanks to federal and state legislation, litigation, parental and professional advocacy, and more effectively trained teachers, students with disabilities are more likely to realize a free appropriate public education. Still there exists room for improvement and better programming. Developing and implementing intervention programs based solely on clinical labels may result in some students receiving inappropriate programs. This text helps prepare special education teachers to implement effective intervention programs for students with mild disabilities.

The authors of this textbook believe in certain tenants of categorical services, noncategorical services, and the regular education initiative. We do not view the solution to providing the best possible services to children with disabilities as simple. The primary premise we utilize in determining appropriate programming for these students is individualization. We adhere to the principle that all children differ from each other, that all children have individual strengths and weaknesses, and that no two children learn the same way or need the same intervention strategies.

It is our opinion that students' programs should not be dictated by categorical labels. Yet at the same time, we believe that many students within particular traditional categories do benefit from similar programs. Our viewpoint is that while clinical categories can give ideas related to appropriate programs, they cannot and should not be considered the single most important factor considered in developing programs.

The most important factors in developing and implementing programs are individual strengths and weaknesses. We advocate comprehensive assessment of students with special focus on future-based assessment. Future-based assessment projects the likely futures of individual students in the areas of post-secondary training, living options, and social skills. Once these general goals are established and the skills necessary for success are established, a comparison is made between necessary skills for success and current functioning. From the discrepancy determined in the comparison comes the individual education program for the student.

Chapters in this textbook will detail the methods used to develop and implement programs for students with mild disabilities. The key in developing such programs is to consider each student on an individual basis, not on the basis of clinical or categorical label. In elementary grades, it is likely that students who are considered mildly disabled, will need to and can benefit from similar intervention programs. Intervention strategies in reading, math, written expression, and other basic skills are similar for most young elementary children with learning problems. The similarity of program needs will likely become less as students matriculate through public school programs.

By the time students with disabilities enter middle school and high school, more focus has to be placed on the students' futures. A determination needs to be made as soon as possible regarding whether or not a student has the potential and motivation to attend post-secondary educational programs, has the potential for independent living, and will be capable of getting along with peers and assimilating into a community setting. Based on these assertions, programs of intervention need to be developed that will truly individualize training and facilitate a successful transition from school to post-secondary school environments.

The content of this textbook is related to instructionally relevant learner characteristics. For example, information provided about teaching strategies for students with disabilities will be related to the characteristics of individual students, not to a clinical label that may be thought of when discussing the strategies approach. There may be instances when students with the same categorical label need the same intervention strategy, but there will also be times when students with the same label need significantly diverse interventions. Likewise, some students with different categorical classifications will benefit from similar instructional strategies, while others will need diverse approaches.

Our primary philososphy, as previously noted, is to provide whatever instructional program is needed to students with disabilities, regardless of clinical classification. If the bureaucratic system requires schools to use categorical groups to determine eligibility, then schools must go beyond this initial classification to determine appropriate educational programs. The simple statement, "base educational interventions on the unique needs of each child" is the framework of the textbook.

ACKNOWLEDGMENTS

We would like to gratefully acknowledge several individuals who were instrumental in the development of this textbook. Foremost is our appreciation for our families who consistently supported our long hours of writing, rewriting, and rewriting. Thank-yous also go to Mel Knight, Arleen Lewis, Judy Johnson, and Wes Shafner, who helped with photographs. Thanks also go to the editorial and production staff at Harcourt Brace Jovanovich, especially to Ms. Jo-Anne Weaver, our editor and primary source of encouragement. We would also like to thank Ms. Daphnie Beaman, whose secretarial and editorial support made the process move much more efficiently than would have been possible without her. And finally, a word of thanks to the numerous reviewers who provided suggestions that made the text significantly better. These individuals included: Scott Sparks, Ohio University; Virginia Brown, Quincy College; Stan Morris, McNeese State; Edward Shultz, University of Maine-Farmington; Tom Lovitt, University of Washington; Belinda Dunnick Karge, San Diego State University; John Miazga, Angelo State University; Dona Icabone, Western Michigan University; and Doris Williams, Indiana State University

Contents

Teaching Students

with Mild Disabilities

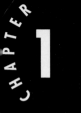

Introduction

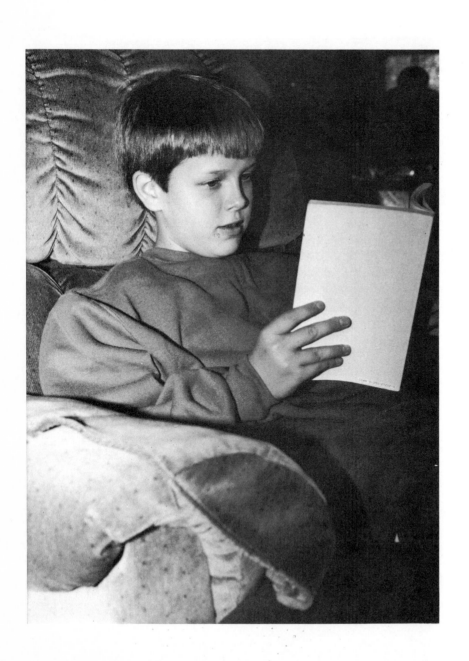

Outline

Introduction

Services for Children with Disabilities
Historical Overview
Current Special Education Services
Status of Services to Children with
Disabilities
Parental Involvement
Multicultural Special Education

Classification of Disabilities
Categorical Classification System
Noncategorical or Generic
Classification System

Current Service Delivery Models
Integrated Services
Typical Services in the 1990s

Current Developments in Services for
Students with Mild Disabilities
The Regular Education Initiative
Consultation/Collaboration Model
Transition Programming

Outline of the Textbook

OBJECTIVES

After reading this chapter, you will be able to:

- define special education;

- define disabled children;

- describe the historical treatment of persons
  with disabilities;

- discuss the role of the civil rights movement
  to special education;

- describe the major components of Public Law
  94-142;

- list the changes in Public Law 94-142 made
  by the Individuals with Disabilities
  Education Act (IDEA);

- define the major categories of disabilities
  served in special education programs;

- discuss the noncategorical approach to services;

- discuss the major service delivery approaches
  used in special education today;

- define the regular education initiative;

- discuss the transition movement.

Introduction

Public education in the United States has been a reality for most citizens for nearly one hundred years. In fact, the provision of twelve years of a free public education is frequently taken for granted here. Not only is this education provided without charge, but by most standards, it is is of very high quality. Although the public education system in this country has come under major criticisms since the late 1970s, overall the system is extremely sound. There is no other country that provides such a high quality of education to its citizens, rich or poor, capable or not capable, as does the United States (Smith, 1990).

Although the availability of a free, quality public education has been expected for the majority of citizens during the twentieth century, not all children have had equal access to these programs. In the 1950s, members of racial minorities began demanding their right to equal public educational opportunities. The result, after many years of struggle, was the Civil Rights Act and integrated schools. Still another group of children who were frequently denied equal access to public educational programs were those who differed from the majority of students either physically, sensorially, or mentally, to such an extent that special education programs were necessary. This group of children, frequently classified as handicapped or disabled, has recently secured their right to equal educational opportunities through litigation and legislation (Smith, Price, & Marsh, 1986).

The result of the movement to secure the rights of children with disabilities to equal educational opportunities was a major expansion of special education services. Special education can be described as instruction that is designed to meet the unique needs of students who differ from other children in ways that require specialized methods and materials. It includes assessment, placement, instruction, and evaluation (Ysseldyke & Algozzine, 1990). Some children with various types of problems need special education services in order to receive an appropriate education.

There are several terms that are used to describe children served through special education programs. The terms most often used include exceptional, handicapped, disabled, and impaired. Exceptional children can be defined as "those who require special education and related services if they are to realize their full human potential." (Hallhan & Kauffman, 1991, p. 6) Handicapped is the term that was used by the federal government in legislation that mandated services, and is therefore used in many states. The term handicapped can be defined as having one of several identified conditions, such as mental retardation, learning disabilities, emotional disturbance, visual impairment, hearing impairment, orthopedic impairment, traumatic brain injury, autism, or other health impairment.

An impairment is generally associated with a physical, mental, or medical problem. For example, if something is wrong with a person's vision, it could be referred to as a visual impairment. The term disability is the most functional of the terms used to describe atypical individuals. Disability results from an impairment; it is the manifestation of the impairment. For example, a visually impaired person may be disabled related to driving a car, but the visual problem may not result in a disability in the area of listening to a lecture and remembering what was said. Disabilities, therefore, are the manifested results of impairments or handicaps. There is generally a positive correlation between the level of disability and the degree of handicap. For example, although not always the case, more significant disabilities usually result in more severe handicaps.

Individuals classified with these terms would prefer not to be labeled. Unfortunately, the current system of services requires the classification of individuals with clinical labels before services can be provided. Children are not allowed to access special education and related services from schools unless they are determined to be eligible based on specific criteria associated with different handicapping conditions. Since labels must be used, they should be applied in a manner that results in the least negative stigma. For the most part, individuals who are classified prefer the label "disabled." The most normalizing manner of referring to these individuals is to say "person with a disability." This places the "disability" in proper perspective. First there is the person, a regular person. It just so happens that the person has some type of disability. Recently the federal government adopted "disability" as the preferred label (National Association of State Directors of Special Education, 1990).

Public schools are now required to provide children with disabilities a free, appropriate education. This mandate resulted from Public Law 94–142, the Education for All Handicapped Children Act, passed in 1975. Prior to this federal legislation, some schools provided appropriate programs for students with disabilities, but many others did not. This legislation has been reinforced and expanded by litigation. Schools are now required to provide educational services to children with disabilities in the most normal setting appropriate. This means that regular classroom teachers must share the responsibility of educating these children with special education teachers.

A key element in providing appropriate educational services to students with disabilities is parental involvement. Public Law 94–142 mandated that schools involve parents in each step of the educational process. Schools must now inform parents of their intentions for children in special education programs, as well as invite parents to participate in the decision-making process. Parents must have the opportunity to be full partners in the education of their children with disabilities.

Services for Children with Disabilities

HISTORICAL OVERVIEW

Persons with disabilities have not always received appropriate services. In the Greek city-states of Sparta and Athens, individuals with disabilities were either killed or allowed to die. Later, disabled persons were used as court fools and jesters to entertain royalty and their guests. In the Middle Ages, various churches began providing services to persons with disabilities. Although these were simply providing the basic necessities of life, and did not result in any educational or habilitative programs, it was a positive step for this group of individuals. From this early effort evolved the multitude of services that currently are available for this population (Smith, Price, & Marsh, 1986).

Even in the United States, appropriate educational services for children with disabilities have only recently been available. Dunn (1973) noted that even with compulsory school attendance laws, local public schools avoided serving students with disabilities. Many were institutionalized, some laws were passed to exclude students with disabilities from school, and day schools were developed to provide services outside the school. As recent as the early 1970s, public school services for children with disabilities were limited. Before Congress passed Public Law 94–142, the Education for All Handicapped Children Act, in 1975, they found that of the eight million school-age children with disabilities, four million were receiving inadequate services, while as many as one million were totally denied educational programs in public schools.

While some of the special education programs that were available prior to the passage of Public Law 94–142 were meeting the needs of students with disabilities, many could be characterized as isolated. Most programs were in self-contained classrooms or other segregated facilities. There was limited interaction between special education students, special education teachers, and students and teachers in regular educational programs. The result was that students served in special education programs were stigmatized and separated from the rest of their peers. Even more disturbing, prior to the passage of Public Law 94–142 many children were simply denied services by public schools. Principals used the excuses that there were no teachers at the school trained to serve a particular type of child or that there was not enough money to support programs for certain children. In view of this resistance, many parents simply kept their children at home or enrolled them in private day schools or institutions.

CURRENT SPECIAL EDUCATION SERVICES

The passage of Public Law 94–142, subsequent amendments to the law, and litigation that has helped interpret the law, have all resulted in a major overhaul of our educational system for children with disabilities. None of these actions came easily. In fact, the passage of Public Law 94–142 was the result of significant efforts on the part of parent advocacy groups and professionals. Forces that led to the passage of this act included the civil rights movement, parent advocacy groups, professional advocacy, litigation, and federal and state legislation (Smith et al., 1986).

The Civil Rights Movement

Although not thought of as a movement that affected services for children with disabilities, the civil rights movement had a strong influence on parents of these children. During the 1950s, parents of black children went to court and lobbied state and federal legislative bodies for equal educational opportunities. The *Brown v. Board of Education* court case in 1954 and the subsequent civil rights legislation passed in the 1960s laid to rest the question of whether or not racial minority children had a legal right to equal educational opportunities. Parents of children with disabilities observed the success of the Civil Rights movement and used it as a blueprint for their own activism.

Parent and Professional Advocacy Groups

Parents acting alone for their children had limited power to effect change. However, as members of advocacy groups, their power increased substantially. Parent advocacy groups for children with disabilities began to exert themselves in the 1970s. Groups such as the National Association for Retarded Citizens (formerly the National Association for Retarded Children), the United Cerebral Palsy Association, and the Association for Children with Learning Disabilities were the leaders that brought pressure to bear in the courts and in Congress and state legislatures (Salend, 1990).

In addition to parents advocating for children with disabilities, various professional groups also rallied to support equal educational opportunities for these children. The foremost group was the Council for Exceptional Children (CEC), established in 1922. For many years CEC was a unit in the National Education Association, but in 1974 it became an independent organization. CEC and its different divisions have become an extremely powerful advocacy for children with disabilities; it currently has approximately 55,000 members nationwide (Hallahan & Kauffman, 1988). Primarily composed of special education teachers and university personnel, CEC worked closely with Congress to write the legislation necessary to secure equal educational opportunities for children with special needs and lobbied strongly for its passage.

Litigation

Parent advocacy groups, modeling the tactics of groups seeking racial equality in the 1960s, began taking their cause to the courts. Several landmark court cases during the early 1970s proved to be the beginning of litigation that resulted in right to education rulings. The success of the civil rights activists in the *Brown* case showed special education advocacy groups that the courts could pave the way for improved services.

The first case of national significance was *PARC v. Pennsylvania* (1973). In this case, the Pennsylvania Association for Retarded Citizens (PARC) filed suit on behalf of several children classified as mentally retarded who were seeking equal access to public education. In a consent decree approved by the court, Pennsylvania agreed to provide appropriate services to children classified as mentally retarded.

Following the *PARC* case was *Mills v. Board of Education, District of Columbia*. In this case, the court ruled that children with disabilities had a right to equal access to educational programs. Furthermore, the court ruled that schools could not use limited financial resources as an excuse for not providing these services. These two cases were quickly followed by many more that supported the right to education for this group of children. In addition to *PARC* and *Mills*, there have been numerous court cases that have helped interpret Public Law 94–142. Table 1–1 (pages 8–9) briefly summarizes several of these cases.

Federal and State Legislation

Several legislative acts passed in the late 1960s and early 1970s laid the ground work for the passage of the Education for Handicapped Children Act. Two of the more important acts were Section 504 of the Rehabilitation Act of 1973, and Public Law 93–380. Section 504 of the Rehabilitation Act of 1973 was basic civil rights legislation for persons with disabilities. The section prohibited discrimination toward persons in employment, housing, and public transportation based on disability. It afforded protections for all persons considered disabled, regardless of age. Public Law 93–380 was passed in 1973. This law contained many of the provisions of Public Law 94–142, but it did not include funds to support their implementation. Still, this act is considered the immediate predecessor to the Education for All Handicapped Children Act.

TABLE 1-1 Summary of Significant Court Cases

CASE	SUMMARY
PARC v. Pennsylvania 1971	Filed by the Pennsylvania Association for Retarded Citizens on behalf of all children with mental retardation in Pennsylvania.
	Sought equal educational opportunities for students with mental retardation.
	Consent decree resulted in students with mental retardation in Pennsylvania being afforded appropriate educational programs.
Mills v. Board of Education	Filed by parents of students with mental retardation to gain access to public education programs.
	Ruling in favor of parents resulting in access to educational programs for students with mental retardation and other disabilities.
	Court ruled that schools could not use limited finances as a reason for denying programs to students with disabilities.
Diana v. State Board of Education 1970	Filed by parents of Spanish-speaking students to challenge placement in classes for students with educable mental retardation.
	Resulted in ruling against discriminatory testing.
	Mexican-American and Chinese students were to be tested in their native language for eligibility for special education.
Larry P. v. Riles 1977	Filed on behalf of black children in California who had been placed in classes for students labeled educable mentally retarded to challenge testing procedures.
	Resulted in the requirement to 1. stop using standardized IQ tests to place black students in classes for mentally retarded children; 2. eliminate disproportionate number of black children in EMR classes; and 3. retest every black student in EMR classes to determine appropriate placement.
Armstrong v. Kline 1979	Filed by parents of a student with disabilities denied summer programming.
	Directly challenged Pennsylvania's law prohibiting funding educational programs beyond 180 days per year.
	Ruling found in favor of parents and required schools to provide extended school year programs (summer programs) to students with disabilities who would regress significantly without summer programs.

continued

TABLE 1-1 Summary of Significant Court Cases (cont'd.)

CASE	SUMMARY
Board of Education v. Henrick Hudson Central School District Board of Education 1983	Parents of a student with hearing impairment filed suit requesting an interpreter.
	First case dealing with Public Law 94-142 to reach U.S. Supreme Court.
	U.S. Supreme Court overturned all previous rulings and stated that Public Law 94-142 requires schools to provide an appropriate education to students with disabilities, not an educational program to maximize the education for these students.

Public Law 94–142 has proven to be a great success. The law has resulted in appropriate services for many children with disabilities who had previously been unserved, or who were receiving inappropriate services. In 1986 Madeline Will, then Assistant Secretary for the Department of Education and head of the Office of Special Education and Rehabilitation Services, concluded that ten years of Public Law 94–142 had:

- redefined the concept and practice of individualized instruction;
- redefined the role of parents in the education of the child;
- made education possible for 500,000 children previously unserved;
- improved services for several million children with disabilities (411–412).

There is no doubt that the passage of Public Law 94–142 had an enormous impact on the education of children with disabilities. Not only did the number of children served increase significantly, but the services became more individualized and were provided in regular classrooms as much as possible. Succinctly stated, Public Law 94–142 mandated a free appropriate public education for all school-age children with disabilities. It also gave parents legal rights to be active partners in the planning and implementation of services for their children.

Key components of the legislation included:

1. educating children in the least restrictive environment
2. mandating individualized educational programs (IEPs) for all children with disabilities
3. utilizing nondiscriminatory assessment procedures to identify children
4. requiring schools to involve parents in the special education process

5. due process rights for children and parents. Table 1–2 summarizes some of the key provisions of the legislation.

In 1986 another major federal act, Public Law 99–457, was passed by Congress. This legislation mandates educational services through the public schools for children with disabilities ages three to five beginning in 1991–1992. Originally the legislation mandated the law take effect in 1990–1991 unless certain federal appropriations were not made. Since the specified level of funding was not appropriated, the mandate year was delayed until 1991–1992. The law effectively lowers the requirements of Public Law 94–142 to the new age category. This legislation will have a major impact on public schools by requiring them to serve children not previously served by most school districts.

An additional component of Public Law 99–457 was the establishment of a financial incentive program to state and local education agencies that provide services to children with disabilities, ages birth to two years (Ysseldyke & Algozzine, 1990). Schools opting to serve children in this age category are required to develop an individual family service plan (IFSP), which is an individual program that includes the entire family unit. This program could result in a major effort to provide services to children from birth through the school years.

In the 1990 reauthorization of Public Law 94–142 (Public Law 101–476), several important areas were changed. For one thing, the name of the legislation was changed from the Education of All Handicapped Children Act to the Individuals with Disabilities

TABLE 1–2 Key Provisions of Public Law 94–142

PROVISIONS	DESCRIPTION
Least Restrictive Environment	Children are educated with nondisabled children as much as possible.
Individual Education Program	All children served in special education must have an individual education program (IEP).
Due Process Rights	Disabled children and their parents must be involved in decisions about special education.
Due Process Hearing	Parents and schools can request an impartial hearing if there is a conflict over special education services.
Nondiscriminatory Assessment	Students must be given a comprehensive assessment that is nondiscriminatory in nature.
Related Services	Schools must provide related services, such as physical therapy, counseling, and transportation, if needed.
Free Appropriate Public Education	The primary requirement of Public Law 94–142 is the provision of a free, appropriate public education to all school-age children with disabilities.

Education Act (IDEA). In keeping with the trend to "normalize" the language concerning students receiving special education services, all references to "handicapped children" in the legislation were changed to "children with disabilities" (National Association of State Directors of Special Education, 1990).

IDEA added two new handicapping categories to the legislation, traumatic brain injury (TBI) and autism. Prior to these changes, autism was included in the "other health impaired" category. As a result of the change, autism is now considered a separate handicapping condition. A final major addition to IDEA was the requirement for transition services to be specific in students' individual education programs (IEPs) (National Association of State Directors of Special Education, 1990). Transition services include all activities covered in the student's program designed to facilitate movement from high school to post-school adjustment.

In 1990, probably the most important civil rights legislation passed for more than two decades was signed into law by President Bush. Called the Americans with Disabilities Act (ADA), the legislation guarantees equal opportunities and access to the more than 40 million Americans with various disabilities. "The scope of this Act is broad and deep, extending detailed protection against discrimination on the basis of disability to all persons with disabilities in almost all daily life situations." (Linthicum, Cole, & D'Alonzo, 1991, p. 1) Specific provisions include 1. accessibility to restaurants, stores, offices, and other businesses and services; 2. nondiscriminatory employment practices for businesses with more than fifteen employees; 3. accessibility to public transportation; and 4. telephone accommodations for persons with hearing and speech impairments. This legislation should do for persons with disabilities what the Civil Rights Act of 1964 did for members of racial minority groups. Although it will not impact public school programs significantly, since Public Law 94–142 already guaranteed equal educational opportunities for students with disabilities, it does expand the opportunities for all ages of individuals with disabilities.

STATUS OF SERVICES TO CHILDREN WITH DISABILITIES

The number of children with disabilities served by public school programs has increased substantially since the passage of Public Law 94–142. The Twelfth Annual Report to Congress on the Implementation of the Education of the Handicapped Act (U.S. Department of Education, 1990) revealed that approximately 4.5 million students, ages three to twenty-one, received special educational services in schools and community programs in the 1988–1989 school year. The number of children served increased 2.1 percent over the number served in 1987–1988, the largest increase since 1980–1981. The number of students served in 1988–1989, represents an increase of more than 700,000 students since 1977. The average number of new students added to special education programs each year since 1977 has been approximately 70,000 (U.S. Department of Education, 1989). Table 1–3 (page 12) summarizes the numbers of students served in special education between 1977 and 1989.

Children served in special education programs range from those who are intellectually capable, but have physical limitations, to those with significant cognitive deficits. The major categories served include children with mental retardation, learning disabilities, emotional problems, vision or hearing problems, physical disorders, or other health impairments. Although students with learning disabilities compose the newest recognized

TABLE 1-3 Number of Students Served in Special Education between 1977 and 1989

SCHOOL YEAR	PERCENTAGE CHANGE IN TOTAL NUMBER SERVED FROM PREVIOUS YEAR	TOTAL SERVED
1988–89	2.1	4,587,370
1987–88	1.6	4,494,280
1986–87	1.2	4,421,601
1985–86	0.2	4,370,244
1984–85[b]	0.5	4,363,031
1983–84	1.0	4,341,399
1982–83	1.5	4,298,327
1981–82	1.3	4,233,282
1980–81	3.5	4,177,689
1979–80	3.0	4,036,219
1978–79	3.8	3,919,073
1977–78	1.8	3,777,286
1976–77	—	3,708,913

[a]These numbers include children 0–21 years counted under Chapter 1 of ESEA (Elementary and Secondary Education Act) State Operated Programs (SOP) and children 3–21 years counted under EHA-B (Education for Handicapped Act, Part B). The totals do not reflect infants and toddlers 0–2 years served under Part H of EHA (Education for Handicapped Act).

[b]Beginning in 1984–85, the number of handicapped children reported reflects revisions to State data received by the Office of Special Education Programs following the July 1 grant award date, and includes revisions received by October 1. Previous reports provided data as of the grant award date.

Source: U.S. Department of Education, (1990) Office of Special Education Programs, Data Analysis System (DANS).

disability category, they currently represent the largest single group of children served. Table 1–4 summarizes the number of students, by disability, receiving special education services.

PARENTAL INVOLVEMENT

When Public Law 94–142 was passed in 1975, it mandated parental involvement in the special education process. Prior to this mandate, some special education professionals actively involved parents of students with disabilities, but many did not. Some professionals continued with the assumption that they were the experts and were therefore in a position to make the decisions about children with disabilities. Although Public Law 94–142 required schools to involve parents, some professionals remained skeptical about the parent's legitimate role in the special education process (Shea & Bauer, 1991).

Although there is no one section of Public Law 94–142 that focuses on parental involvement in the special education process, the requirements to involve parents permeate

TABLE 1-4 Number of Children with Disabilities Served in Special Education
Programs in 1988–1989*

HANDICAPPING CONDITION	NUMBER	PERCENTAGE	PERCENT OF TOTAL SCHOOL POPULATION
Learning Disabled	1,998,422	47.7	4.5
Speech or Language Impaired	968,908	23.1	2.3
Mentally Retarded	581,465	13.9	1.2
Emotionally Disturbed	377,295	9.0	0.85
Multihandi-capped	84,870	2.0	
Hard of Hearing and Deaf	57,555	1.4	0.13
Orthopedically Impaired	47,392	1.1	0.10
Other Health Impaired	50,349	1.2	0.11
Visually Handicapped	22,743	0.5	0.05
Deaf-Blind	1,516	0.0	0.01
All Conditions	4,190,515	100.0	9.5

*Percentages are within column.

Source: U.S. Department of Education, (1990) Office of Special Education Programs, Data Analysis System (DANS).

the regulations. The following requirements of the law relate to parental involvement (Gearheart, Weishahn, & Gearheart, 1988).

1. Schools must use the native language of the home in informing parents about special education activities.

2. Schools must secure parental permission before conducting an individual comprehensive assessment.

3. Parents must be informed and invited to conferences where assessment results are presented and discussed.

4. Schools must invite parents to participate in the development of the student's individual educational program.

5. Schools must make student records available to parents.

6. Parents may seek an independent evaluation of their child if they want additional assessment data.

7. Parents have a right to request an administrative review of decisions made regarding their child.

While some special education professionals and administrators may consider the requirements to involve parents of students with disabilities in the special education process as unnecessary, there are many benefits that can result from parent-teacher collaboration. For example, benefits for the students include 1. their understanding that their parents are interested in their educational program, 2. increased likelihood that they will experience success, and 3. consistent expectations for parents and teachers (Shea & Bauer, 1991).

There are also advantages for the parents and teachers that result from teacher-parent collaboration. These include development of mutual trust and respect, access to information from both parties that can be beneficial in the school and home setting, and a mutual understanding of the goals and objectives for the educational program (Shea & Bauer, 1991). Schools can easily meet the requirements of Public Law 94–142 by making weak attempts to involve parents in the educational process. However, they should do more than simply getting parents' signatures on documents; schools should make a thorough attempt to bring parents into the special education process. With parents "on board," the educational program for students with disabilities can only improve.

MULTICULTURAL SPECIAL EDUCATION

Special education serves all students with disabilities, those from the majority culture as well as those from minority cultures. The "melting pot theory" prevalent in the 1960s and 1970s projected that individuals from minority cultures would eventually become assimilated into the majority culture; this simply did not become a reality. In fact, rather than holding on to this theory, most educators today believe in "cultural pluralism," the realization that cultural diversity exists and will continue to exist in our society (Smith, 1990).

Multicultural education emerged from the racial chaos of the 1960s and 1970s. Grant (1982) stated that multicultural education "is a concept predicated upon a fundamental belief that all people must be accorded respect, regardless of age, race, sex, economic class, religion, physical or mental ability." (p. 485) It is therefore based on the uniqueness of individual students and the acknowledgment that our schools are not composed of a homogeneous group of students. Rather than becoming more and more homogeneous, students in public schools are becoming more and more diverse.

An unfortunate reality is that students from minority cultural groups have traditionally been overrepresented in special education classes (Polloway & Smith, 1992). This could be the result of discriminatory assessment practices, difficulties that result from poverty, language-different environments, or a combination of both. Regardless of the reason, for special education professionals there are numerous factors that complicate the provision of appropriate services to minority students. These include:

- *Lack of assessment personnel*   There is a lack of skilled personnel who can test children in their native language and who are qualified to interpret performance in light of children's linguistic and cultural characteristics. As a result, modifications in assessment procedures, for example, the introduction of an interpreter into the testing environment, often have significant effects upon standardization.

- *Inadequate procedures*   Assessment instruments and procedures are inadequate for the purpose of identifying handicapping conditions among culturally diverse children. Inadequacies of such instruments and procedures are often not considered when reaching decisions related to school problems and educational programming.

- *Lack of trained personnel*   Many culturally diverse handicapped children cannot be provided an appropriate education due to the lack of special education personnel who are uniquely trained to serve this population. Of particular concern is the lack of personnel who can provide instruction in a child's native language.

- *Limited knowledge base*   Research in the area of special education for culturally diverse handicapped children is almost nonexistent. The evidence that is available is basically deductive or generalized from studies in bilingual education, special education, or general theories of learning. Yet, without legitimate data and knowledge specific to this population, efforts to provide appropriate services will continue to be based upon assumptions and intuitions.

- *Lack of instructional materials*   Few materials are specifically designed for handicapped children from linguistically and culturally diverse backgrounds. Instructional personnel usually adapt materials or create their own—a difficult task, given the absence of a theoretical basis for modification, adaptation, or creation.

- *Bilingual education*   There is growing concern that bilingual education has become an alternative to special education placement. Education personnel who make placement decisions may hope that, by putting a child in a class with a teacher who speaks the child's native language, a remedy for the child's handicapping condition will emerge. However, bilingual educators often find that they do not have the necessary training to determine whether a child is handicapped or to provide educational interventions to help exceptional children. Further, bilingual teachers are unable to prevent the inappropriate placement of exceptional children in their classes. (Ortiz & Yates, 1984, pp. 117–118)

These problems related to providing special education programs for students from minority cultural groups point out the difficulties faced by special educators. Hallahan and Kauffman (1991) note three areas that school personnel must address to consider the complications of serving students from minority backgrounds. These include 1. assessment, 2. instruction, and 3. socialization. There are methods for dealing with each of these issues involving minority students. Teachers must consider special approaches to ensure the appropriateness of the intervention programs provided (Polloway & Smith, 1992).

Public Law 94–142 requires schools to use nondiscriminatory assessment practices when evaluating students from minority cultural backgrounds. Schools are required to assess students in their native language and to use more than single tests to determine eligibility. While these requirements should help limit discrimination, they do not guarantee fair assessment. It remains easier to mandate nondiscriminatory assessment than to implement it.

Classification of Disabilities

Children and adults with disabilities can be classified in several ways. The traditional classification system was organized around clinical groups with similar characteristics. The primary groups include those that result in mental, physical, sensory, or emotional problems. These groups traditionally include mental retardation, learning disabilities, emotional disturbance, visual impairment, hearing impairment, orthopedic impairments, and other health impairments.

The unfortunate aspect of classification is labeling. Although many professionals and advocates do not like labeling, the fact is, it is a practice that, under the current system, enables students to access services (Smith *et al.*, 1986). There are probably more disadvantages than advantages of labeling. Among the disadvantages are 1. stereotyping, 2. negative effects on self concepts, 3. establishment of certain expectations for teachers, parents, and peers, and 4. the difficulty of removing labels once they have been attributed to a child.

On the other side of the issue are some advantages of labeling. First, labeling helps identify which students can access services authorized by legislative bodies to serve specific types of children. Although not a particularly good reason to label children with deviant names, under the current system it is the only way students can access special education services. Labels also help group children with similar needs and provide a focal point for advocacy. For example, the Association for Children with Learning Disabilities, and the Association for Retarded Citizens were started to focus on a particular group of children. Finally, labels help researchers identify similar subjects that facilitate understanding about certain groups of children.

Although labels are an unfortunate feature of the system of special education, their negative impact may be decreasing. As states and local schools move to implement noncategorical service systems and the regular education initiative, the need and frequency of negative labels should decrease. Providing appropriate services to all children without labels would be an ideal situation and one that all professionals and advocacy groups should work toward.

CATEGORICAL CLASSIFICATION SYSTEM

The traditional system of classifying persons with disabilities has been popularly used for many years. Schools began serving students based on their categorical labels; advocacy groups were initiated for specific categorical groups; research funds have typically been provided for investigations into certain categories of disabilities; and teacher preparation and certification frequently target one or more specific groups of children. Public Law 94–142 identifies ten groups of disabilities as the basis for determining eligibility for services under the Act.

Mental Retardation

Mental retardation is the categorical group that includes individuals with limited intellectual abilities. Individuals classified as "mentally retarded" are determined to have less intellectual abilities than is considered "normal." The determination of intellectual level is made by intelligence tests that reveal an intelligence quotient (IQ) score. The definition used by the federal government and the majority of states in their special education and adult service programs comes from the American Association on Mental Retardation (AAMR): "Mental retardation refers to significantly subaverage general intellectual functioning resulting in or associated with concurrent impairments in adaptive behavior and manifested during the developmental period." (Grossman, 1983, p. 11)

Although this definition is the most widely accepted, without interpretation it appears to be a lot of meaningless words. In lay terms, the AAMR definition defines mental retardation as an IQ of about 70 or below in conjunction with an inability of the individual to adapt to cultural and chronological age expectations. These factors could have a limited relationship to what is needed in the classroom (Patton, Bierne-Smith, & Payne, 1990).

Within the overall category of mental retardation are subgroupings. There are several different ways to subclassify this group of individuals; the AAMR divides mental retardation into mild, moderate, severe, and profound. Many educators are accustomed to the terms *educable mental retardation (EMR)* and *trainable mental retardation (TMR)*. In general, EMR overlaps with the mild category and TMR overlaps with the moderate category. Table 1–5 depicts these categories and the intelligence quotient range associated with each level. What must be considered is that individual IQ scores are fluid and vary a few points from testing to testing. Also, some IQ tests discriminate against certain cultural and socio-economic groups (Luftis, 1989). Therefore, teachers, parents, and other

TABLE 1–5 IQ Criteria for Sub-Groups of Students with Mental Retardation

CATEGORY	IQ CRITERIA
Mild Mental Retardation	50–55 to approximately 70
Moderate Mental Retardation	35–40 to 50–55
Severe Mental Retardation	20–25 to 35–40
Profound Mental Retardation	Below 20 or 25

Source: Grossman, 1983.

consumers of test information must not jump to too many conclusions simply based on an IQ score. Additional information, such as observations, interviews, and test scores generated from other types of assessment instruments, should be considered.

Learning Disabilities

Prior to the 1990 reauthorization of Public Law 94–142, learning disabilities (LDs) was the newest category of disabilities recognized by the federal government and many states serving students in special education programs. The category was included in the definition of handicapped in Public Law 94–142 in 1975, and was further defined and described in federal regulations issued in 1977. The definition that was provided is still used by the federal government and most states.

> "Specific learning disability" means a disorder in one or more of the basic psychological processes involved in understanding or in using language, spoken or written, which may manifest itself in an imperfect ability to listen, think, speak, write, spell, or to do mathematical calculations. The term includes such conditions as perceptual handicaps, brain injury, minimal brain dysfunction, dyslexia, and developmental aphasia. The term does not include children who have learning problems which are primarily the result of visual, hearing, or motor handicaps, or mental retardation, or emotional disturbance, or of environmental, cultural, or economic disadvantage. (U.S. Office of Education, 1977, p. 65083)

As with the AAMR definition for mental retardation, the LD definition is confusing. Basically, students are considered learning disabled when they do not achieve commensurate with their abilities, and the discrepancy cannot be explained by other conditions. Students' abilities are determined with IQ tests and other measures of aptitude; achievement is measured with achievement tests. As a result of different definitions of LD being used, and the definitions lacking specific criteria for determining eligibility, the prevalence rates of LD children and adults varies a great deal.

Another problem in the learning disabilities category is the different terms used to describe the condition. School dysfunction, school failure, learning disorders, and specific learning disabilities have often been used to describe similar conditions (Kosc, 1987). Other terms that have been used include brain damage, brain dysfunction, neurological impairment, and more specific terms, such as dyslexia. Although the term learning disabilities has consolidated many of these terms, there still exists different labels that only add confusion to identification and services to this group.

Emotional Disturbance

Professionals and advocates who serve students with emotional and psychological problems cannot agree on a label, much less a definition. Among the labels advocated and used to identify this group of children are seriously emotionally disturbed, emotionally disturbed, behavior disordered, emotionally conflicted, severely behavior handicapped, and socially maladjusted. These labels reveal specific biases found among certain groups regarding identifying and serving students with these disabilities. For example, advocates of the term *socially maladjusted* would serve many more and different kinds of children than those simply labeled *seriously emotionally disturbed*. Public Law 94–142 uses the label seriously emotionally disturbed (SED). As a result, this category is the one most often served by states, which use the federal definition of SED to determine eligibility of students.

The federal definition of SED states that these are children who "exhibit one or more of the following characteristics over a long period of time and to a marked degree:

1. An inability to learn which cannot be explained by intellectual, sensory, or health factors;

2. An inability to build or maintain satisfactory interpersonal relationships with peers and teachers;

3. Inappropriate types of behavior or feelings under normal circumstances;

4. General pervasive mood of unhappiness or depression; or

5. A tendency to develop physical symptoms, pains, or fears associated with personal or school problems (Federal Register, 1977, p. 42478)."

Visual Impairment

There are two major groups subsumed in the category of visual impairment—blind and partially sighted or low vision. Individuals are classified as blind if they have a visual acuity of 20/200 or less in the better eye with best correction, or a field of vision of 20 degrees or less. Partial sightedness is defined as a visual acuity of 20/70 to 20/200 in the better eye with best correction. These definitions reflect the legal or medical definitions of visual impairment. The more functional definitions preferred by some educators and service providers are as follows. Blind persons are those who cannot learn to read using print; they must read using alternative means. Partially sighted students are those whose visual loss is such that they need some intervention services but they can learn to read using print. Often these individuals simply need large print materials or the ability to enlarge print.

Students served in special education programs as visually impaired make up an extremely small number. The number of children served under this category in 1986–1987 was 27,049, or 0.61 percent of the total school population (Tenth Annual Report to Congress, 1988). This small prevalence rate makes the provision of services very difficult because of a lack of any concentration of students with similar needs to justify employing a specialist in this area.

Hearing Impairment

Like the category of visual impairment, children classified as hearing impaired can fit into one of two groups: deaf and hard-of-hearing. Traditionally, individuals have been classified into these two categories based on their degree of hearing loss, as measured by decibels (Db). Decibels are units of relative loudness of sounds (Hallahan & Kauffman, 1991). For example, a whisper is approximately 10 dB, pencil writing 30 dB, door slamming 70 dB, chainsaw 100 dB, and jackhammer, 130 dB (Hardman, Drew, Egan, & Wolf, 1990). Individuals are considered deaf if they have at least a 90 decibel loss; hard-of-hearing persons have a loss of 26–89 decibels. During the past several years, a movement to make the definitions more functional have resulted in defining deaf and hard-of-hearing based on the ability to process linguistic information through audition (Lowenbraun & Thompson, 1990). This approach is very similar to the functional, educational definition of blind and partially sighted.

Hearing impairment is a low incidence disability. In the 1987–1988 school year, only 66,761 children were served in this category in public school special education programs. This only accounts for 1.5 percent of the school-age population (U.S. Department of Education, 1989). The low incidence nature of hearing impairments, associated with the need for specialized intervention, creates problems for schools trying to provide services to this population.

Orthopedically Impaired

Public Law 94–142 defines orthopedically impaired as children with "disabilities that relate primarily to disorders of the skeleton, joints, and muscles, including 1. clubfoot, the absences of some member, or other congenital anomalies; 2. impairments caused by diseases such as poliomyelitis or bone tuberculosis; 3. impairments caused by cerebral palsy; 4. amputations; and 5. contractures caused by fractures or burns (Federal Register, 1977).

This category is very broad and composed of many varied groups of children. For example, a child with severe cerebral palsy differs significantly from one who has a congenital amputation of one arm. Very often children with orthopedic impairments exhibit other problems, such as a learning disability. This only further limits any generalizations that can be made about the overall category. To better understand children classified as orthopedically impaired, individual students and specific categories, such as cerebral palsy, must be examined. Table 1–6 briefly describes the major conditions included in this category.

Traumatic Brain Injury (TBI)

Along with autism, traumatic brain injury (TBI) is the newest category recognized by IDEA. The Executive Committee of the Board of Directors of the National Head Injury Foundation defines TBI as

> an insult to the brain, not of a degenerative or congenital nature but caused by an external physical force, that may produce a diminished or altered state of consciousness, which results in impairment of cognitive abilities or physical functioning. It can also result in the disturbance of behavioral or emotional functioning. These impairments may be either temporary or permanent and cause partial or total functional disability or psychosocial maladjustment. (Savage, 1988, p. 13)

TBI can obviously result in significant problems for students, especially in school settings. The damage or insult to the nervous system can manifest itself in many different areas, including attentional deficits, memory deficits, and behavior problems. Students classified as TBI compose a very heterogenous group. Although TBI is considered a separate disability category, some professionals argue that interventions for this group of students are no different than they are for students classified as learning disabled or emotionally disturbed.

Autism

The category of autism was initially included in the federal definition of seriously emotionally disturbed, but later moved to the "other health impaired" category. The 1990 reauthorization of Public Law 94–142 made autism a separate category. The result is that children can now be classified as handicapped under IDEA based on a diagnosis of autism. Autism

TABLE 1-6 Descriptions of Students Classified as Orthopedically Impaired

CLASSIFICATION	DESCRIPTION
Spina Bifida	Condition caused by a birth defect when the spinal column does not close properly. Most severe form, myelomeningocele, results in paralysis. Hydrocephalus is present in large percentage of cases with myelomeningocele.
Cerebral Palsy	Nonprogressive disorder of movement or posture. Caused by brain damage. Results in a variety of levels of involvement, ranging from mild to severe. Mental retardation present in the majority of cases; however, individuals with CP can have above average intelligence.
Muscular Dystrophy	Genetically transmitted disease characterized by a "wasting away" of the muscles. Muscle tissue is replaced by fat tissue. Duchenne type, most severe, only affects boys and usually begins as the child begins to walk; by adolescence, wheel chairs are usually necessary. Total disability or death is the normal outcome.
Arthritis	Diseases with pain in and around joints. Varies greatly in severity. Rheumatoid arthritis is the most common form affecting children. Outcome can be major disability remission.

Source: Hallahan & Kauffman, 1991.

is considered an organic disorder with unknown etiology that affects children before the age of thirty months. Children with autism are characterized by limited interactions with other individuals. They frequently do not have expressive language and have a tendency to display repetitive, self-stimulating behaviors (Hallahan & Kauffman, 1991).

Other Health Impaired

Children classified as "other health impaired" also make up a very heterogeneous group. Conditions included in this category are heart problems, hemophilia, cystic fibrosis, epilepsy, tuberculosis, asthma, sickle cell anemia, rheumatic fever, nephritis, lead poisoning, leukemia, AIDS, or diabetes. The category is so broad that an endless list of specific conditions could result and be classified as other health impaired. Prior to the reauthorization of Public Law 94–142 in 1990, autism was also considered a condition within this category.

Children in the "other health impaired" category need a variety of services, ranging from complicated medical interventions to minimal classroom accommodations. Because there is such wide variance among the population, assessment procedures, instructional interventions, and placement options vary considerably from student to student. As medical technology increases the likelihood that children with serious illnesses live longer and attend school programs, special education and other school personnel will have to be prepared to meet the unique needs of individual students.

Attention Deficit Hyperactive Disorder

Another disability category that was considered for inclusion in IDEA was attention deficit hyperactive disorder (ADHD). ADHD is currently defined by the *Diagnostic and Statistical Manual of Mental Disorders* (DMS-III-R) as a condition where children exhibit "developmentally inappropriate degrees of inattention, impulsivity, and hyperactivity." (p. 50). ADHD is the new label for the group of children that were previously classified as "brain injured" and "minimal brain dysfunction" (MBD) (Reeve, 1990).

Rather than formally including ADHD as a separate disability category, Congress required the Secretary of Education to publish a Notice of Inquiry in the *Federal Register* to solicit information concerning the addition of ADHD as a new category of disabilities under IDEA (National Association of State Directors of Special Education, 1990). Although there is some support for including ADHD as a separate category, some professional groups, such as the Council for Exceptional Children (CEC), have gone on record as opposing this step. The argument against including ADHD as a separate category is that children who experience attention and hyperactive problems are already being appropriately served under existing categories.

NONCATEGORICAL OR GENERIC CLASSIFICATION SYSTEM

Beginning in the mid-1970s, professionals began questioning the efficacy of grouping children with disabilities based on clinical labels. Professionals have lined up on both sides of this issue. Advocates of the noncategorical classification system generally group students who have mild disabilities into one general category. Children with mild disabilities can be defined as "the large group of students who differ from nonhandicapped students in cognitive-academic, sensoriphysical, and socioemotional characteristics to such an extent that special education and related services are required, but not to the degree that segregated special class placement is necessary." (Smith *et al.*, 1986, p. 50) In many states, this category includes students who traditionally were classified as learning disabled, mildly or educable mentally retarded, and behaviorally disordered. However, using the above definition, the category could include students with physical or sensory deficits who do not need self-contained settings.

Children classified as mildly handicapped or mildly disabled differ from children with more severe disabilities in the services they need. By definition, an appropriate education can be provided to children with mild disabilities in integrated settings. This could be total regular classroom placement or regular classroom with resource room assistance. Some states actually define the category "mildly handicapped" by the service needs of children. For example, Alabama guidelines indicate that children served in noncategorical, mildly handicapped classrooms should only be those who require resource room assistance. This provision is made to prevent the dumping of severely disabled, low incidence children into classrooms with a teacher certified to deal with more than one category of disabled children.

Children with more severe disabilities frequently need services that are appropriately provided in more restrictive, segregated settings. These could include self-contained classrooms, special schools, or even residential placements. We do not advocate these restrictive settings for any children unless there are obvious, unique needs that cannot be provided in less restrictive settings. It is our belief that there are only a few children who would need such restrictive placements, and that many children placed in these environments could be more appropriately served in more "normalized" settings.

The general argument supporting the noncategorical classification system in that traditional categories do little to facilitate the provision of an appropriate education to students with disabilities (Algozzine, Morsink, & Algozzine, 1988). Proponents of a noncategorical system note that not only do categorical labels not help teachers instruct children, but that many children classified as mildly mentally retarded, learning disabled, and emotionally disturbed actually have similar characteristics (Katims, 1988). Often the unfortunate effect of classifying children with categorical labels is the "typing" of children into groups that may have little relevance for special education (Smith *et al.*, 1986).

Professionals who advocate serving children using a noncategorical model suggest that children's individual educational programs be developed based on specific strengths and weaknesses, not on clinical labels. Specific reasons given for the noncategorical classification model include (Marsh, Price, & Smith, 1983):

- similarities among students from different traditional categories are greater than are differences;

- teaching should be based on individual student's strengths and weaknesses; and

- intervention methods and materials should be based on individual needs, not categorical labels.

Stainback and Stainback (1987) sum up the argument supporting noncategorical services by stating that "what is appropriate servicing is directly dependent on a student's specific interests, needs, and capabilities rather than crude, imprecise labels." (p. 67) Research also supports the noncategorical approach. After reviewing two studies that investigated the success of students from different categorical groups receiving instruction in the same classroom, Jenkins, Pious, and Peterson (1988) concluded that there is no educational rationale for separating groups of students based on categorical label. Other studies have substantiated this conclusion and note that teachers do not differentiate instruction significantly with different groups of students (Algozzine *et al.*, 1988).

Although these reasons may seem very defensible, there are some professionals who continue to support categorical classification and services (Algozzine *et al.*, 1988). Reasons to support this position include the notion that categories do relate to specific instructional techniques, categories group children with similar characteristics, and teachers can only be trained to deal effectively with one specific type of disabled child.

There currently is no concensus concerning the categorical versus noncategorical debate. Even so, many states have moved to the noncategorical model during the past several years, and currently certify teachers and serve students using a noncategorical model (Friend & McNutt, 1984; Smith *et al.*, 1986). In order to prepare professionals to meet this new certification, colleges and universities have developed noncategorical teacher training programs. These are often called mildly handicapped teacher education programs and are designed to prepare teachers to work with children in resource settings who have been classified as having learning disabilities, mild mental retardation, or mild emotional problems.

To date there has been limited research concerning the effectiveness of these training programs. In one of the few studies that focused on the competencies of teachers in non-categorical programs, Marston (1987) found that "LD and EMR pupils, when taught by teachers with certification matching child label, did not make significantly greater gains than LD and EMR children instructed by teachers with licenses not matching pupil label." (p. 423) Still, there is disagreement related to the preparedness of teachers trained to serve a variety of different types of disabled children (Cobb *et al.*, 1989). Additional research focusing on this issue needs to be completed.

Current Service Delivery Models

Special education services for students with disabilities have changed dramatically as a result of Public Law 94–142. Whereas they used to be characterized as self-contained, isolated programs for the most obviously disabled children, they currently can be described as integrated, individualized, comprehensive, and continuing to expand.

INTEGRATED SERVICES

Special education programs are currently integrated with regular education as much as possible. One of the key components of Public Law 94–142 was the "least restrictive environment" requirement. The law states that students with disabilities shall be educated with nondisabled children as much as possible. This one requirement did as much to revolutionize special education as any other action. Although not mentioned in the legislation or the regulations that implemented the legislation, the term "mainstreaming" became the operationalizing term for least restrictive environment.

The least restrictive mandate resulted from the philosophy of "normalization." Normalization "simply implies that the handicapped ought to be able to live a life as equal as possible to a normal existence and with the same rights and obligations of other people." (Juul, 1978, p. 326) The philosophy can be implemented in several ways, including deinstitutionalization and community-based services (Ysseldyke & Algozzine, 1990) and competitive employment. In schools normalization is operationalized through mainstreaming, educating children with disabilities with nondisabled children as much as possible.

Deinstitutionalization is the movement of individuals from institutions to community-based settings. As a result of this movement, the population of institutions for persons with mental retardation and other disabilities has decreased significantly since the early 1970s. For example, during the decade of the seventies, the number of persons in public residential facilities for persons with mental retardation dropped from nearly 200,000 to approximately 125,000, a nearly 40 percent decrease (Scheerenberger, 1982). Although the rate of deinstitutionalization has slowed, the trend through the 1980s and into the 1990s has been to continue to reduce the number of persons residing in institutions.

Many individuals residing in institutions in the past were only mildly disabled and could function very well in community-based programs. Some were actually institutionalized because community-based services were simply not available, while others were placed in institutions because parents were told that there were limited services for children in communities. As a result of Public Law 94–142 requiring educational services in public schools and the normalization philosophy advocating deinstitutionalization, most individuals with mild and moderate levels of mental retardation have been placed in community-based programs.

Concomitant with the deinstitutionalization movement has been the expansion of community-based services (Salend, 1990). These include living arrangements, such as group homes and apartments, community training programs, and work experiences in competitive, community settings. With many disabled individuals leaving institutions and others not entering them, programs in communities had to be developed to provide normalized opportunities and prevent the reinstitutionalization of many persons with disabilities.

Without ample numbers of group homes and other supported living options, persons leaving institutions had no place to live. Also, without work options for individuals with disabilities, community living was only an extension of the institution where persons with disabilities would live but would not be integrated into the community. The increase in number of group homes and other community living options, as well as the supported employment movement and efforts to facilitate vocational success, have all enabled deinstitutionalization to be successful.

Least Restrictive Environment

Although deinstitutionalization and community-based programs are important to schools, the primary component of integration that schools must contend with is the requirement to serve children in the least restrictive environment. Public Law 94–142 defines least restrictive environment as educating children with disabilities in settings with nondisabled children as much as possible. Unfortunately, the interpretation of least restrictive environment has varied a great deal from district to district and state to state. The key element in determining the least restrictive environment for an individual student is that student's individualized educational program (IEP). The placement of the student must be based on the student's IEP. The individual educational program is a plan, specifically designed for an individual student, that takes into consideration the student's strengths, weaknesses, and designs an individual intervention program for the student.

Schools determine the program needs of a student and develop an IEP accordingly. In order to place the students in the least restrictive environment based on the IEP, schools must have available a variety of placement options. While there are several models to describe placement options that should be available, most are based on Deno's model (1970). This placement options model ranges from least restrictive, full-time regular classroom, to most restrictive, institution or hospital. A thorough discussion of the continuum of services will be presented in a later chapter; various levels of the continuum are discussed below.

Level I Regular classroom placement This option places the child in the regular classroom for all instructional purposes. Students in this option may receive all services from the regular classroom teacher, or may receive additional services from support staff or consulting teachers. The key factor is that the children remain with nondisabled peers all day.

Level II Regular classroom/resource room   Students placed in level II option receive a portion of their instruction in regular classrooms with regular teachers and are pulled out to receive some instruction in a resource room. This option is the most common placement option currently used by public schools (Friend & McNutt, 1984; Smith *et al.*, 1986; Smith, 1990). The amount of time spent in the resource room varies from child to child. Some children may need extensive resource time (several hours daily) while others may need very minimal resource services.

Level III Self-contained special education   Students who receive services in self-contained classrooms remain in the special education classroom all day with the special education teacher. This option, which was the most popular prior to the mainstreaming movement, is now reserved for children who need more intensive interventions than would be received in a regular classroom/resource room setting.

Level IV Special school   A still more restrictive setting than self-contained options is a special school or program that is physically segregated from regular schools. Although the number of these programs has diminished dramatically since Public Law 94–142 was passed, there are still some that serve children with severe disabilities. Proponents for integrating students with disabilities into mainstreamed settings are strongly opposed to special school options.

Level V Residential option   For children with very debilitating conditions, residential options are available. As a result of deinstitutionalization, many residents of institutions have been returned to communities. There still are approximately 90,000 individuals residing in large institutions (White, Lakin, & Bruininks, 1989). The majority of residential programs currently only serve individuals with very severe disabling conditions.

The goal of special education and other intervention programs is to move students with disabilities toward less restrictive service options. Therefore, although a child may be placed in a self-contained classroom, the goal for that child would likely be to move into a normalized, regular classroom for at least a portion of each school day. Children would be moved into more restrictive environments only if evidence indicated that the child needed a more structured, intensive educational program than could be provided.

The exact placement of students should occur only after the IEP has been developed. The IEP indicates goals and objectives for student's which are developed only after extensive evaluations have been conducted. Part of the IEP indicates the services that should be provided in order to help the child achieve the goals and objectives. These services dictate placement. Decisions regarding placement should never be made before the IEP is developed, nor should they be made based on clinical labels. Children placed in the same handicapping category, such as learning disabilities, may need a variety of placement options.

TYPICAL SERVICES IN THE 1990s

The service delivery model for children with disabilities has evolved significantly since the 1960s. The predominant model was the self-contained special education classroom. In this approach, one special education teacher taught a group of children with disabilities for the majority of each school day. The same children in the self-contained program, identified by categorical labels, had limited opportunities for interaction with nondisabled children. Other regular classroom teachers had limited contact with the special education students or their teachers. This resulted in a very isolated program, where the students with disabilities along with their teachers were literally cut off from the rest of the school program.

As a result of Public Law 94–142 and professionals realizing the importance of integrating children with disabilities into regular classrooms as much as possible, the predominant service delivery option currently used is the resource room. In this option, children with disabilities remain in regular classes with their nondisabled peers for a portion of each school day and are pulled out for intensive assistance in the resource room for part of the school day. This model gives students the benefits of being with nondisabled peers and also receiving individualized intervention by a special education teacher. The Twelfth Annual Report to Congress (1990) revealed that the resource room is the most popularly used placement option for students in special education. Placement in regular classrooms with support services is the next most common.

One of the reasons for the movement to integrate students with disabilities into regular classrooms for part of the day was the results of efficacy studies. A series of studies that investigated the effectiveness of self-contained special education programs resulted in major questions about segregating them. Probably the one article that did more to question the efficacy of educating students with disabilities in self-contained classrooms was authored by Dunn (1968). This article, entitled "Special Education for the Mildly Retarded—Is Much of it Justifiable?" summarized the results of various studies of the effectiveness of special education programming and concluded that special education students progress as much in regular classes as in special classes.

In a later article, Dunn (1973) summarized conclusions related to the efficacy of self-contained, special classes for students with mental retardation. These included the following.

1. These students perform as well academically in regular classes as their mental age peers do in special classes.

2. Mental age capacity is not reached by these students regardless of their educational setting.

3. Members of this group with higher intellectual levels actually dislike special class placement.

4. Students who make the greatest gains in regular classes are from minority ethnic groups.

The results of the efficacy studies suggested that if isolated, special classes were no more effective than regular classes in educating students with disabilities, then the students might as well be integrated into regular classrooms, at least part of the day, to achieve any benefits derived from associating with nondisabled peers. These conclusions fueled the mainstreaming movement, bringing professional reasons to support the legislation and litigation that mandated serving children with disabilities in the least restrictive environment.

Therefore, the typical service model currently used is the resource room. Every state uses some form of the resource room model in serving students with mild disabilities (Friend & McNutt, 1984). Some states and local education agencies use categorical resource rooms, while others provide services through noncategorical resource rooms or multicategorical resource rooms. The categorical resource room serves children with one specific type of disability, such as learning disabilities or mental retardation. Noncategorical resource rooms usually serve a combination of children who would traditionally be labeled mildly mentally retarded, learning disabled, or behaviorally disordered. These children are frequently grouped together for instructional purposes. The multicategorical resource room is a setting that provides services to children from several different categorical groups, but usually with only one group being served at any one time. Comingling more than one disability is frequently discouraged.

Rich and Ross (1989) studied the amount of time students with disabilities spend on tasks in different settings. The results indicated that on-task time is greater for students in resource rooms than in regular classes, special classes, or special schools; the lowest on-task behaviors were recorded for students in special classes and special schools. While the results of this study appear to support the resource room, the fact that some students appear to be "on-task" does not guarantee that they are attending and learning.

In a study investigating the effectiveness of resource rooms, Jenkins and Heinen (1989) found that when given a clear choice for service delivery model, the majority of students with disabilities preferred the pull-out program over in-class services. The results revealed that the older the students, the more likely they were to desire a pull-out over an in-class program. Ysseldyke *et al.* (1990) surveyed teachers in over 200 schools across the United States to determine the instructional arrangements for students with mild disabilities. Their findings concerning the education of this group included:

- students spend between thirty minutes and three hours in resource rooms;

- direct instruction was the method used by sixty percent of the teachers when dealing with these students;

- secondary teachers dealt with more disabled students than elementary teachers;

- holding students accountable and altering instruction to enable success were the two most desirable adaptions;

- fifty percent of the elementary teachers had adult assistance in their classrooms compared to thirty-five percent of the secondary teachers;

- the majority of teachers made no changes in their instructional settings because of mainstreamed students with disabilities.

Although students with mild disabilities access services through the resource room approach, some children with more severe disabilities continue to receive special education services in self-contained classrooms with a single teacher providing the majority of their instruction. These types of programs, while they continue to exist, are used much less frequently than they were prior to the mainstreaming movement. Currently approximately 25 percent of all students served in special education programs receive services in self-contained, special classes (U.S. Department of Education, 1990).

Current Developments in Services for Students with Mild Disabilities

While the resource room model is the service delivery model used for the majority of students with mild disabilities, there are several developments that are currently impacting special education. Some of these developments may make headlines in journals but never have a significant impact on the field, while others will undoubtedly result in permanent changes. Some of the developments include the regular education initiative, emphasis on transition services, and the consultation/collaboration model.

The 1970s and 1980s will be remembered as the decades when children with disabilities received the right to appropriate educational services. Public Law 94–142, Public Law 99–457, and the American with Disabilities Act passed in 1990, guarantee access to educational programs by students with disabilities. The 1990s will see new areas of emphases. Primarily, the focus of the 1990s will be services. Moving to a future based assessment model where students' programs are based on their future (Dowdy & Smith, 1991; Smith & Dowdy, 1992), focusing on appropriate curricula (Polloway *et al.*, 1989), and adopting new instructional models, such as consultation and collaboration will be the focus. The trend in the 1990s will be "to look away from the traditional arena of change—public policy and legislation—and refocus on curriculum and teaching." (*Special education in the 1990s*, 1990). Major initiatives in the curriculum and teaching area include the regular education initiative, consultation and collaboration model, and transition programming.

THE REGULAR EDUCATION INITIATIVE (REI)

In 1986, Madeline Will proposed the merger of special education and regular education into one educational system. She noted several problem areas affecting the current special education system in the schools.

1. Special education services are fragmented into numerous categorical programs.

2. Special education and regular education are a dual system of education where the responsibility for students with disabilities is passed to the special education professionals.

3. Special education students in segregated programs are often stigmatized by their chronological age peers.

4. Eligibility criteria are often so rigid that disputes between parents and schools develop and impact negatively on the student's education.

Since Will's call for the merger of regular and special education, several noted special education professionals have become strong proponents of this movement, referred to as the regular education initiative (REI).

The regular education initiative is extremely controversial, sparking more debate than was present when mainstreaming was first proposed as the best method of serving children with disabilities. Lilly (1988) believes that REI is not simply a passing fad, but a movement that has evolved from more than twenty-five years of research into the efficacy of providing educational programs to children with disabilities. As early as 1984, Wang and Birch noted that research supported the feasibility of restructuring regular education to better serve students with disabilities.

The regular education initiative focuses on integrating regular education and special education. The movement advocates "that the general education system assume unequivocal, primary responsibility for all students." (Braaten, Kauffman, Braaten, Polsgrove, & Nelson, 1988, p. 21) Regular educators would have to assume the primary responsibility for educating all students under the REI (Jenkins, Pious, & Jewell, 1990). Although controversial, there are many arguments that have been made supporting REI (Davis, 1989).

1. Approximately ten percent of the more than 40 million public school students are classified as disabled and receive special education.

2. Approximately ten percent to twenty percent of public school students need some special attention but are not eligible for special education services.

3. Approximately twenty percent to thirty percent of the school population, or a minimum of 7.8 million students are having problems and need assistance.

4. Efforts need to be made collaboratively to provide appropriate services to all of these children.

5. The current system identifies students as "disabled" or "nondisabled"; there is no in-between.

6. The system of education as it now exists is a dual system.

7. The dual system is discriminatory, cost ineffective, and programmatically inefficient.

Reynolds, Wang, and Walberg (1987), strong advocates for REI, state that "unless major structural changes are made, the field of special education is destined to become more of a problem, and less of a solution, in providing education for children who have special needs." (p. 391) Among the problems cited include an increased number of referrals for special education, the realization that many children in need fail to receive services because they do not fit into one of the categorical conditions served by special education, and the amount of time spent on the process of securing appropriate services for children with disabilities.

Although the regular education initiative has garnered a great deal of support among some parents and professionals, it remains to be seen whether REI will be implemented to the degree that its proponents advocate. The movement has sparked a great deal of reflection among providers and consumers of special education services, and has created an atmosphere where new service delivery models, such as the cooperative teaching and consultation model, are being developed as alternatives to the more traditional resource room approach.

CONSULTATION/COLLABORATION MODEL

One of the intervention strategies that has been a result of the regular education initiative is the consultation/collaboration model. Using this strategy, "multidisciplinary planning support is given to classroom teachers to improve the quality of instruction provided to learning disabled and other exceptional and low achieving students presently receiving educational services in general education settings." (Bauwens, Hourcase, & Friend, 1990, p. 17) This approach enables regular teachers and special educators to collaborate in determining appropriate teaching methods for students served in regular classes (Tateyama-Sniezek, 1990). Donaldson and Christiansen (1990) suggest that a primary focus of this model is to use the "least intrusive" methods possible to provide appropriate instruction. The key elements in the consultation/collaboration model include the regular classroom teacher, special education teacher, and student with special needs (Tindal, Shinn, & Rodden-Nord, 1990).

The consultation/collaboration model facilitates the regular education initiative. It provides a mechanism for regular and special education teachers to deal with problems that develop as a result of students with disabilities receiving services in regular classrooms. Proponents of this approach realize that regular classroom teachers will not be able to provide appropriate instruction to students with disabilities without assistance from special education personnel. Special education teachers, therefore, become "consultants" for regular classroom teachers; instruction is provided in a collaborative approach.

Special education teachers using the consultation/collaboration teaching model do not assume the role of an authoritative expert. Rather, they genuinely collaborate with regular education personnel to provide appropriate instruction. The consulting special education teacher and regular classroom teacher share an equal status in the instructional process (Salend, 1990). Specific differences between this model and a model where the special education teacher assumes the role of an expert are summarized in Table 1–7 (page 32).

If the consultation/collaboration teaching model is successful, certain basic tenets must be accepted. These include:

1. joint responsibility for problems (i.e., all professionals share responsibility and concern for all students);

2. joint accountability and recognition for problem resolution;

3. belief that pooling talents and resources is mutually advantageous, with the following benefits:
   a. increased range of solutions generated;
   b. diversity of expertise and resources available to engage problem;
   c. superiority and originality of solutions generated;

4. belief that teacher or student problem resolution merits expenditure of time, energy, and resources;

5. belief that correlates of collaboration are important and desirable (i.e., group morale, group cohesion, increased knowledge of problem-solving processes and specific alternative classroom interventions). (Phillips & McCollough, 1990, p. 295)

TABLE 1-7 Comparison of Consultation/Collaberation with Traditional Resource Room Model

DIMENSION	COLLABORATION MODEL	RESOURCE MODEL
Objectives/Goals	Resolve problem/ improve consulting skills	Resolve problem
Target for Change	Student and teachers	Student
Relationship with Regular Teachers	Equal	Superior/ subordinate
Responsible for Student	Regular teacher	Regular teacher
Responsible for Intervention	Regular teacher	Special ed. teacher
Regular Teacher Involvement in Solving Problems	Extensive	Minimal
Alternatives Developed	Numerous	Minimal to numerous
Assumptions about Regular Teacher Involvement	Wants to be involved	Wants special ed. teacher to solve problems
Time Involved	Greater	Less
Professional with Expertise to Solve Problems	Consulting and regular teacher	Special ed. teacher

Source: Zins, J. E., Curtis, M. J., Graden, S. G., & Ponti, C. R., 1988.

TRANSITION PROGRAMMING

Although not new, programming for students with disabilities to make a smooth, successful transition from school to post-secondary school environments continues to be emphasized. Transition can be defined as the movement from one service delivery system to another. Traditionally it has been thought of as moving from the public school service system to the adult service system. However, transition can also be applied to the movement of children from preschool programs to school programs, and elementary programs to secondary programs. Transition developed rapidly as a major service need when follow-up studies of students with disabilities revealed their limited success following their exit from secondary special education programs. For example, follow-up studies of students formerly served in special education programs revealed that many students were unemployed, underemployed, or that these individuals experienced chronic social problems (Hasazi, Gordon, & Roe, 1984; Mithaug, Horiuchi, & Fanning, 1985; Wehman, Kregel, & Seyfarth, 1985; Rusch, & Phelps, 1987). (Chapter 11 also discusses transition programing.)

In 1983, Public Law 98–199 was passed by Congress. This federal legislation was the first effort to emphasize transition as a national priority. The legislation provided $6.6 million annually for projects related to the successful transition of students from high school to post-secondary environments (Rusch & Phelps, 1987). Although there are many different models to implement transition programs, there are also many barriers to the implementation of programs (Mitgaug, Martin, & Agran, 1987). Schools and service providers must take steps to circumvent and overcome these obstacles in order to provide appropriate transition programming to young adults with disabilities.

Public Law 101–475, IDEA, mandates that schools include transition programming in students' individual education programs. IDEA defines transition as:

> . . . a coordinated set of activities for a student, designed within an outcome-oriented process, which promotes movement from school to post-school activities, including post-secondary education, vocational training, integrated employment (including supported employment), continuing and adult education, adult services, independent living, or community participation. The coordinated set of activities shall be based upon the individual students' needs, taking into account the student's preferences and interests, and shall include instruction, community experiences, the development of employment and other post-school adult living objectives, and, when appropriate, acquisiton of daily living skills and functional vocational evaluation. (National Association of State Directors of Special Education, 1990).

Outline of the Textbook

The textbook is divided into five major sections. Section one, which includes the introductory chapter and the chapter on characteristics of students considered to have mild disabilities, provides an overview of services to students with disabilities in public school settings. Content in this section provides a description of the types of students considered mildly disabled. Although most of the research cited relates to categories of disabilities because a sound research base does not exist with subjects simply classified as "mildly handicapped," the readers should realize that instructional programs for students must be based on individual characteristics that impact instruction; categorical labels should not dictate programming decisions.

Section two of the text deals with a general overview of the teaching process for students with mild disabilities. Chapters on the instructional setting and instructional processes are included. The content in this section provides a basis for specific instructional strategies provided in section three, which focuses on basic skills instruction. Chapters include topics on teaching reading, written and oral expression, and math. Basic instructional techniques for students with various types of learning characteristics are presented.

Section four, teaching strategies, includes chapters on supporting students in regular classrooms, behavior management strategies, and teaching social skills. The content in this section provides information that will enable teachers to include strategies and accommodative techniques in their repertoire of skills. The final section includes information in other curricular areas. Specific topics include career and transition programming and technology and instruction. These areas are included because of their current relevance to intervention programs for students with mild disabilities, and the importance of these areas in the future.

SUMMARY

This chapter has provided an overview of children with mild disabilities. The first section presented a general overview of special education and disabilities. It was noted that the identification and labeling of school-age children is required in order to provide appropriate educational services. The history of how persons with disabilities were treated was presented to describe the major gains made in serving this population. It was pointed out that individuals with disabilities were literally eliminated from society in the early stages of recorded history. The treatment and services provided to disabled individuals were traced to the 1990s.

The legislation and litigation that resulted in current services to students with disabilities were described. Public Law 94–142, the Education for All Handicapped Children Act, now referred to as the Individuals with Disabilities Education Act (IDEA) was discussed. Specific components of this legislation were described, along with a description of court cases that had a major impact on the current special education delivery system.

The next major section of the chapter targeted the classification of disabilities. Specific disabling categories, including mental retardation, learning disabilities, emotional problems, visual and hearing disorders, other health impairments, and orthopedic impairments, were all defined and described. Traumatic brain injury and autism, the two most recently identified separate categories of disabilities recognized in federal legislation, were also discussed. Finally, a discussion on the movement to serve students based on general characteristics, rather than clinical labels, was presented.

Current service delivery systems for students with disabilities was the next major section of this chapter. The self-contained model, resource room model, and collaboration/ consultation model were highlighted. It was noted that students with disabilities have varying service needs and should be considered individually when trying to determine the most appropriate service approach. The final section of the chapter targeted current developments in services to students with mild disabilities. Topics included in the chapter were the regular education initiative, a movement to combine regular and special education programs, the consultation/collaboration model, and transition programming. Each of these new developments was described to provide an overview of current developments in the field of special education.

REFERENCES

Algozzine, B., Morsink, C.V., & Algozzine, K.M. (1988). What's happening in self-contained special education classrooms? *Exceptional Children, 55*, 259–265.

Bauwens, J., Hourcade, J.J., & Friend, M. (1989). Cooperative teaching: A model for general and special education integration. *Remedial and Special Education, 10*, 17–22.

Braaten, S., Kauffman, J.M., Braaten, B., Polsgrove, L., & Nelson, C.M. (1988). The regular education initiative: Patent medicine for behavioral disorders. *Exceptional Children, 55*, 21–27.

Brown v. Board of Education, Topeka, Kansas.

Cobb, H.B., Elliott, R.N., Powers, A.R., & Voltz, D. (1989). Generic versus categorical special education teacher preparation. *Teacher Education and Special Education, 12*, 19–26.

Donaldson, R., & Christiansen, J. (1990). Consultation and collaboration: A decision-making model. *Teaching Exceptional Children, 22*, 22–25.

Dowdy, C.A., Carter, J., & Smith, T.E.C. (1990). Differences in transition needs between students with learning disabilities and without learning disabilities. *Journal of Learning Disabilities, 23*, 343–348.

Dunn, L.M. (1968) Special education for the mildly retarded—Is much of it justifiable? *Exceptional Children, 35*, 5–22.

Dunn, L.M. (1973). *Exceptional children in the schools: Special education in transition.* New York: Holt, Rinehart, and Winston.

Friend, M., & McNutt, G. (1984). Resource room programs: Where are we now? *Exceptional Children, 51*, 150–155.

Gearheart, B.R., Weishahn, M.W., & Gearheart, C.J. (1988). *The exceptional student in the regular classroom,* 4th Ed. Columbus, OH: Merrill.

Grossman, H.H. (1983) (Ed.). *Classification in mental retardation.* Washington, D. C.: American Association on Mental Deficiency.

Hallahan, D.P., & Kauffman, J.M. (1991). *Exceptional children,* 5th Ed. Englewood Cliffs, NJ: Prentice Hall.

Haring, N.G. (1990). Overview of special education. In Haring, N.G., & McCormick, L. (Eds.). *Exceptional children and youth,* 5th Ed. pp. 1–37. Columbus, OH: Merrill.

Hasazi, S.B., Gordon, L.R., & Roe, C.A. (1985). Factors associated with the employment status of handicapped youth exiting high school from 1975 to 1983. *Exceptional Children, 51*, 455–469.

Jenkins, J.R., & Heinen, A. (1989). Students' preference for service delivery: Pull out, in-class, or integrated models. *Exceptional Children, 55*, 516–523.

Jenkins, J.R., Pious, C.G., & Jewell, M. (1990). Special education and the regular education initiative: Basic assumptions. *Exceptional Children, 56*, 479–491.

Jenkins, J.R., Pious, C.G., & Peterson, D.L (1988). Categorical programs for remedial and handicapped students: Issues of validity. *Exceptional Children, 55*, 147–158.

Juul, K.D. (1978). European approaches and innovations in serving the handicapped. *Exceptional Children, 44*, 322–330.

Katims, D.S. (1988). Effective teaching and learning in the noncategorical classroom. *Academic Therapy, 24*, 199–206.

Kosc, L. (1987). Learning disabilities: Definition or specification? A response to Kavale and Forness. *Remedial and Special Education, 8*, 36–41.

Lilly, M.S. (1988). The regular education initiative: A force for change in general and special education. *Education and Training in Mental Retardation, 23,* 253–260.

Linthicum, E., Cole, J.T., & D'Alonzo, B.J. (1991). Employment and the Americans with Disabilities Act of 1990. *Career Development for Exceptional Individuals, 14,* 1–13.

Luftig, R. (1989) *Assessment of learners with special needs.* Boston: Allyn & Bacon.

Marsh, G.E., Price, B.J., & Smith, T.E.C. (1983). *Teaching mildly handicapped children.* St. Louis: C. V. Mosby.

Mithaug, D.E., Horiuchi, C.N., & Fanning, P.N. (1985). A report on the Colorado statewide follow-up survey of special education students. *Exceptional Children, 51,* 397–404.

Mithaug, D.E., Martin, J.E., & Agran, M. (1987). Adaptability instruction: The goal of transitional programming. *Exceptional Children, 53,* 500–505.

National Association of State Directors of Special Education. (1990). *Education of the Handicapped Act Amendments of 1990 (P. L. 101–476): Summary of Major Changes in Parts A through H of the Act.* Washington, D. C.: National Association of State Directors of Special Education.

Ortiz, A.A., Yates, J.R. (1984). Linguistically and culturally diverse handicapped students. In R.S. Podemski, B.J. Price, T.E.C. Smith, & G.E. Marsh. (Eds.), *Comprehensive administration of special education,* (pp. 114–140). Rockville, Maryland: Aspen.

Patton J.R., Bierne-Smith, M., (1990). *Mental retardation,* 3rd Ed. Columbus, OH: Merrill.

Phillips, V. & McCullough, L. (1990). Consultation-based programming: Instituting the collaborative ethic in schools. *Exceptional Children, 56,* 291–304.

Polloway, E.A. & Smith, T.E.C. (1992). *Language instruction for students with disabilities,* 2nd Ed. Denver: Love.

Polloway, E.A., Patton, J.R., Payne, J., & Payne, (1989). *Strategies for teaching learners with special needs,* 4th Ed. Columbus, OH: Merrill.

Polloway, E.A., Patton, J.R., Epstein, M.A., & Smith, T.E.C. (1989). Comprehensive curriculum for students with mild handicaps. *Focus on Exceptional Children, 21,* 1–12.

Reeve, R.E. (1990). ADHD: Facts and fallacies. *Intervention in School and Clinic, 26,* 70–78.

Reynolds, M.C., Wang, M.C., & Walberg, H.J. (1987). The necessary restructuring of special and regular education. *Exceptional Children, 53,* 391–398.

Rich, H.L., & Ross, S.M. (1989). Students' time on learning tasks in special education. *Exceptional Children, 55,* 508–515.

Rusch, R.R., & Phelps, L.A. (1987). Secondary special education and transition from school to work: A national priority. *Exceptional Children, 53,* 487–492.

Salend, S.J. (1990). *Effective mainstreaming.* New York: Macmillan.

Savage, R.C. (1988). Introduction to educational issues for students who have suffered traumatic brain injury. In R.C. Savage & G.F. Wolcott (Eds.), *An educator's manual: What educators need to know about students with traumatic brain injury,* 1–9. Southborough, MA: National Head Injury Foundation, Inc.

Shea, T.M., & Bauer, A.M. (1991). *Parents and teachers of children with exceptionalities,* 2nd Ed. Boston: Allyn & Bacon.

Smith, T.E.C. (1990). *Introduction to education,* 2nd Ed. St. Paul: West Publishing.

Smith, T.E.C., & Dowdy, C.A. (1989). The role of study skills in the secondary curriculum. *Academic Therapy, 25,* 479–490.

Smith, T.E.C., Dowdy, C. A., & Finn, D.L. (in press). Teacher training issues for secondary special education. *Teacher Education and Special Education.*

Smith, T.E.C., Price, B.J., & Marsh, G.E. (1986). *Mildly handicapped children and adults.* St. Paul: West Publishing.

Special education in the 1990s: Return to curriculum, teaching. (1990). *Education of the Handicapped. 16,* 1+.

Stainback, S., & Stainback, W. (1987). Integration versus cooperation: A commentary on "educating children with learning problems: A shared responsibility." *Exceptional Children, 54*, 66–68.

Tateyama-Sniezek, K.M. (1990). Cooperative learning: Does it improve the academic achievement of students with handicaps? *Exceptional Children, 56*, 426–437.

Tindal, G., Shinn, M.R., & Rodden-Nord, K. (1990). Contextually based school consultation: Influential variables. *Exceptional Children, 56*, 324–336.

U.S. Department of Education. (1988). *Tenth annual report to Congress on the implementation of Public Law 94–142*. Washington, D. C.: U. S. Government Printing Office.

U.S. Department of Education. (1989). *Eleventh annual report to Congress on the implementation of Public Law 94–142*. Washington, D. C.: U. S. Government Printing Office.

U. S. Department of Education. (1990). *Twelfth annual report to Congress on the implementation of Public Law 94–142*. Washington, D. C.: U. S. Government Printing Office.

Wang, M.C., & Birch, J.W. (1984). Comparison of a full-time mainstreaming program and a resource room approach. *Exceptional Children, 51*, 33–40.

Wehman, P. Kiregel, J., & Seyfarth, J. (1985). Transition from school to work for individuals with severe disabilities: A follow-up study. pp. 47–61. In P. Wehman & J. W. Hill (Eds.), *Competitive employment for persons with mental retardation: From research to practice*. Richmond: Virginia Commonwealth University.

White, C.C., Lakin, K.C., & Bruininks, R. H. (1989). *Persons with mental retardation and related conditions in state-operated residential facilities: year ending June 30, 1988 with longitudinal trends from 1950 to 1988*. (Report No. 30). Minneapolis: University of Minnesota Center for Residential and Community Services.

Will, M.C. (1986). Educating children with learning problems: A shared responsibility. *Exceptional Children, 52*, 411–415.

Ysseldyke, J.E., & Algozzine, B. (1990). *Introduction to special education*. Boston: Houghton Mifflin.

Ysseldyke, J.E., Thurlow, M.L., Wotruba, J.W., & Nania, P.A. (1990). Instructional arrangements: Perceptions from general education. *Teaching Exceptional Children, 22*, 4–8.

Zins, J.E., Curtis, M.J., Graden, S.G. & Pontin, C.R. (1988). *Helping students succeed in the regular classroom*. San Francisco: Jossey-Bass, Inc.

Characteristics of Students with Mild Disabilities

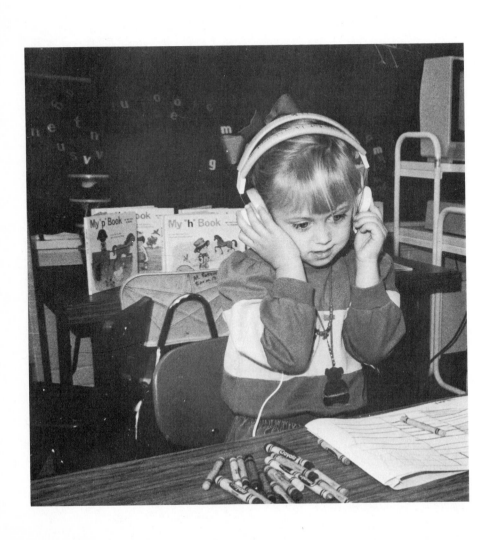

Outline

OBJECTIVES

After reading this chapter you will be able to:

- discuss importance of knowing the characteristics of students with mild disabilities;

- describe reasons for labeling students with categorical labels;

- discuss the cognitive characteristics of students with mild disabilities;

- describe the general intellectual ability of students with mild disabilities;

- discuss cognitive styles and how they relate to students with mild disabilities;

- list characteristics that suggest attention problems in students with mild disabilities;

- describe the memory skills of students with mild disabilities;

- summarize the general and specific academic problems experienced by students with mild disabilities;

- describe the self-concepts of students with mild disabilities;

- discuss the behavior problems experienced by students with mild disabilities;

- describe the social skills of students with mild disabilities.

Introduction

The number one characteristic of students classified as mildly disabled is that they need special education and related services and are capable of benefiting from these services in a normalized school setting. This is the one primary distinguishing factor between students with mild disabilities and those with more severe problems. There are many other characteristics that apply to students classified as mildly disabled. As with any category of disabilities, some students will display some of these characteristics, while other students display others. Although students placed in this category vary significantly, they display characteristics that are more similar than dissimilar (Marsh, Price, & Smith 1983; Smith, Price, & Marsh, 1986).

One of the key reasons for labeling students with disabilities is to group those with similar characteristics for instructional purposes. While it is the contention of those who advocate classification along categorical lines that students in the traditional categories display unique characteristics, professionals who support the noncategorical, or generic classification systems, believe that the characteristics of students in several categorical groups, namely mild mental retardation, learning disabilities, and mild emotional problems, overlap significantly. Advocates for the "mild disability" category believe that students with mild disabilities exhibit similar characteristics, even though several traditional categories of students are included in the broad "mild" group (Marsh *et al.*, 1983; Smith *et al.*, 1986; Cobb, Elliott, Powers, & Voltz, 1989).

Another reason for categorical labels is to group students who need a unique instructional intervention strategy. However, a recent study confirms that students grouped according to categorical label for instructional purposes are not taught with techniques unique to that category. In the study, data were collected through observations in self-contained classrooms for students classified as emotionally handicapped, learning disabled, and educable mentally retarded. After extensive data analysis, the authors concluded that the "Observations of teachers in self-contained classrooms containing LD, EH, or EMR students did not support conclusions about differentiated instruction on the basis of category." (Algozzine, Morsink, & Algozzine, 1988, p. 264)

If students classified as mildly mentally retarded, learning disabled, and mildly emotionally disturbed display similar characteristics and if instructional approaches for different groups of children with disabilities are similar, the rationale for categorical groups is severely limited. This chapter will provide information about the characteristics of students traditionally labeled mildly mentally retarded, learning disabled, and mildly emotionally disturbed. The philosophy of this text suggests classifying these students as mildly disabled because of the similar characteristics and similar instructional approaches. The information presented will mostly come from research using categorical groups for subjects, because only limited research has been completed that focuses on the generic, noncategorical label, mildly disabled.

Cognitive Characteristics

Cognitive characteristics include a variety of different skills related to information processing (Torgesen, 1988a). Cognition can generally be defined as "the mental processes (perceiving, remembering, using symbols, reasoning, and imagining) that human beings use to acquire knowledge of the world." (Scarr, Weinberg, & Levine, 1986, p. 133) These include general intellectual ability, cognitive styles, attention, memory, problem solving, and organizing.

Skills in these cognitive areas are required for individuals to be successful in academic, social, and intellectual areas. "Examples of such processing activities might include coding information for storage in working memory, comparing incoming information with the contents of long-term memory to check for similarities and discrepancies, and selecting an appropriate strategy to enhance performance on a task." (Torgesen, 1988a, p. 587) For students to succeed in many school tasks, their cognitive skills must be intact. Limitations in any of these areas can result in major academic and adjustment problems.

Students with mild disabilities display a variety of deficits related to cognitive functioning. These include below average general intellectual ability, field-dependent cognitive styles, attention deficits, problems with memory, poor problem-solving skills, and deficits in planning and organizing. Deficits in these areas are frequently the primary reason for the initial referral of the student for special education services.

GENERAL INTELLECTUAL ABILITY

One factor associated with the area of cognitive functioning is general intellectual ability. Intelligence is a term that we routinely use in everyday conversation (Lutwig, 1989). People say their children are "bright" (meaning very intelligent), that they make intelligent decisions, and that some people "are not very smart" (meaning not very intelligent). Although the term is used a great deal, intelligence is a complex, difficult-to-define concept that has been defined in many different ways.

Early definitions of intelligence relied heavily on scores obtained from intelligence tests to describe levels of intellect. The scores that resulted from these tests were converted to intelligence quotients (IQs) (Lutwig, 1989). IQ refers to a statistical ratio between a person's mental age and chronological age. IQ tests are designed so that the mean score is 100, and the standard deviation is 15 or 16. When a representative sample of the population is tested, a normal distribution results. In a normal distribution, there are an approximate equal number of persons who score on the positive side of the mean as on the negative side of the mean. When describing intellectual levels of persons, IQ test scores still are used primarily.

The major individual IQ tests currently used include the Wechsler scales and the Stanford-Binet test (Scarr *et al.*, 1986). An individually administered IQ test takes about one to one and a half hours to complete and is administered to only one person at a time.

Persons who administer individual IQ tests must have specialized training and are generally licensed or certified by state agencies or psychological associations.

Determining the IQ scores is important because there is generally a positive correlation between IQ score and academic achievement. Persons who score in the average IQ range usually perform near their grade level or age equivalent. Individuals who have high IQs are usually performing above their grade or age peers; those with low IQ scores perform lower than their grade or age peers on academic tasks (Smith *et al.*, 1986).

The primary characteristic of students with mental retardation is deficient cognitive skills. This is the one characteristic, above all others, that distinguishes this group of individuals. By definition, students must have an intelligence quotient of about seventy or below to be classified as having mental retardation. Students in the mild category of mental retardation have IQs in the general range of fifty-five to seventy (Grossman, 1983). This means this group of individuals is functioning at the second percentile.

For children with learning disabilities and behavior problems, below average IQ scores are not as obvious. However, various studies have determined that students in these two categories typically have below-average IQ scores. For example, in one study of 200 elementary students classified as having learning disabilities, twenty-eight percent had IQ scores between eighty and eighty-nine, and fifteen percent had IQs between seventy and seventy-nine (Rivers, 1986; Rivers & Smith, 1989). In another study, more than 900 students with learning disabilities who had completed high school were surveyed one year after their exit from school. The mean IQ for the group was 94.43 (Sitlington & Frank, 1990). While this fits in the average range, it still reflects a mean IQ score nearly 6 points below the mean score obtained by students without disabilities.

Margalit (1989) studied the academic competence of students with learning disabilities and behavior problems and concluded that "special attention should be devoted to the similarity found between the learning disabled and the behavior disordered boys with regard to their cognitive competence and functioning." Traditionally, authors have assumed that students with behavior disorders functioned in the normal intellectual range. However, studies over the past twenty-five years have determined that individuals with mild to moderate behavior and emotional problems have IQ scores in the low average range (Kauffman, 1989).

After reviewing research on the intellectual functioning level of students with emotional problems, Kauffman (1989) concluded that "although the majority of mildly and moderately disturbed students fall only slightly below average in IQ, a disproportionate number, compared to the normal distribution, score in the dull normal and mildly retarded range, and relatively few fall in the upper ranges." (p. 183) Figure 2–1 depicts the intellectual range of students with emotional problems, compared to nondisabled students.

COGNITIVE STYLES

Cognitive styles refer to how individuals think. There are two general cognitive styles that relate to how individuals use environmental cues in making judgments—field dependence/field independence and impulsivity/reflectivity (Wallace & McLoughlin, 1988). Individuals who have a field dependent style have a tendency to operate in a global manner and are distracted by nonessential elements in their environments. On the other hand,

FIGURE 2-1 Hypothetical frequency distributions of IQ for mildly to moderately, and severely to profoundly disturbed as compared to a normal frequency distribution.

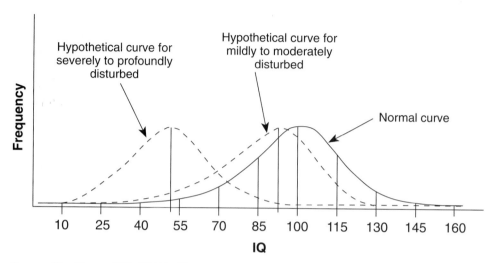

Source: Kauffman, J.M. (1989). *Characteristics of behavior disorders of children and youth*, 4th Ed. Columbus, OH: Merrill. p. 142. Used with permission.

field-independent individuals overcome distracting elements in the environment and focus on relevant information (Bice, Halpin, & Halpin, 1986).

Students who experience achievement problems too often display a field-dependent cognitive style (Wallace & McLoughlin, 1988). Bice *et al.* (1986) compared the cognitive strategies of eighty students with mild mental retardation to eighty students who were not disabled. The results revealed that the students with mental retardation were more field-dependent, while nondisabled students were more likely to be field-independent. Students with learning disabilities and behavior problems also display field dependence (Patton, Payne, & Beirne-Smith, 1986; Kauffman, 1989). On a related issue, Day and Hall (1988) compared the way students with mental retardation and nonretarded students learn. Results indicated that students with mental retardation need more assistance in learning than their nonretarded peers, and they also have more problems transfering their learning than nondisabled students.

Students with learning disabilities, mental retardation, and behavior problems have a tendency to be impulsive in their responses; they often react or respond without a great deal of thought (Polloway *et al.*, 1985; Patton *et al.*, 1986; Mercer, 1987; Kauffman, 1989). This response pattern can create problems for students with disabilities by increasing their chances of making errors. Research has shown that these students can be taught to use a more reflective response approach and thus enhance their chances for academic success (Mercer, 1987).

ATTENTION

Attention can be defined as selectively focusing the senses on external stimuli. We are routinely bombarded with more information than we can possibly process, especially in an academic setting. What we attend to determines what information we process (Woolfolk, 1990). For students in school, what is attended to results in what is learned (Polloway & Smith, 1992). Students cannot learn if they do not attend to appropriate stimuli. "Focusing attention is a critical first step in the learning process." (Patton, Payne, & Beirne-Smith, 1986, p. 328)

While most people think of attention as representing a simple construct, it is really a very complex process composed of many different skills. Recently there has been a great deal of interest in the negative impact of attention problems. In fact, some professionals and parents advocate a new category of children identified as attention deficit disorder (ADD) or attention deficit hyperactivity disorder (ADHD).

Children who experience attention deficit/hyperactivity disorders display the following behaviors.

- inattention

- impulsiveness

- difficulty remaining seated

- difficulty organizing and completing work

- failure to follow instructions

- failure to complete tasks

- difficulty in following rules

- excessive jumping and moving (DSM-III-R, 1987).

Attention has been shown to be directly related to learning and language problems (Shames & Wiig, 1990). Many children classified as mentally retarded, learning disabled, and emotionally disturbed display attention problems (Krupski, 1985). In a recent study, Roberts, Pratt, and Leach (1991) reported that a group of students with mild disabilities were "off task" nearly twice as often as nondisabled students. This "off task" behavior, which is related to attention, only adds to the learning problems experienced by students with disabilities.

Teachers who have taught students with learning disabilities attest to the attention problems experienced by this group of students (Fleisher, Soodak, & Jelin, 1984). Indeed, attention deficits as a characteristic of students with learning disabilities is confirmed by most textbook authors (Houk, 1984; Wallace & McLoughlin, 1988; Reid, 1988; Mercer, 1987; Lerner, 1989; Myers & Hammill, 1990). In reviewing the records of 200 elementary students with learning disabilities, Rivers (1986) determined that twenty-one percent experienced problems in listening comprehension, a skill that depends heavily on attention.

Students with mild mental retardation also have a tendency to have problems with attention (Forness & Polloway, 1987). Polloway, Eptstein, and Cullinan (1985) found that students in this category displayed attention deficits, were inattentive, distractible, and had shorter attention spans than their nondisabled peers. In the sample of more than 600 students with mild mental retardation, over half had problems related to attention-deficit disorders.

In another study investigating the attention of students with mental retardation, it was determined that lowered intellectual levels correlated positively with inattention; the lower the intellectual level, the lower the attention level (Siegel, Crawford, & Evelsizer, 1985). Students with mental retardation cannot afford the problems presented by attentional deficits. They need to be trained to focus their attending to selectively process information.

Students with behavior disorders have traditionally been characterized as being distractible and having short attention spans. This distractibility results in these students shifting their attention from academic tasks, often to activities related to acting out behaviors. Hyperactivity is often associated with the distractibility and short attention span in children with behavior problems (Kauffman, 1989). The combination of distractibility, short attention span, and hyperactivity makes it very difficult for students with behavior disorders to perform well in academic tasks.

MEMORY

Memory is the ability to store and recall information. The importance of memory in academic activities is obvious. Students have to remember sounds and letters, spelling rules, math facts and functions, rules of grammar, and facts related to content courses, such as history, literature, and biology.

Memory can be broken into short-term memory and long-term memory. Short-term memory has been called the "working memory," because it contains what you are currently thinking about. Information in short-term memory is kept for about twenty seconds. Storing information longer than twenty seconds requires rehearsal or some other activity. Information retained for longer periods of time is stored in long-term memory. Whereas information is stored in short-term memory rather easily, more effort is required to store information in long-term memory. Information can also be stored in long-term memory for an indefinite period of time in contrast to the very restrictive length of time that it can be kept in short-term memory (Woolfolk, 1990).

Students with mild disabilities frequently experience problems in memory (McDaniel, Einstein, & Waddill, 1990; Cornoldi, 1990). Memory deficits are common among students classified as learning disabled. In fact, "deficits in memory are among the most frequently demonstrated psychological consequences of a learning disability." (Swanson & Trahan, 1990, p. 82). The incredible thing about memory deficits in students with learning disabilities is that these are students with average to above average intellectual abilities who perform in the mentally retarded range on activities that require immediate recall (Torgesen, 1988b).

Hallahan, Kauffman, and Lloyd (1985) reviewed studies that investigated the memory skills of students with learning disabilities. The following summarizes their conclusions.

- Compared to students without disabilities, students with learning disabilities experience memory problems.

- A failure to use certain strategies results in memory problems among students with learning disabilities.

■ Strategies that nondisabled students use in memory can be effectively taught to students who have learning disabilities.

Problems in memory have also been routinely found in studies with students who have mental retardation. Ellis, Deacon, and Wooldridge (1985) conducted several studies to investigate the memory of persons with mental retardation. Their results revealed that 1. individuals with mental retardation forget more easily than nonretarded persons when there is limited time for encoding; 2. additional encoding time increases memory for persons with mental retardation, but not to a normal level; and 3. persons with mental retardation have more difficulty remembering letters than pictures.

PROBLEM SOLVING

Problem solving can be defined as "formulating new answers, going beyond the simple application of previously learned rules to create a solution." (Woolfolk, 1990, p. 267) Problem solving occurs when persons are faced with situations that do not have an obvious solution. Students in school must have problem-solving skills in order to be successful on academic tasks. While many students have difficulties with problem solving, those with mild disabilities are more likely to have deficits.

Numerous sources have revealed the deficient problem-solving skills found among students with learning disabilities (Zimmerman, 1988; Wallace & McLoughlin, 1988), mental retardation (Polloway *et al.*, 1986; Patton *et al.*, 1986; Ferretti & Butterfield, 1989) and behavior disorders (Kalfus, Hawkins, & Reitz, 1984; Kauffman, 1989). In a recent study, the problem-solving skills of elementary-aged students classified as gifted, normal, and mildly mentally retarded were compared. Results indicated that the students with mild mental retardation had the poorest problem-solving abilities of the three groups. The general conclusion of the study was that "the sophistication of children's scientific problem-solving strategies is related to intelligence." (Ferretti & Butterfield, 1989, p. 431)

PLANNING AND ORGANIZING SKILLS

Planning and organizing skills are necessary for students to experience academic and social success in school. Without these skills, students will likely not be effective in using their time, studying, and completing tasks efficiently. Kops and Belmont (1985) studied the planning and organizing skills of students with average intellectual abilities who were experiencing academic achievement problems. Results revealed that lower achieving students have a tendency to be poor planners and organizers. These deficiencies result in lowered achievement levels.

Academic Problems

Students with mild mental retardation, learning disabilities, and behavior disorders frequently display academic deficits (Leigh, 1987; Patton, Payne, & Beirne-Smith, 1986;

Mercer, 1987). When using the federal criteria for determining eligibility for special education services, the disability must adversely affect educational performance. Therefore, academic achievement problems are actually a requirement for special education services provided through Public Law 94–142. Beyond the school years, many persons with mild disabilities continue to experience problems related to academic skills (Hoffman *et al.*, 1987).

Deficits in academic achievement are found in most persons with disabilities. Students with mild mental retardation, learning disabilities, and behavior disorders all display certain levels of academic deficits. It is the academic deficit that drives the educational intervention program for most of these students (Polloway & Smith, 1992).

A common problem experienced by students with learning disabilities is academic deficits. Zimmerman (1988) found that one group of students with learning disabilities had a mean score on the Science Research Associates (SRA) Achievement test of 81 compared to a mean score of 105 obtained by a group of nondisabled students. In a study that compared achievement levels of students with emotional problems, Morgan (1986) determined that these students who were mainstreamed into regular classrooms, where the majority of students with mild emotional problems are placed, experienced problems in academic achievement.

While describing how to limit the number of students with disabilities from dropping out of high schools, deBettencourt and Zigmond (1990) noted that the overall grades received by these students was significantly below the grades received by their nondisabled classmates. While some students with mild disabilities experience academic deficits across the board, others perform well in some areas, while displaying deficits in others. The following describes the performance of students with learning disabilities, mild mental retardation, and emotional problems in specific academic areas.

READING PROBLEMS

Students with mild disabilities are classified and served in special education programs because they are experiencing academic problems. The academic area that most often causes problems for these students is reading. Since most students with mild disabilities receive a portion of their educational program in general education classrooms, their ability to process information through reading is critical (Polloway & Smith, 1992).

Students with learning disabilities frequently experience reading problems (Santos, 1989). Rivers (1986) found that, out of a sample of 200 elementary students with learning disabilities, 54.5 percent had educational deficits in basic reading and reading comprehension skills. In another study, elementary students with learning disabilities scored a mean percentile rank of 7.74 on the Wide Range Achievement Test-Revised (WRAT-R) (Wiener, Harris, & Shirer, 1990). This means that they scored as well or better than only seven percent of their age peers.

Reading problems for students with learning disabilities frequently continue into high school. In a study of older students, the performance of high school sophomores with learning disabilities and that of their nondisabled peers on reading and writing competencies were compared. The results revealed that between eighty and ninety percent of the nondisabled students exhibited competence in reading and writing skills, compared to between forty and eighty percent of the students with learning disabilities (Algozzine, O'Shea, Stoddard, & Crews, 1988).

Adults with learning disabilities continue to have problems with reading (Rogan & Hartman, 1990). A survey of more than 900 high school graduates who were learning disabled revealed a mean reading grade equivalency of 6.68 (Sitlington & Frank, 1990). Hoffman et al. (1987) found that seventy-five percent of the adults with learning disabilities involved in a survey wanted assistance with their reading problems.

Problems in reading are also inherent in persons with mental retardation. On the Florida State Student Assessment Test, students with mild mental retardation performed very poorly on the reading component. The percentage of the students with mental retardation who passed the reading subtests ranged from a low of 5.6 percent on the facts/opinion and diagram/tables subtests, to a high of twenty-three percent on the identify/inform sources subtest (Crews, 1988). (See Table 2–1)

WRITTEN LANGUAGE PROBLEMS

The ability to express yourself with written language is extremely important for students in academic settings. Teachers routinely require written assignments and written responses on tests; also, students need to be able to take written notes in classes where lecturing is the primary source of information dissemination. Students with disabilities often have problems with written language. Unfortunately, many of these students may be able to deal effectively with the content in a classroom but fail the course because of poor writing abilities (McLaughlin, Mabee, Byram, & Reiter, 1987; Polloway & Smith, 1992).

For students with learning disabilities, problems in handwriting are a common feature (Blandford & Lloyd, 1987; Polloway & Smith, 1992). Algozzine *et al.* (1988) reported that students with learning disabilities are much less likely to demonstrate competence in writing skills than their nondisabled peers. In one study, students with learning disabilities were compared to a group of nondisabled students and another group of nondisabled students who were matched to the LD students in IQ scores and reading ability. Results of the paragraph-writing task showed the students with learning disabilities scoring significantly lower than both nondisabled groups in writing skills (Thomas, Englert, & Gregg, 1987).

Adults with learning disabilities continue to experience problems with writing. Written expression for adults is critical in personal activities, such as letter writing, making lists, and keeping diaries, as well as vocational tasks. Therefore, adults with written language problems are at a major disadvantage compared to their nondisabled peers. In one study, eighty-eight percent of the adults with learning disabilities who were surveyed indicated a desire for help with writing skills (Hoffman *et al.*, 1987).

Students with mild mental retardation also experience difficulties in written language. Crews (1988) noted that only 12.4 percent of the individuals with mild mental retardation taking the Florida State Student Assessment Test passed some sections of the writing test. Table 2–1 summarizes this information.

SPELLING SKILLS

Spelling is a subcomponent of written expression that is important for school-age students. Spelling is one of those skills that often presents problems for many people. For students with disabilities, such as mental retardation and learning disabilities, spelling is even more

TABLE 2-1 Performances of Students with Mental Retardation on the Florida State
Student Assessment Test

	FREQUENCY			
Skill	Passed	Failed	Percentage Passed	Mean Number of Items Correct
Reading				
Main Idea (stated)	21	261	7.0	1.44
Who, What, When	58	224	20.5	2.12
Cause/Effect	36	246	12.7	1.89
Written Directions	33	249	11.7	1.55
Main Idea (implied)	26	256	9.2	1.53
Paragraph Conclusion	32	250	11.3	1.76
Facts/Opinion	16	266	5.6	1.40
Pictures, Maps, Signs	46	236	16.3	2.00
Diagrams/Tables	15	267	5.6	1.56
Indexes/Dictionary	42	240	14.8	1.92
Identify Inform Sources	65	217	23.0	1.92
Writing				
Request Inform/Messages	69	213	24.4	2.13
Letter	35	247	12.4	1.74
Complete Forms	80	202	28.3	2.32
Money Order/Check	102	180	36.1	2.60

Source: Crews, W.B. (1988). Performance of students classified as educable mentally handicapped on Florida's state student assessment test, Part II. *Education and Training in Mental Retardation, 23*, p. 189. Used with permission.

difficult (Matson, Esveldt-Dawson, & Kazdin, 1982; Vallecorsa, Zigmond, & Henderson, 1985). Luenberger and Morris (1990) described spelling for students with learning disabilities as a "seemingly impossible" task. Wiener *et al*. (1990) found that students with learning disabilities had a mean percentile rank of 7.52 on the spelling subtest of the WRAT-R.

Students with learning disabilities often continue to have problems with spelling after high school (Hoffman *et al*, 1987). Leuenberger and Morris (1990) compared the spelling abilities of students with learning disabilities and nondisabled students who were enrolled in a university. The results revealed that the disabled students had significantly more problems with spelling than their nondisabled peers. The fact that students with learning disabilities in college continue to have spelling problems was also noted by Rogan and Hatman (1990) in a ten-year follow-up study of students.

MATH PROBLEMS

The academic success and vocational potential for students is dependent on proficiency in math (Mattingly & Bott, 1990). Skills in the area of math are very important for students during their school years since math is a common component of the elementary and secondary curricula for most schools (Smith, 1990). Also, students need math skills after they exit the school system. Simple skills such as matching numbers required for using the telephone are important for adults with disabilities in order to function independently (Lalli, Mace, Browder, & Brown, 1989). Other functional purposes of math for adults include money management, computing taxes, and working through simple problems, such as determining how much floor covering is needed for a specific size room.

Students with mild disabilities frequently experience problems in math. In one study, students with learning disabilities scored a mean 10.68 percentile on the math subtest of the WRAT-R (Wiener, Harris, & Shirer, 1990). Former graduates from a secondary program for learning disabled students scored a mean math grade equivalency of 7.5 (Sitlington & Frank, 1990). In a ten-year follow-up of students with learning disabilities, Rogan and Hartman (1990) found significant problems in math, even for students who attended college. In still another study of adults with learning disabilities, seventy-four percent of the sample indicated a need for help with math skills (Hoffman *et al.* 1987).

Students with mental retardation also have problems with math. Crews (1988) studied the performance of students with mild mental retardation on the Florida State Student Assessment Test. In the area of math, the number of students with mental retardation who passed specific skill areas ranged from a low of 2.4 percent on the subject of perimeter to a high of 35.5 percent on the subject of dollars and coins. Table 2–2 summarizes the results of students on the math subtest.

Social and Behavioral Problems

Social and behavioral problems are common among students with disabilities. The ability to get along with peers, feel good about yourself, and control behaviors to conform to classroom expectations are all vitally important in the success for all students. For students with disabilities, competence in these areas is even more important, however; there has been a great deal of data to suggest that these students frequently experience problems in these areas (Sabornie & Beard, 1990).

SELF-CONCEPT

The self-concepts of students are very important for academic and social success. A person's self-concept develops out of "the complex interaction between the capabilities of the individual, the social environments in which self-evaluations occur, and cognitive development . . ." (Coleman, 1985, p. 26). For students, these environments where self-evaluations occur usually include the classroom and social settings around the school and neighborhood.

The self-concepts of students with mild disabilities are important for several reasons. First, self-concepts are related to students' general mental health. Secondly, self-concepts

TABLE 2-2 Performances of Students with Mental Retardation on the Florida State Student Assessment Test in Math

Skill	FREQUENCY		Percentage Passed	Mean Number of Items Correct
	Passed	Failed		
Averages 10 Numbers	14	270	4.9	1.16
One or Two Whole Number Operations	27	257	9.5	1.35
Add/Subtract Proper Fractions	18	266	6.3	1.06
Decimals/Percents	29	264	10.9	1.70
Equivalent Dollars-Coins	76	214	35.5	2.25
Comparison Shopping	11	273	3.8	1.59
Simple Interest	13	271	4.5	1.45
Purchases and Sales Tax	11	273	3.8	1.35
Rate of Discount	21	263	7.3	1.52
Time	30	254	10.5	1.76
Perimeter	7	277	2.4	1.20
Length, Width, Height	12	272	4.2	1.58
Capacity, Measurement	8	276	2.8	1.35
Mass/Weight Measurement	11	273	3.8	1.37
Graphs/Tables	22	262	7.7	1.50

Source: Crews, W.B. (1988). Performance of students classified as educable mentally handicapped on Florida's state student assessment test, Part II. *Education and Training in Mental Retardation, 23*, p. 189. Used with permission.

can directly affect performances in academic settings. And finally, a student's self-concept will affect expectations (Cooley & Ayres, 1988). Students with mild disabilities already experience social and academic problems. Negative self-concepts can contribute to failures, while positive self-concepts can result in improved academic and social performances.

Students with disabilities have been shown to have lowered self-concepts when compared to their nondisabled peers. Students with learning disabilities (Cooley & Ayres, 1988), mental retardation (Polloway *et al.*, 1985), and behavior problems (Kauffman, 1989) generally have lowered self-concepts. These negative self-concepts make remediation and improved social skills more difficult.

In one study of adults with mild mental retardation, Zetlin and Turner (1988) found that conformity and dependency were the two most frequent comments made during the survey. Respondents made statements such as "I will do things you want me to do" and "I should learn to take teasing," which reflect the external rather than internal controls in these persons' lives.

Negative self-concepts are also found in students with learning disabilities. When you consider the failure and frustration experienced by students in this population, it is not surprising to find lowered self-concepts. Continued failures, pressure from parents, and questions from teachers and peers about their failures only facilitate lowered self-concepts (Mercer, 1987).

MOTIVATION

Motivation can be defined as the "general process by which behavior is initiated and directed toward a goal." (Woolfolk, 1990, p. 302) It is the desire to be successful and not fail (Scarr *et al.*, 1986). Without adequate motivation, students have a more difficult time achieving success in school. Teachers, both regular and special education, face daily questions regarding the motivation of their students. What factors motivate their students and how teachers can increase the motivation of students are common concerns (Mehring & Colson, 1990). Students with disabilities often exhibit poor motivation because of their histories of failure (Raschke, Dedrick, & Thompson, 1987).

There are numerous factors that influence the motivation of students. These include 1. anxiety, 2. self-concept, 3. teacher expectations, 4. the learning process, 5. goal structure, and 6. incentives for learning (Mehring & Colson, 1990). Unfortunately, for many students with disabilities, these factors result in poor motivation. For example, students who have learning problems are likely to be anxious about the entire learning process. Also, the self-concepts of these students will be lower than self-concepts for nondisabled students, and teachers are likely to expect less of students in the disability group. Students with mild disabilities, therefore, frequently display motivational problems.

Beckman and Weller (1990) noted that students with learning disabilities often lack the motivation that they need to complete specific tasks independently. These students rely on others, such as teachers or parents, to provide the motivation necessary. Often, special education teachers do this through the use of concrete positive reinforcers. In another study, Heavey *et al.* (1989) concluded that students with learning disabilities displayed less motivation than their nondisabled peers on a variety of tasks that related to academic success.

BEHAVIOR PROBLEMS

Students classified as behaviorally disordered or emotionally disturbed frequently display behavior problems. Conduct disorders, characterized by acting out behaviors, compose one of the major categories of behavior disorders (Kauffman, 1989). Teachers expect these students to display inappropriate behaviors because that is a key characteristic for the group. In addition to students with behavior problems displaying inappropriate behaviors, students classified as learning disabled and mentally retarded also exhibit problems maintaining appropriate behaviors.

Problems with behavior are common occurences among students with learning disabilities. The misbehavior in these students may be the result of problems in learning, or it might actually lead to the learning problems. In one recent study, students with learning disabilities were compared to nondisabled students in the areas of anger and behavior problems. As hypothesized, parents and teachers of the learning disabled group rated them as having more behavior problems than did the parents and teachers of nondisabled students (Heavey, Adelman, Nelson, & Smith, 1989).

Russell and Forness (1985) studied behavior problems in nearly 400 students who were classified as mildly mentally retarded. The results of the study revealed the following:

1. Relationships between intellectual level, behavioral problems, and etiology are complex and not clear.

2. Approximately five percent of the students exhibited behavioral problems.

3. Behavior problems increased as intellectual levels declined.

4. Approximately eight to nine percent of a small group of students with mental retardation exhibit significant behavioral problems.

In another study, students with mild mental retardation who were referred to a mental retardation center for related services were evaluated for behavioral and emotional problems. The results indicated that 13.1 percent had conduct or attentional problems, 12.5 percent displayed personality disorders, and 9.4 percent had affective disorders. Of the sample, only 22.7 percent had no psychiatric diagnosis (Forness & Polloway, 1987).

HYPERACTIVITY

Hyperactivity can be defined as "an excess of nonpurposeful motor activity (e.g., out of seat, finger and foot tapping, asking questions incessantly and often repeating the same question, inability to sit or stand still)" (Mercer, 1987, p. 43). Hyperactivity may be related to academic deficits and can also cause social problems for students. The exact nature of hyperactivity is not known; however, a large number of professionals believe that it is caused by receiving too much stimuli. For some reason, students with hyperactivity have a problem filtering out some of the stimuli making it difficult to focus on specific input (Wallace & McLoughlin, 1988). When students are incapable of attending to the important incoming stimuli, they frequently become distracted by extraneous stimuli (Mercer, 1987).

Students with mild disabilities frequently display hyperactivity, along with impulsivity and distractibility. Although not all students with learning disabilities have hyperactivity, it occurs in this population more prevalently than in nondisabled groups and is frequently listed as a characteristic of this group (Mercer, 1987).

Hyperactivity is also a characteristic of students with mental retardation. Polloway *et al.* (1986) analyzed data collected on 234 students with mild mental retardation and determined that the rate of hyperactivity ranged from a high of 21.4 percent in younger boys to a low of 14.3 percent in older girls. The percentage of older boys with hyperactivity was 18.5 percent; 17.8 percent of younger girls were considered hyperactive. The rates of hyperactivity found in students with mental retardation was significantly higher than found among students without disabilities.

Students with behavior disorders and emotional problems frequently exhibit hyperactive behaviors. There is considerable overlap between hyperactivity and conduct disorders. In fact, the characteristics that describe students with conduct disorders closely reflect hyperactivity (Kauffman, 1989). Regardless of the overlap, most authorities include hyperactivity as a characteristic of students with behavior problems.

SOCIAL SKILLS

Social skills can be defined as "those skills that enhance and facilitate a student's ability to interact successfully with peers and adults" (Blackbourn, 1989, p. 28). This ability is vitally important to the success of all students but especially to those with disabilities. Unfortunately, students with mild disabilities frequently experience problems with their social skills. In one study, teachers indicated that a majority of students with mild disabilities in their classrooms experienced problems in social interactions with peers. Teachers reported that 81.8 percent of students with behavior problems, 57.5 percent of the learning disabled students, and 33.3 percent of the students with mental retardation and physical problems experience problems with social interactions (Ray, 1985).

Students with disabilities are more likely to be integrated into regular classrooms for part of their school days now than prior to the passage of Public Law 94–142 and the implementation of the least-restrictive-environment mandate. If students with disabilities are to succeed in their regular classes, several competencies must be present. These include academic competence, behavior control, and social skills (Fad, 1990). Too often poor social skills lead to limited success in mainstream placements (Nelson, 1988).

Students with learning disabilities typically have social problems. Studies for numerous years have documented the fact that these students have social status problems (Wiener, Harris, & Shirer, 1990). In one recent study, the social status of learning disabled students in mainstream physical education classes was measured using sociometric surveys. The results appear to confirm earlier research findings: "LD students, as a group, were unaccepted and rejected among their mainstream peers." (Sabornie, Marshall, & Ellis, 1990, p. 320)

The social perception of students with learning disabilities was studied to determine if older students have more accurate social perceptions than younger students. Although the results indicated that the social perceptions of students with learning disabilities increase with age, the differences between their social perceptions and the social perceptions of nondisabled children remained the same (Jackson, Enright, & Murdock, 1987). These negative social perceptions can result in negative self-concepts (Ness & Price, 1990). When comparing the adaptive behavior of students with learning disabilities to their nondisabled peers, Leigh (1987) found the learning disabled group below average in all areas, including social skills.

Adults with learning disabilities continue to have social problems. In one study, 381 adults with learning disabilities, 948 service providers for adults with learning disabilities, and 212 consumers, or advocates for persons with learning disabilities were surveyed regarding characteristics and needs of adults with learning disabilities. The results revealed that there are many social problems present among adults, including making and keeping friends and making conversations (Hoffman et al., 1987). Table 2–3 summarizes these data. While students with learning disabilities have a tendency to exhibit problems in social skills, intervention programs that focus on the development and generalization of appropriate social skills can be effective (Blackbourn, 1989).

The behavior of students also appears to influence their social acceptability. Van Bourgondien (1987) used videotapes of children to determine the social acceptability of students with obvious behavior and learning problems. The results indicated that inappropriate behaviors leads to social rejection. Since inappropriate behaviors are common

TABLE 2–3 Social Problems of Adults with Learning Disabilities

Problem	PERCENTAGE		
	LD Adults (N = 381)	Service Provicers (N = 948)	Consumers (N = 212)
Making and Keeping Friends	17	29	50
Dating	27	7	11
Making Conversation	24	26	26
Using Free Time	16	22	21
Knowing about Sex	7	5	7
Dependence on Others	18	38	37
Shy	31	25	17
Talking or Acting before Thinking	33	47	57
Don't Know	—	19	16

[a]Question on the adult survey asked respondents to check all problems with social skills they were having while service provider and consumer surveys asked respondents to check the three major social problems of learning disabled adults.

Source: Hoffman, F.J., Sheldon, K.L., Minskoff, E.H., Sautter, S.W., Steidle, E.F., Baker, D.P., Bailey, M.B., & Echols, L.D. (1987). Needs of Learning Disabled Adults. *Journal of Learning Disabilities, 20*, p. 48. Used with permission.

among students with behavior and emotional problems, this category of disabilities often includes those with problems in social acceptability.

Just as social skills intervention programs can be effective in improving the social skills of students with learning disabilities, intervention can also aid students with behavior and emotional problems. In one study, students with emotional and behavior problems were taught appropriate social skills in an integrated structured setting. The results suggest that this type of intervention can facilitiate the development of appropriate social skills by students with behavior and emotional problems (Anderson, Rush, Ayllon, & Kandel, 1987).

Students with mental retardation also are likely to be rejected by their nondisabled peers. Sabornie and Kauffman (1987) used sociometric ratings to determine the social acceptability of students with mild mental retardation. Results indicated that these students received more negative classroom ratings than their nondisabled classmates.

Teachers of 234 students classified as mildly mentally retarded were surveyed to determine the social and behavioral characteristics of the students. The findings indicated that students with mental retardation were often rejected by their age peers. Table 2–4 (page 56) summarizes the findings. A key fact in the data is that twenty to twenty-nine percent of the students with mental retardation were either rejected or neglected by their peers (Polloway, Epstein, Patton, Cullinan, & Luebke, 1986). Intervention programs to improve the social skills of students with mental retardation can be effective (McEvoy, Shores, Wehby, Johnson, & Fox, 1990).

TABLE 2–4 Social and Behavioral Ratings of Students with Mental Retardation

	YOUNGER GIRLS	YOUNGER BOYS	OLDER BOYS	OLDER GIRLS
Social Status				
Popular (percent)	10.5	15.2	5.3	3.6
Accepted (percent)	50.9	54.3	48.0	47.3
Rejected (percent)	5.3	4.3	4.0	12.7
Accept-Reject (percent)	17.5	8.7	24.0	20.0
Conners ATRS				
Percent Hyperactive[a]	21.4	17.8	18.5	14.3
Mean Score	10.3	8.0	8.8	5.7
SD	6.8	5.6	6.9	6.6

[a]Based on a cutoff score of 15.

Source: Polloway, E.A., Epstein, M.H., Patton, J.R., Cullinan, D., & Luebke, J. (1986). Demographic, social, and behavioral characteristics of students with educable mental retardation. *Education and Training in Mental Retardation, 21,* p. 30. Used with permission.

SUMMARY

This chapter has described students with mild disabilities. The first section of the chapter focused on the cognitive characteristics of these students. It was noted that they have below average IQ scores, and deficits in memory, attention, problem-solving abilities, and organizational and planning skills. Students from the categorical groups of mild mental retardation, learning disabilities, and behavior disorders/emotional problems all display these characteristics to various degrees.

The second section dealt with the academic characteristics of mildly disabled students. It was noted that these students experience problems in most academic areas, including reading, writing, spelling, math, and content subject areas. Section three focused on the behavioral and social characteristics of students with mild disabilities. Self-concept, which impacts performance in many different areas, is generally low among these students. Also, they experience problems with motivation, have a tendency to be hyperactive, and display acting out and other behavior problems more than their nondisabled peers.

Finally, the social skills of students with mild disabilities was discussed. It was noted that these students have a tendency to be rejected by their peers and to have problems simply getting along with their teachers and fellow students. These social skills not only affect the academic performance of students, but can carry over into adulthood and present significant vocational problems.

The final section of the chapter dealt with the overlap of characteristics among the three traditional categories mild mental retardation, learning disabilities, and emotional/behavioral disorders. It was noted that many characteristics of students with mild mental retardation are also experienced by students with learning disabilities and behavioral/emotional problems. With the overlap of characteristics among these three categories being so significant, it was suggested that students with mild disabilities be grouped together for educational purposes, when their needs are similar.

One major rationale for providing special education services to students based on categorical labels is the unique similarity of characteristics exhibited by children in each group. This chapter has pointed out the significant overlap among these characteristics. Educating students with mild disabilities based on their characteristics and needs is much more justified than doing so on the basis of clinical labels.

REFERENCES

Algozzine, B., Morsink, C.V., & Algozzine, K.M. (1988). What's happening in self-contained special education classrooms? *Exceptional Children, 55,* 259–265.

Algozzine, B., O'Shea, D.J., Stoddard, K., & Crews, W.B. (1988). Reading and writing competencies of adolescents with learning disabilities. *Journal of Learning Disabilities, 21,* 154–160.

Anderson, C.G., Rush, D., Ayllon, T., & Kandel, H. (1987). Training and generalization of social skills with problem children. *Child and Adolescent Psychiatry, 4,* 294–298.

Beckman, P., & Weller, C. (1990). Active, independent learning for children with learning disabilities. *Teaching Exceptional Children, 22,* 26–29.

Bice, T.R., Halpin, G., & Halpin, G. (1986). A comparison of the cognitive styles of typical and mildly retarded children with educational recommendations. *Education and Training of the Mentally Retarded, 21,* 93–97.

Blackbourn, J.M. (1989). Acquisition and generalization of social skills in elementary-aged students with learning disabilities. *Journal of Learning Disabilities, 22,* 28–34.

Blandford, B.J., & Lloyd, J.W. (1987). Effects of a self-instructional procedure on handwriting. *Journal of Learning Disabilities, 20,* 342–346.

Cobb, H.B., Elliott, R.N., Powers, A.R., & Voltz, D. (1989). Generic versus categorical special education teacher preparation. *Teacher Education and Special Education, 12,* 19–26.

Coleman, J.M. (1985). Achievement level, social class, and the self-concepts of mildly handicapped children, *Journal of Learning Disabilities, 18,* 26–30.

Cooley, E. J., & Ayres, R.R. (1988). Self-concept and success-failure attributions of nonhandicapped students and students with learning disabilities. *Journal of Learning Disabilities, 21,* 174–178.

Cornoldi, C. (1990). Metacognitive control processes and memory deficits in poor comprehenders. *Learning Disability Quarterly, 13,* 245–255.

Crews, W.B. (1988). Performance of students classified as educable mentally handicapped on Florida's state student assessment test, part II. *Education and Training in Mental Retardation, 23,* 186–191.

Day, J.D., & Hall, L.K. (1988). Intelligence-related differences in learning and transfer and enhancement of transfer among mentally retarded persons. *American Journal on Mental Deficiency, 93,* 125–137.

deBettencourt, L.U., & Zigmond, N. (1990). The learning disabled secondary school dropout. *Teacher Education and Special Education, 13,* 17–20.

Dupont, H. (1989). The emotional development of exceptional students. *Focus on Exceptional Children, 21,* 1–10.

Ellis, N.R., Deacon, J.R., & Wooldridge, P.W. (1985). Structural memory deficits of mentally retarded persons. *American Journal of Mental Deficiency, 89,* 393–402.

Fad, K.S. (1990). The fast track to success: Social-behavioral skills. *Intervention in School and Clinic, 26,* 39–43.

Ferretti, R.P., & Butterfield, E.C. (1989). Intelligence as a correlate of children's problem solving. *American Journal on Mental Deficiency, 93,* 424–433.

Fleisher, L.S., Soodak, L.C., & Jelin, M.A. (1984). Selective attention deficits in learning disabled children: Analysis of data base. *Exceptional Children, 51,* 136–141.

Forness, S.R., & Polloway, E.A. (1987). Physical and psychiatric diagnoses of pupils with mild mental retardation currently being referred for related services. *Education and Training in Mental Retardation, 22,* 221–228.

Heavey, C.L., Adelman, H.S., Nelson, P., & Smith, D.C. (1989). Learning problems, anger, perceived control, and misbehavior. *Journal of Learning Disabilities, 22,* 46–50.

Hoffman, F.J., Sheldon, K.L., Minskoff, E.H., Sutter, S.W., Steidle, E.F., Baker, D.P., Bailey, M.B., & Echols, L.D. (1987). Needs of learning disabled adults. *Journal of Learning Disabilities, 20,* 43–52.

Horton, S. (1985). Computational rates of educable mentally retarded adolescents with and without calculators in comparison to normals. *Education and Training of the Mentally Retarded, 20,* 14–24.

Houck, C.K. (1984). *Learning disabilities.* Englewood Clliffs, NJ: Prentice Hall.

Jackson, S.C., Enright, R.D., & Murdock, J.Y. (1987). Social perception problems in learning disabled youth: Developmental lag versus perceptual deficit. *Journal of Learning Disabilities, 20,* 361–364.

Kalfus, G.R., Hawkins, R.P., & Reitz, A.L. (1984). A program for teaching problem solving in a school for disturbed-delinquent youth. *Child and Adolescent Psychotherapy, 1,* 26–29.

Kauffman, J.M. (1989). *Characteristics of behavior disorders of children and youth,* 4th Ed. Columbus, OH: Merrill.

Kops, C., & Belmont, I. (1985). Planning and organizing skills of poor school achievers. *Journal of Learning Disabilities, 18*, 8–14.

Krupski, A. (1985). Variations in attention as a function of classroom task demands in learning handicapped and CA-matched nonhandicapped children. *Exceptional Children, 52*, 52–56.

Lalli, J.S., Mace, F.C., Browder, D., & Brown, D.K. (1989). Comparison of treatments to teach number matching skills adults with moderate mental retardation. *Mental Retardation, 27*, 75–83.

Leigh, J. (1987). Adaptive behavior of children with learning disabilities. *Journal of Learning Disabilities, 20*, 557–562.

Lerner, J., (1989). *Learning disabilities*, 5th Ed. Boston: Houghton Mifflin.

Leuenberger, J., & Morris, M. (1990). Analysis of spelling errors by learning disabled and normal college students. *Learning Disabilities Focus, 5*, 103–118.

McDaniel, M.A., Einstein, G.O., & Waddill, P.J. (1990). Material-appropriate processing: Implications for remediating recall deficits in students with learning disabilities. *Learning Disability Quarterly, 13*, 258–269.

McLaughlin, T.F., Mabee, W.S., Byram, B.J., & Reiter, S.M. (1987). Effects of academic positive practice and response cost on writing legibility of behaviorally disorderd and learning-disabled junior high school students. *Child and Adolescent Psychotherapy, 4*, 216–221.

Margalit, M. (1989). Academic competence and social adjustment of boys with learning disabilities and boys with behavior disorders. *Journal of Learning Disabilities, 22*, 41–45.

Matson, J.L., Esveldt-Dawson, K., & Kazdin, A.E. (1982). Treatment of spelling deficits in mentally retarded children. *Mental Retardation, 20*, 76–81.

Mattingly, J.C., & Bott, D.A. (1990). Teaching multiplication facts to students with learning problems. *Exceptional Children, 56*, 438–449.

Mehring, T.A., & Colson, S.E. (1990). Motivation and mildly handicapped learners. *Focus on Exceptional Children, 22*, 1–14.

Mercer, C.D. (1987). *Students with learning disabilities*, 3rd Ed. Columbus, OH: Merrill.

Morgan, S.R. (1986). Locus of control and achievement in emotionally disturbed children in segregated classes. *Child and Adolescent Psychotherapy, 3*, 17–21.

Morris, M. & Leuenberger, J. (1990). A report of cognitive academic, and linguistic profiles for college students with and without learning disabilities. *Journal of Learning Disabilities, 23*, 355–361.

Myers, P.I., & Hammill, D.D. (1990). *Learning Disabilities*, 4th Ed. Austin, TX: Pro-Ed.

Nelson, C.M. (1988). Social skills training for handicapped students. *Teaching Exceptional Children, 20*, 19–22.

Ness, J., & Price, L.A. (1990). Meeting the psychosocial needs of adolescents and adults with LD. *Intervention in School and Clinic, 26*, 16–21.

Polloway, E.A., Epstein, M.H., & Cullinan, D. (1985). Prevalence of behavior problems among educable mentally retarded students. *Education and Training of the Mentally Retarded, 20*, 3–13.

Polloway, E.A., & Smith, T.E.C. (1992). *Teaching Language Skills to Students with Disabilities*. Denver: Love Publishing.

Polloway, E.A., & Epstein, M.H. (1985). Prevalence of behavior problems among educable mentally retarded students. *Education and Training of the Mentally Retarded, 20*, 3–13.

Polloway, E.A., Epstein, M.H., Patton, J.R., Cullinan, D., & Luebke, J. (1986). Demographic, social, and behavioral characteristics of students with educable mental retardation. *Education and Training of the Mentally Retarded, 21*, 27–34.

Polloway, E.A., Patton, J.R., Epstein, M.H., & Smith, T.E.C. (1989). Curriculum. *Focus on Exceptional Children, 21*, 1–12.

Ray, B.M. (1985). Measuring the social position of the mainstreamed handicapped child. *Exceptional Children, 52,* 57–62.

Raschke, D., Dedrick, C., & Thompson, M. (1987). Reluctant learners: Innovative contingency packages. *Teaching Exceptional Children, 19,* 18–21.

Reid, D.K. (1988). *Teaching the learning disabled.* Boston: Allyn & Bacon.

Rivers, D. (1986). *Labeling learning disabled children: The implications of variability.* Unpublished Doctoral dissertation. University of Arkansas.

Rivers, D., & Smith, T.E.C. (1988). Traditionally eligibility criteria for identifying students as specific learning disabled. *Journal of Learning Disabilities, 21,* 642–644.

Rogan, L.L., & Hartman, L.D. (1990). Adult outcome of learning disabled students ten years after initial follow-up. *Learning Disabilities Focus, 5,* 91–102.

Roberts, C., Pratt, C., & Leach, D. (1991). Classroom and playground interaction of students with and without disabilities. *Exceptional Children, 57,* 212–224.

Russell, A.T., & Forness, S.R. (1985). Behavioral disturbance in mentally retarded children in TMR and EMR classrooms. *American Journal of Mental Deficiency, 89,* 338–344.

Sabornie, E.J., & Beard, G.H. (1990). Teaching social skills. *Teaching Exceptional Children, 23,* 35–38.

Sabornie, E.J., & Kauffman, J.M. (1987). Assigned, received, and reciprocal social status of adolescents with and without mild mental retardation. *Education and Training in Mental Retardation, 22,* 139–149.

Sabornie, E.J., Marshall, K.J., & Ellis, E.S. (1990). Restructuring of mainstream sociometry with learning disabled and nonhandicapped students. *Exceptional Children, 56,* 314–323.

Santos, O.B. (1989). Language skills and cognitive processes related to poor reading comprehension performance. *Journal of Learning Disabilities, 22,* 131–133.

Siegel, P.S., Crawford, K.A., & Evelsizer, Z. (1985). Attention in discrimination learning in relation to certain teacher-rated behavior anomalies. *American Journal of Mental Deficiency, 89,* 389–392.

Sitlington, P.L., & Frank, A.R. (1990). Are adolescents with learning disabilities successfully crossing the bridge into adult life? *Learning Disability Quarterly, 13,* 97–113.

Smith, T.E.C. (1990). *Introduction to education,* 2nd ed. St. Paul: West Publishing.

Smith, T.E.C., Price, B.J., & Marsh, G.E. (1986). *Mildly handicapped children and adults.* St. Paul: West Publishing.

Swanson, H.L., & Trahan, M. (1990). Naturalistic memory in learning disabled children. *Learning Disability Quarterly, 13,* 82–96.

Thomas, C.C., Englert, C.S., & Gregg, S. (1987). An analysis of errors and strategies in the expository writing of learning disabled students. *Rural and Special Education, 8,* 21–30.

Torgesen, J.K. (1988a). The cognitive and behavioral characteristics of children with learning disabilities: An overview. *Journal of Learning Disabilities, 21,* 587–589.

Torgeson, J.K. (1988b). Studies of children with learning disabilities who perform poorly on memory span tasks. *Journal of Learning Disabilities, 21,* 605–612.

Vallecorsa, A.L., Zigmond, N., & Henderson, L.M. (1985). Spelling instruction in special education classrooms: A survey of practices. *Exceptional Children, 52,* 19–24.

Van Bourgondien, M.E. (1987). Children's responses to retarded peers as a function of social behaviors, labeling, and age. *Exceptional Children, 53,* 432–439.

Wallace, G., & McLoughlin, J.A. (1988). *Learning disabilities: Concepts and characteristics.* Columbus, OH: Merrill.

Wiener, J., Harris, P.J. & Shirer, C. (1990). Achievement and social-behavioral correlates of peer status in LD children. *Learning Disability Quarterly, 13,* 114–127.

Woolfolk, A.E. (1990). *Educational psychology,* 4th Ed. Englewood Cliffs, NJ: Prentice-Hall.

Zetlin, A.G., & Turner, J.L. (1988). Salient domains in the self-conception of adults with mental retardation. *Mental Retardation, 26,* 219–222.

Zimmerman, S.O. (1988). Problem-solving tasks on the microcomputer: A look at the performance of students with learning disabilities. *Journal of Learning Disabilities, 21,* 637–641.

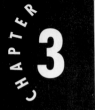
The Instructional Setting

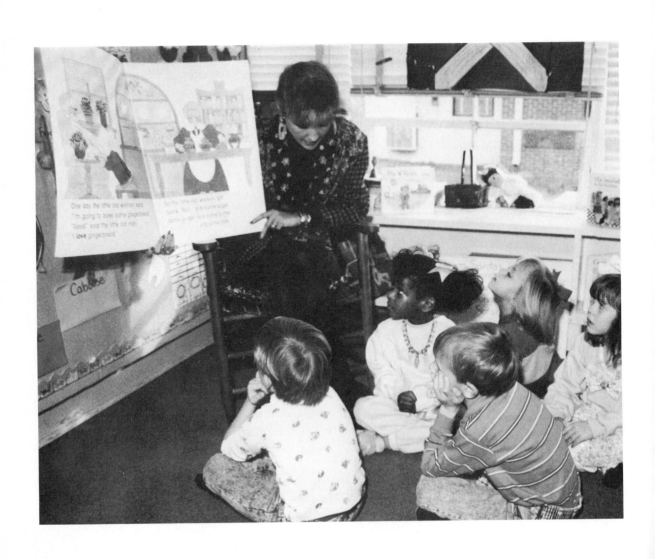

Outline

Introduction
   Importance of the Instructional Setting
   Relationship of the Instructional Setting to Instructional Success

Least Restrictive Setting
   Public Law 94–142 Requirements
   Continuum of Services

Special Classes
   Characteristics of Special Classes
   Advantages of Special Classes for Students with Mild Disabilities
   Disadvantages of Special Classes for Students with Mild Disabilities
   Current Use of the Special Class Model
   Special Class Teachers

Resource Room
   Characteristics of Resource Rooms
   Types of Resource Rooms
   Advantages of Resource Rooms
   Current Use of Resource Rooms
   Resource Room Teachers

Regular Classrooms
   Characteristics of Regular Classrooms
   Advantages of Regular Classrooms for Placement of Students with Mild Disabilities
   Disadvantages of Regular Classroom for Placement of Students with Mild Disabilities
   Classroom Arrangements

The Regular Education Initiative (REI)
   Definition of the Regular Education Initiative
   Pros and Cons of the Regular Education Initiative
   Impact of the Regular Education Initiative on Serving Students with Mild Disabilities

OBJECTIVES

After reading this chapter, you will be able to:

- describe the importance of the instructional setting;

- discuss the importance of the least restrictive environment;

- describe the types of special classes available for students with mild disabilities;

- discuss the advantages and disadvantages of resource rooms;

- describe the responsibilities of regular classroom teachers when dealing with a child with disabilities;

- specify the nature of modifications often made for students with disabilities in the regular classroom;

- discuss the concept of the Regular Education Initiative for student with mild disabilities.

Introduction

The provision of appropriate instruction and related services to students with disabilities requires a complex interaction among several factors. For example, the student's learning style and teacher's teaching style are critical to effective instruction. Also, the materials used to provide the instruction must be appropriate for certain populations of children. They must be grade-appropriate and age-appropriate. If you peruse any methods textbook, a large portion of the content will likely focus on these issues.

Yet, one of the most contemporary issues facing educators of students who have mild disabilities is the setting—where students are provided instruction. The type of instructional setting is important because it sets the stage for interactions among students and their teachers. While a growing number of educators advocate that students with mild disabilities should be educated in regular classes with their age-appropriate peers (Wang & Walberg, 1988; Stainback & Stainback, 1989; and Villa & Thousand, 1990) it is important to keep a variety of options available to meet the unique educational needs of each student. For example, isolating students in a self-contained classroom may yield different results than if the students were integrated into regular classrooms part of the day and grouped together in a resource room the remaining part of the day. The setting where students are expected to learn should be a primary consideration when providing services to students with disabilities. Some students may need the security of a self-contained setting, while others need the opportunities provided in an integrated classroom.

This chapter is organized around three main themes to help teachers understand ways they can successfully address the environmental needs of students who have disabilities. First, readers will be provided with a review of the legal foundations established for making environmental determinations. Second, a variety of instructional settings will be described that are designed to meet the needs of children with various disabilities. In many instances, however, the learning needs of children who have mild mental retardation, learning disabilities, or behavioral disorders can be quite similar. Teachers should also consider the fact that students who have mild disabilities have many of the same needs, wants, and aspirations as do their peers who are not disabled. Finally, suggestions will be presented that will enable teachers to create responsive environments that optimize students' abilities to work productively, learn efficiently, play creatively, and, most importantly, enhance their ability to establish meaningful social networks.

IMPORTANCE OF THE INSTRUCTIONAL SETTING

One of the strongest influences on children is the actual structure of the learning environment. Researchers have well documented the powerful effects of the environment on young children (Skeels & Dye, 1939; Infant Health and Development Project, 1990; Martin, Ramey & Ramey, 1990). Each of those studies has clearly demonstrated that when interventionists (i.e., teachers) carefully plan and implement environmental modifications to meet the unique needs of children at-risk, the outcomes can effect childrens' development on a variety of dimensions including cognitive competence, physical growth, and social/emotional development.

Consider some of your earliest recollections of grammar school. Does the smell from an old book or an open jar of paste conjure up vivid images in your mind and remind you of specific people or perhaps even lessons from long ago? Can you remember your reaction to a particular seating arrangement or who sat next to you in the third grade and how that might have affected your interest in a particular subject or teacher?

In ways that can be both direct and subliminal, teachers must recognize the power of the environment and be able to create positive components to enhance their teaching. The environment has been described, in the broadest sense, as a combination of the "physical, cultural, and social conditions that influence the life of an individual or group" (Yoshida, 1984, p. 406).

RELATIONSHIP OF THE INSTRUCTIONAL SETTING TO INSTRUCTIONAL SUCCESS

Decisions regarding where students with disabilities should be educated have received, "more attention, undergone more modifications, and generated even more controversy than have decisions about how or what these students are taught (Jenkins & Heinen, 1989, p. 516). Over the last twenty years, placement options for students with mild disabilities have gone full circle. Initially students with mild disabilities were served in regular classes, then moved into separate classes, and then in a combination of regular and special education classrooms. The most recent trend regarding placement is the full inclusion of students with disabilities in regular classrooms. Thus, we have come full circle: from a model that espoused total inclusion (because there were limited special services available), to self-contained classrooms, to resource rooms, and back to full inclusion (the regular education initiative—REI). There have been debates, arguments, and the development of bad feelings over the issue of placement options for these students. Often, decisions have been made based not on empirical data, but on politics and new ideas that sound good, but have not been validated.

In spite of this constantly changing picture of where students should be placed, there seems to have always been some professionals advocating for normalized settings for students with mild disabilities (Lilly, 1970; Wang & Birch, 1984; Will, 1984; Smith, Price, & Marsh, 1986; Roberts, Pratt, & Leach, 1991). While there have been and will always be those who advocate for segregated services, the prevailing direction over the past two decades has been providing services to these students in normal environments. Still, there seems to be some resistance to this movement. Is it perhaps that regular classroom teachers have not been adequately trained and prepared to deal with the needs of these students in their classes, or is the resistance primarily the result of special education teachers giving up some of their "control" over special education?

There is no one answer why professionals cannot agree on the appropriate placement for students with disabilities. And, like the disagreement among professionals, parents are also divided over the issue. Some parents advocate for the integration of their children into regular classrooms for status and social interactions; others are opposed to such interaction for fear of ridicule and rejection of their children by other students.

There is no one best instructional setting for all students with disabilities. Some need a very "normalized" classroom, while others may require the structure and level of services provided in self-contained programs. Unfortunately, research does not clarify the picture. This is probably due to difficulty in implementing a research design that can adequately adjust for variables such as quality of teaching, motivation of students, and learning aptitude of students. With no one setting being best, teachers must review placement options and determine which setting provides the best opportunities for specific children.

Least Restrictive Setting

As mentioned earlier, one of the greatest challenges facing educators in today's schools is the notion of *where* special education services should be offered, particularly for children with mild disabilities. Over the last several decades parents, educators, and legislators have been promoting the idea that children who have disabilities should be educated, "to the maximum extent possible," in the least restrictive environment. Least restrictive environment can be defined as the placement option for students with disabilities that allows as much interaction with nondisabled peers as can be beneficial, academically and socially.

Mainstreaming is a term used by educators to help explain "least restrictive environment." However, the word "mainstreaming" is not found in Public Law 94–142, nor is it in the regulations used to implement Public Law 94–142. It is strictly an educator's term and is not synonymous with "least restrictive environment" (Lerner, 1988). Mainstreaming can be defined as the process of including students with disabilities in the regular education process (Lewis & Doorlag, 1987). Wood (1984) defined mainstreaming as "educating handicapped children with their nonhandicapped peers in the least restrictive environment possible" (p. 4). Therefore, mainstreaming is the process of inclusion, whereas the least restrictive environment is the setting where students are placed. When determining the least restrictive environment for a particular student, the issue quickly becomes which setting is the best place.

Some people think that regardless of the severity of a disability, the best educational setting is one where students with disabilities are taught in classes with their nondisabled peers (Stainback & Stainback, 1989; Villa & Thousand, 1990). Advocates of this position support the integration of all students with disabilities into regular classrooms. This philosophy requires teachers to modify the curriculum to accommodate the students. While this approach is considered extreme by many professionals, full inclusion is being implemented in some schools.

On the other hand, some people, often parents of disabled children, may feel that placement of their son or daughter in a "regular" class for any amount of time may place them at-risk for isolation or ridicule. There may also be concern about the potential lack of individualized materials and instruction that their child may require to fully develop certain skills. These parents and professionals support the placement of these students in self-contained settings staffed by professionals specifically trained to work with disabled children. Cruickshank (1977) noted that a more restrictive physical environment does not necessarily imply a negatively compromised psychological setting.

Although there are advocates of both of these extreme views, neither position is always the better choice. Teachers and parents must weigh the pros and cons of various placement options to determine the best setting for a particular child. Since there are no two children who are exactly alike and who require the exact same services, it is likely that the placement needs of children will vary also.

The foundation for determining the least restrictive environment for children with disabilities can be found in existing federal legislation. Public Law 94–142, which ushered in the mandate to provide special education and related services to children with disabilities in the least restrictive environment, provides the framework for determining the appropriate placement for children.

PUBLIC LAW 94–142 REQUIREMENTS

In 1975 Congress passed Public Law 94–142, the Education for All Handicapped Children Act. Since that time, in response to changes in terminology, Congress renamed this bill the Individuals with Disabilities Education Act or "IDEA." While other chapters in this text deal with a number of important concepts relative to that landmark legislation, of particular interest here is the provision of "least restrictive environment" (LRE), which states:

> . . . that special classes, separate schooling, or other removal of handicapped children from the regular educational environment occurs only when the nature or severity of the handicap is such that education in regular classes . . . cannot be achieved satisfactorily (PL 94–142, p.9).

This requirement is often misinterpreted. Many parents and school officials have assumed that the mandate to provide services to disabled children in the least restrictive setting meant to place all children in regular classrooms. However, as Hallahan and Kauffman (1991) point out, the least restrictive environment may not always be the regular classroom. In some instances, the placement of students in regular classrooms could result in negative consequences.

The concept means more than physical placement and integration, it also means a placement where the student can benefit maximally from instruction and social interactions. Hallahan and Kauffman (1991) note that the least restrictive environment provision means that segregating children who have disabilities from their home, family, community, and regular class setting should occur as infrequently as possible. The goal of placing students in the least restrictive environment should be to identify an educational environment that provides maximum assistance to children with special needs (Morse, 1984), and at the same time allow interactions with nondisabled peers.

Unfortunately, some educators and parents have assumed that the least restrictive environment requirements of Public Law 94–142 means to eliminate special education classrooms. In response to mandates within federal and state legislation regarding least restrictive environment, parents and well-intentioned educators placed students with disabilities in regular classes to "mainstream them," thinking this was the best approach for meeting the child's educational and social needs. The end result has not always been positive. In fact, some students may have suffered negative consequences when they were integrated into settings that did not provide sufficient supports to ensure their success.

While this notion of "mainstreaming" all disabled students has been argued, debated, and researched over the last fifteen years (Calhoun & Ellicott, 1977; Forness & Kavale, 1984; Stainback & Stainback, 1984; and Rich & Ross, 1989), a number of questions still remain to be addressed including an investigation of the factors that account for variability in placement rates among states and the number of placements made by noneducational agencies (Danielson & Bellamy, 1989). There appears to be great variability among states and local districts regarding how the least-restrictive-environment mandate is implemented. Some districts totally use a resource room model, while others employ both resource rooms and self-contained special education classrooms, as well as other options along a continuum of possible placements.

The implementation of the least restrictive environment for students has varied a great deal. The next section describes several different service delivery options and the types of classes available for serving children with disabilities.

CONTINUUM OF SERVICES

Just prior to the passage of PL 94–142, a number of service delivery models were developed and are still widely used today to assist in developing a continuum of services for children who require special education services (Deno, 1970; Dunn, 1973; Van Etten & Adamson, 1973; and Berry, 1974). These models emphasized the continuum of service options that schools should provide students. Two of the most popular models include Evelyn Deno's Cascade System (1970) and Lloyd Dunn's Inverted Pyramid (1973). Although approximately twenty years old, both of these models have relevance in the way students with disabilities are served in the 1990s.

Deno's Cascade Model

As depicted in Figure 3–1, Deno's cascade system is based on a hierarchy of levels of service (teaching environments) ranging from segregated settings at the bottom of the model to fully integrated settings at the top. As one of the earliest proposed service delivery models, this approach was very important in understanding the notion of least restrictive environment.

In reviewing the impact this model has had on special education services, Smith, Price, and Marsh (1986) noted several positive and negative outcomes. First, Deno's model provided a conceptual model from which administrators and service providers could actualize their own services (Podemski, Price, Smith, & Marsh, 1984). Consider the dilemma a special education planner might have had in 1975 when trying to address the issue of least restrictive environment when few specialized placements were available at that time. About the only service delivery options available were self-contained special education classrooms, special schools, and residential programs.

The second positive aspect of this model is that the focus of services described are not tied to a physical plant or existing services (Reid & Hresko, 1981). Service options can be developed to meet a child's educational needs without regard to how they fit in with existing classroom space. Many of the options can be implemented with minimal space requirements or modifications to existing programs. This provides a great deal of flexibility to teachers when implementing the model.

The last interesting component of Deno's cascade is that the model is dynamic and implies movement toward the least restrictive environment (Cegelka & Prehm, 1982; Marsh, Price, & Smith, 1983; Smith *et al.*, 1986). This aspect becomes increasingly important as the child's Individualized Education Program (IEP) is reevaluated at the end of each year and the child's placement is reconsidered. The goal for every child with a disability is the provision of services in the least restrictive environment. Placement is not permanent, but

FIGURE 3-1 Deno's Cascade of Educational Placement Options

Exceptional children in regular classes,
with or without supportive services

Regular class attendance plus
supplementary instructional
services

Part-time special
class

Full-time
special
class

Special
stations*

Homebound services

Instruction in
hospital, residential, or total care settings

*Special schools in public school system

Source: Deno, E. (1970). Special education as development capital. *Exceptional Children, 37,* p. 236.

should be reviewed at least annually to determine if the placement could be changed; change is always preferred in the lesser restrictive direction.

A number of negative criticisms of Deno's model have also been identified. First, this approach lacks specificity in addressing different levels of disability. While a majority of students referred for special education services usually end up receiving those services, some children may "fall through the cracks" due to variations in their diagnosis and may not be easily identified for predetermined service slots. Although the model presents a continuum, some teachers and parents only view the options presented in the cascade as being available. Indeed, these stations only represent steps along the continuum; there are numerous other points along the continuum that are not fully described.

A second criticism is that the organizational procedures needed to implement a variety of options may render this model less flexible than originally proposed. School officials may implement the model in a very structured manner and prevent its full potential because of the organizational difficulties in providing all of the options. Finally, critics argue that this model does not discriminate between factors such as length of time in various settings and thus the model may operate "somewhat differently than policy implies" (Peterson, Zabel, Smith, & White, 1983). Even though these criticisms have been voiced repeatedly, even after twenty years Deno's continuum is still widely adapted for structuring services for children with disabilities.

Dunn's Inverted Pyramid

A second and frequently used model was developed by Dunn (1973). Dunn, a long time critic of segregated special classes (1968), modified Deno's cascade model in several ways (Meyen & Skrtic, 1988). He:

- described four different types of exceptionalities;
- arranged levels of exceptionality by severity;
- modified the placement options from 8 to 11;
- named the model the Inverted Pyramid.

The model is referred to as an inverted pyramid because the majority of children who receive special education are those with mild disabilities. These students, identified as type 1 students, are located at the top of the model in the most normalized setting. The continuum ranges from the type 1 students to those identified as type 4, students with severe limitations. This group includes a relatively small number of students, is placed in the most restrictive setting, and receives intensive interventions (see Figure 3–2).

While both the Deno and Dunn models have distinct differences, both prescribe a philosophy wherein a majority of students (especially those who have mild disabilities) should be educated in regular classroom settings with appropriate support services. The objective of the concept of least restrictive environment is to assist children to master content and skills in a setting that is as close to "normal" as possible. This enables them to interact with nondisabled peers and facilitates appropriate role modeling for the acquisition of academic and social skills.

The Dunn and Deno models only represent a continuum of placement options; they are presented to describe the various components of a continuum of services. Realistically, school personnel must consider an infinite number of options along a continuum, from the very least restrictive of total regular classroom placement, to the most restrictive, a residential program. Even in the regular classroom option and residential option, there are various options available that range in levels of restrictiveness. Table 3–1 (page 72) describes some examples of services provided in a regular classroom setting; Table 3–2 (page 72) provides a similar description of services available in residential programs.

Models are good to provide examples. In reality, there are several primary placement options that are used to serve the majority of children with mild disabilities. The next section describes some of the more common service arrangements. Each of those options are described in terms of the characteristics, strengths, and weaknesses of each setting. When reading this section, keep in mind that all children with disabilities differ to such an extent that placement decisions should be made based on the unique strengths and weaknesses of each child. Children with similar IQs, categorical labels, or other characteristics may not need similar placements.

FIGURE 3-2 Dunn's Inverted Pyramid of Educational Placement Options

Type I Exceptional Pupil

Enrolled in the regular class in public schools, but,

Teachers have failed to such a degree that special materials and equipment are necessary.

Special educators used as consultants only and do not provide direct teaching services.

Type II Exceptional Pupil

Received direct education from one or more special educator

Continues to receive part of academic education from regular educators

May be enrolled in either a regular or special class

Type III Exceptional Pupil

No education provided in the regular class

Receives all services in a separate, self-contained class in the public school system

Type IV Exceptional Pupil

Unable to attend any type of day school program

Is in a special boarding school or receives hospital or home instruction

Source: Dunn, L.M. (1973). *Exceptional children in the schools: Special education in transition* (2nd Ed.). New York: Holt, Rinehart & Winston.

TABLE 3-1 Placement/Service Options in Regular Classrooms

- Large Group Instruction
- Small Group Instruction
- Individualized Instruction
- Using the Buddy-System
- Peer Tutoring and Collaboration
- Special Education Services in the Regular Classroom
- Specialized Materials for Use in the Regular Classroom
- Using a Combination of All of the Above Options

TABLE 3-2 Placement/Service Options in Residential Settings

- Large Group Instruction
- Small Group Instruction
- Individualized Instruction
- Reverse Mainstreaming - Integration of Nondisabled Students For Brief Periods
- Community Integration and Community Based Instruction
- Visits to Regular School Settings for Special Occasions
- Peer Instruction and Activities

Special Classes

Special classes are generally thought of as classrooms where students spend the bulk of the school day with the same teacher. They are also referred to as self-contained special education classrooms. The U.S. Department of Education (1990) describes this placement option as including "students who receive special education and related services for more than 60 percent of the school day and are placed in self-contained special classrooms with part-time instruction in regular class or placed in self-contained classes full-time on a regular school campus" (p. 19).

Self-contained special education classes for children who have mild disabilities is not a primary, nor often used option. In fact, according to data collected between 1986 and 1987 regarding trends in educational placements, only about twenty-five percent of all children who received special education services in the United States received those services in separate, self-contained classes (U.S. Department of Education, 1989). The majority of these children are likely those with more significant disabilities. Nonetheless, there have been times when this type of class was used extensively to serve all students with disabilities. From 1950 to 1970, self-contained special education classes for children with mild disabilities was the preferred educational strategy (Reynolds, 1973). In fact, in many school districts, the only placement options available for students with disabilities was the self-contained special education classroom.

CHARACTERISTICS OF SPECIAL CLASSES

Self-contained special education classrooms are physical settings where students with disabilities receive the entire or the majority of their educational services. They are generally staffed by a single special education teacher. Students are grouped homogeneously, frequently based on their categorical label. There are limited opportunities for students served in special classes to interact with their nondisabled peers.

Although self-contained special education classrooms vary in some characteristics, there are several general characteristics usually associated with this service option (Smith *et al.*, 1986).

1. The teacher, certified in special education, has the primary responsibility for directing classroom instruction.

2. Most of the instruction is delivered in a single classroom.

3. Ancillary services (speech, physical therapy/education, etc.) are most often delivered by support personnel.

4. The degree of individualized instruction depends on both the skills and motivation of the teacher and the types of materials and approaches used in the classroom.

Students with disabilities who receive their educational programs in a self-contained, special class, often participate in nonacademic activities including assemblies, athletic events, concerts, and clubs with their nondisabled peers. However, these opportunities for interaction are extremely limited and occur in settings without the necessary structure to facilitate the cooperative activities.

ADVANTAGES OF SPECIAL CLASSES FOR STUDENTS WITH MILD DISABILITIES

Special classes are not all good or all bad; they have advantages and disadvantages. The obvious advantage of placement in a special class is that the student/teacher ratio is usually quite low. Most states limit the number of students, by major handicapping condition, to a manageable number. Table 3–3 (page 74) provides an example of a state's guidelines on the maximum number of students that can be included in a self-contained classroom. This

TABLE 3-3 Maximum Number of Students by Disability Allowed in Special Classes

DISABILITY	MAXIMUM NUMBER
Mild Mental Retardation	15
Moderate Mental Retardation	12
Severe/Profound MR	4
Serious Emotional Disturbance	4
Learning Disabilities	10
Hearing Impaired	10
Visually Impaired	8
Deaf-Blind	5
Orthopedically Impaired	12
Other Health Impaired	12
Multihandicapped	4

Source: Alabama State Department of Education, Administrative Policy Manual (1986).

instructional arrangement allows the teacher, who should be highly qualified to deal with a particular type of student, to spend more time with individualized, one-on-one teaching. Teaching in this setting also allows for a greater degree of scheduling flexibility.

Special classes also facilitate the use of small group instruction. Small group arrangements enable students to better acquaint themselves with their peers and establish friendships. Additionally, children may find this setting to be less threatening and more relaxed, one where the student feels more competent than in a larger group.

The special classroom is considered a safe haven for students; children who function differently than their peers may feel unduly challenged in regular classrooms where everyone else in their environment is able to perform better than they do. From their perspective, the self-contained environment is a place where they can work on their skills without regard to the fact that their readers are of a different color, content, or length, and without worry of stigmatization as a result of their academic deficiencies. On the other hand, some students may indeed feel stigmatized as a "special ed kid" when they attend classes that are different than those their regular peers attend. Regular and special education teachers should collaborate together with their classes to develop positive attitudes toward students who have disabilities so as to avoid the negative effects that can occur when children of a similar age group are educated in separate educational settings.

Teaching students in a self-contained setting also has benefits for parents. When children are taught by one teacher instead of many, it becomes easier for the parents to establish a relationship with that teacher as opposed to when they deal with several (Cegelka & Prehm, 1982). Parents also like special classes because they are more assured that their child will not be ridiculed and rejected by the nondisabled students. A major fear of parents when their children are integrated into regular classes is that their children will be the objects of ridicule.

One additional advantage of the special class is that the special education teacher has as the opportunity to get to know the students very well. As a result of students being in the same setting with the same teacher all day, their individual strengths and weaknesses can be accurately determined. Special classroom teachers are thus in a position to:

- understand specific strengths, weaknesses, and learning styles of students;

- gear instruction to the unique needs of students;

- provide a great deal of support to students; and

- take into consideration all of the factors that need to be accounted for in planning for the students' futures.

DISADVANTAGES OF SPECIAL CLASSES FOR STUDENTS WITH MILD DISABILITIES

Placement of children who have mild disabilities in self-contained classrooms may be a temporary harbor from the inquisitive remarks by their peers, but it may be a poor training setting, over the long haul, for preparing those students to deal with the challenges of independent living. The gestalt of a child's school experience includes far more than a series of academic tasks and lessons. By restricting interactions with their peers, students with disabilities have few nondisabled models to imitate. Access to appropriate modeling is critically important in the acquisition of adequate communication and social skills (Sargent, 1989).

Isolation of the teacher is another negative consequence. Teachers in self-contained classrooms have few, if any, opportunities to interact with other professionals, in spite of the fact that they are in close proximity to them. This limited opportunity results in the special classroom being isolated from the "mainstream" of what happens throughout the school. The special classroom teacher becomes associated with the special education students by other teachers and by other students. This only makes it more difficult for students with mild disabilities to become assimilated into the activities of the school.

CURRENT USE OF THE SPECIAL CLASS MODEL

The special classroom model is used less frequently today than before the movement to integrate students into regular classrooms, which really became strong with the passage of Public Law 94–142 in 1975. Currently the special class model is primarily used to serve children who have severe disabilities. Fewer than half the children classified as mentally retarded are currently served in segregated settings, including special classes (U.S. Department of Education, 1989). Since students classified as mildly mentally retarded form the largest group of mildly disabled students likely served in special classes, this means that the majority of children with mild disabilities are being educated in lesser restricted settings. Teachers should be cautious about the use of this model and should, therefore, clearly document the need for such services.

In the *Twelfth Annual Report to Congress on the Implementation of the Education of the Handicapped Act* (1990), it was reported that 24.7 percent of all students served in special education programs were placed in separate classes. The percentage of students in different handicapping categories ranged from a low of 3.8 percent for students with speech impairments to a high of 57.6 percent for students with mental retardation. Table 3–4 summarizes the percentages of different disability categories served in special classes.

TABLE 3–4 Percentage of Students Receiving Services in Special Classes

Learning Disabled	21.7%
Speech Impaired	3.8%
Mentally Retarded	57.6%
Emotionally Disturbed	34.6%
Hearing Impaired	35.2%
Multihandicapped	45.9%
Orthopedically Impaired	31.8%
Other Health Impaired	18.7%
Visually Impaired	20.8%
Deaf-Blind	35.1%

Source: U.S. Department of Education (1990). *Twelfth Annual Report to Congress on the Implementation of The Education of the Handicapped Act.*

SPECIAL CLASS TEACHERS

Role of the Teacher

There are several roles for teachers in a special class setting. The primary role, of course, is to teach. In special education settings, goals for teaching are guided and monitored via the students' IEPs. The actual content of the IEP varies with each child. Although there may be two or more children in a special class with similar needs, it is unlikely that their IEPs will be identical.

The special classroom teacher is responsible for implementing the IEP. With the exception of the physical therapist, counselor, or other persons providing related services to the student, the special classroom teacher is responsible for the entire IEP. The advantages of this are that teachers are in full control; they can make sure that students' programs are individualized and that the IEP is implemented properly. The downside of this total responsibility is that the teacher may not have all of the skills necessary to implement everything in the IEP as effectively as some other professionals.

A second role of the special class teacher is to work toward moving students to a lesser restrictive environment. To accomplish this, teachers must take an ecological view of the environments that child is (or will be) functioning in. This process helps to identify barriers (social, physical, academic) that might prevent successful integration of that student at a later date. For example, if a student has been placed in a self-contained special class due to behavioral problems, the teacher needs to identify the antecedents or consequences of peer interactions that child might face in a variety of settings, including the classroom, lunchroom, or in the line waiting for the bus.

Relationships with Other School Personnel

As mentioned earlier, teachers serving children in segregated settings have certain responsibilities within the mainstream of the school setting. They are primarily responsible for the students in their program. However, they also need to interact with other teachers and programs as much as possible. As noted, special class teachers may become associated with the special education students and have difficulty getting involved in other school activities. Regardless of the difficulties in doing this, they need to make a strong effort. Volunteering for helping to sponsor activities that primarily involve nondisabled students is one good way of doing this. Other actions that special class teachers can take include:

- participating on school committees;

- encouraging special class students to get involved with school-wide activities;

- taking an active role in the parent-teacher organization (PTO) or parent-teacher association (PTA); and

- socializing with teachers from outside special education.

In addition to these activities, teachers in self-contained settings can fulfill a real need in regular settings by assisting regular classroom teachers and nondisabled students to understand the nature of disabilities. Young children in particular, and students who have had limited exposure to children with disabilities often approach the issue of handicaps with an open mind—inquisitive, curious, and interested. A sensitive and astute teacher can mediate those early learning experiences and develop strong, positive, lifelong attitudes regarding special education in children who do not have disabilities.

There are numerous activities that the teacher in a self-contained class do to foster healthy attitudes toward children who have disabilities. The story presented on page 78 describes a real situation and provides a base from which we can address that concern.

Unfortunately, Phillip's situation is all too common. Yet, by following a few key suggestions and principles, situations such as this can be reversed. The activities described on page 79 reveal some steps that can be taken to improve such situations.

The Resource Room

The least restrictive environment for students who have mild disabilities is the regular classroom. However, some students may require more intensive one-on-one teaching. Often, that type of educational requirement is delivered through the resource room. These classes have been defined by Wiederholt, Hammill, and Brown (1983) as "any instructional setting in which a person (usually the resource teacher) has the responsibility of providing supportive educationally related services to students and/or to their teachers" (p. 3). The U.S. Department of Education (1990) describes a resource room as a setting where

PART I Teaching an Old Dog New Tricks
Mrs. B. Meets Mr. Special Ed.

At 7:30 A.M. it was already hot and sticky. The tie around this young teachers' neck was for looks; not a bit comfortable on this August morning. But Phillip Winters was beginning his first day as a public school teacher of special education, and he was excited. The principal was busy greeting returning teachers and handling a multitude of tasks common on the first day of school. Mr. Winters was given a polite, "Hello" and then quickly assigned to his classroom.

Realizing that Phillip was a bit unsure of procedures, Mrs. B., a veteran teacher of fifteen years, took him aside and extended a hearty welcome. "I know your class is empty, and I have a few extra tables and chairs to share with you. Our rooms are right next to each other! Just let me know what you need. By the way what will you be teaching?" "Special education," he said with a wide smile. Mrs. B. seemed to lose her posture. "Oh, that's nice," she said with an odd look, and off she went.

Passing by Mrs. B.'s 5th grade class, Phillip noted a room full of excited children, many of whom were anxious to know who the new "male" teacher was. The morning flew by. So much to do! IEPs to review, emergency contact forms to update, supplies to obtain, and bulletin boards to put up. He was so busy he hardly noticed the clock. 11:45! Lunch period . . . and those rolls smell so good!

Passing by Mrs. B.'s class, Phillip was surprised to see a now empty room. What happened? He knew the class was full at 8 a.m. Phillip hurried toward the lunchroom and ran right in to Mrs. B. Awkwardly she mentioned that a bigger room was available at the opposite end of the hall and she had taken advantage of it.

Somehow, the rolls weren't quite as good as he hoped. Actually, he had a lump in his stomach. Did Mrs. B. really want a larger room, or was it the "special ed" part that bothered her? Phillip knew most of the kids coming into his class . . . he had taught them previously in a class located in a church basement. PL 94–142 had just been passed and Phillip and the parents thought the fight for services was over. Phillip's thoughts quickly turned to Rene, one of his favorite students. "If the teachers don't want to be near my students, how can I expect other students in the school to accept my kids?"

students "receive special education and related services for 60 percent or less of the school day and at least 21 percent of the school day. This may include resource rooms with part-time instruction in the regular class" (p. 19). While no one advocates determining the exact percentage a student remains in regular and special classes, the notion is that a significant portion of the day is spent in a combination of regular and special education classrooms.

The movement to educate students with mild disabilities in resource rooms grew after the passage of Public Law 94–142 and the requirement to educate these students in the least restrictive environment. A key factor in the movement away from special classes to resource rooms was efficacy studies that were conducted in the 1960s and early 1970s (Yoshida, 1984). These studies revealed that students with disabilities who were educated in self-contained classrooms did not generally fare any better than their peers who remained in regular classrooms (Dunn, 1968; Dunn, 1973; Marsh, Price, & Smith, 1983; Podemski, Price, Smith, & Marsh, 1984; Smith, Price, & Marsh, 1986; Hallahan &

PART II Mr. Winters Takes Action
Suggestions for Enhancing Integration in the Public Schools

1. Adhere to the Professional Code of Ethics suggested by the Council for Exceptional Children (Council for Exceptional Children, 1991). (see appendix)

2. Exhibit good basic work behaviors (punctuality, responsibility, etc.).

3. Implement a "Disability Awareness Program" for children at all grade levels and ensure that staff (administrative, instructional, support, custodial and nutrition) have an opportunity to participate.

   Be sure to cover the nature of disabilities that may be present in your school and highlight the strengths of the students.

   Make sure you don't violate the confidentiality of students with disabilities. If in doubt, ask the students' parents and double check with your supervisor.

4. Participate in regular school day activities including bus/playground duty and lunchroom supervision.

5. Get involved in regular extracurricular activities (athletic events, clubs, PTA, etc.).

6. Encourage parents in your class to support extracurricular activities, as well.

7. Provide opportunities for nonhandicapped children to become active in your class. Activities such as peer tutoring and a free-play buddy system will help students outside your class understand the strengths and weaknesses of the students in your class.

Kauffman, 1991). As a result of these studies, professionals started questioning the reasons for separating students from their nondisabled peers on a full-time basis.

CHARACTERISTICS OF RESOURCE ROOMS

Resource rooms are typically equipped with a wide variety of materials designed to augment the curriculum in the regular class. Some resource rooms are quite small; only allowing for small instructional groups. Other resource rooms may have a variety of learning areas, including a listening center, reading center, small group work areas, and areas for individual study. There are several purposes for the resource room. One purpose of this class is to provide an intensive instructional setting so that the student can maintain the pace of the regular class. Still another purpose is to remediate basic skills that may be deficient, such as reading, written expression, spelling, or math. By using the resource room model, these purposes can be achieved without the total isolation of the child from nondisabled peers.

The actual arrangement of the resource room and the manner in which students are served within that resource room environment can vary considerably. Several models are described below.

TYPES OF RESOURCE ROOMS

There are a variety of different types of resource rooms used. Wiederholt, Hammill, and Brown (1983) have identified five.

1. Categorical resource room.
2. Cross-categorical resource room.
3. Noncategorical resource room.
4. Specific skill resource room.
5. Itinerant model.

A number of other types of resource rooms have also been established to address noninstructional purposes, including assessment, counseling, and for mental health services. Our discussion will focus on resource rooms that impact directly on the daily instruction for students with mild disabilities.

The **categorical resource room**, as the name implies, serves children with specific disabilities, such as mental retardation, specific learning disabilities, serious behavior disabilities, sensory impairments (vision/hearing), communication disorders, and children who have physical disabilities. The notion behind this approach is that these groups of children have similar learning needs which can best be met in a common setting.

This model is attractive to school administrators, and is one of the more popular approaches. School personnel like this approach because it enables students with specific disabilities to be grouped for instructional purposes. Parents often prefer this resource room model because it separates students with different disabilities. A parent may feel more comfortable accepting the fact that her child has a specific learning disability and is being taught in a resource room with children who have similar learning needs as opposed to being educated with children who are mentally retarded.

Regardless of its popularity, there are problems with this model because it is based on a diagnostic label. The idea that children who have learning disabilities, mild mental retardation, mild behavior problems, and other conditions that result in mild disabilities learn under very different conditions has been challenged (Marsh et al., 1983; Smith et al., 1986; Polloway et al., 1989; Hallahan & Kauffman, 1991).

The **cross-categorical** or **"interrelated"** program is another popular resource room model used today. In this approach, teachers may serve children from more than one disability category. Students may be taught in distinct groups during the day (i.e., children with mental retardation during first period, and then students who have learning disabilities in the second period); or students may be grouped together (students with learning disabilities, mental retardation, and behavior disorders) so they can work on common instructional goals (like reading) (Wiederholt et al., 1983).

Similar to the cross-categorical model, the **noncategorical model** was designed to serve children with different disabilities who have similar learning and behavior characteristics. This model may be preferred by some professionals due to the absence of labeling. Many administrators prefer this model because it is often a more cost-efficient way of serving small numbers of students with different disabilities. Unfortunately, some parents oppose this approach because they do not want their children comingled with children who have different types of disabilities.

The **specific skill resource program** is unique in that the training provided under this model is specific to a content area, often math, reading, or speech. This approach is less frequently used since it was primarily designed for children who do not have disabilities. Teachers in this program usually have special certifications in the area of remedial math, reading, or speech. Since this model typically serves nondisabled children, the cost for these services must be paid by the school district and are not usually reimbursable by federal monies (Wiederholt *et al.*, 1983).

The itinerant resource room model differs from the others in that teachers move from location to location to provide services to students in resource rooms. An example would be a small district with a few children who had mild disabilities spread throughout several elementary schools. Rather than requiring all of the students to attend the same school, or employing a teacher for each school to instruct only three or four students, one teacher travels from school to school providing resource services. This model is extremely effective with children who have low-incidence disabilities, such as visual impairments and hearing impairments. Advantages of the itinerant model include:

- one teacher can serve many children;

- low-incidence disabilities can be served cost efficiently;

- students are able to remain in their "home" school.

The major disadvantage to the itinerant model is that itinerant teachers often feel like they do not belong to any school. By traveling from school to school they have a difficult time establishing collegial relationships. Also, students may need assistance from the itinerant teacher when she is at another school.

Although each of the five types of resource rooms described are unique, there are some commonalities found in all five (Marsh & Price, 1980).

- Students spend part of the day in regular classrooms and part in the resource room.

- Resource rooms serve small groups of students at any one time.

- Individualized instruction is the primary mode used in the resource room.

- Extensive collaboration between the special education teacher and regular classroom teachers is critical.

ADVANTAGES OF RESOURCE ROOMS

The greatest advantage of the resource room model lies in its flexibility. A child may only need a resource teacher for a specific subject or project. For some students, resource teachers can work side-by-side with teachers in the regular classroom, thereby enabling students to benefit from a decreased need for segregated services and the opportunity to practice skills in a more natural setting with their peers. Table 3–5 (page 82) lists some specific advantages of resource rooms.

TABLE 3-5 Advantages of Resource Rooms

1. Students receive specialized instruction and related services from special education professionals.
2. Students receive portions of their educational services in regular classrooms with nondisabled peers.
3. Students with disabilities have nondisabled role models.
4. Students with disabilities have opportunities for developing appropriate social skills in a natural setting (regular classroom).
5. Students without disabilities have the opportunity to interact with students who are disabled.
6. Regular classroom teachers and special education teachers share the responsibility of students with disabilities.

The resource room model also has some disadvantages. These include:

- Some students may require more intensive services than are provided in a resource room.
- Scheduling students in and out of regular classes often presents problems.
- Close collaboration between the resource room teacher and regular classroom is difficult to accomplish and may result in confusion for the student.
- Students may feel stigmatized by having to leave the regular classroom for services.

CURRENT USE OF RESOURCE ROOMS

The resource room model is the most popular service delivery model currently used in schools (Smith *et al.*, 1986). The *Twelfth Annual Report to Congress on the Implementation of the Education of the Handicapped Act* (1990) reported that forty percent of all students served in special education programs receive those services in resource rooms. This number includes nearly sixty percent of students with learning disabilities, which is the largest category of students receiving special education services. Table 3–6 shows the percentage of students in each disability category that receive services in resources room settings.

RESOURCE ROOM TEACHERS

Role of the Teacher

The primary function of a resource room teacher is to identify alternative instructional strategies so that a student can be successful with the mainstream curricula. Hallahan and Kauffman (1991) have identified five distinct roles for resource room teachers regardless of the types of disabilities represented in the class. These roles and responsibilities include:

1. assess the students' need for instruction and management;

2. provide individual and small group instruction either in the regular class or in a separate resource room;

3. offer advice and demonstrate specific teaching techniques or materials to regular teachers;

4. make referrals to other agencies when a student requires additional services; and

5. work toward total integration of the student.

TABLE 3-6 Percentage of Students with Disabilities Receiving Services in Resource Rooms

Learning Disabled	59.2%
Speech Impaired	19.7%
Mentally Retarded	24.0%
Emotionally Disturbed	32.9%
Hearing Impaired	20.9%
Multihandicapped	13.3%
Orthopedically Impaired	18.0%
Other Health Impaired	20.8%
Visually Impaired	25.6%
Deaf-Blind	7.2%

Source: U.S. Department of Education (1990). *Twelfth Annual Report to Congress on the Implementation of The Education of the Handicapped Act.*

A major role of the resource room teacher is to interface and communicate with regular classroom teachers. The critical factor in the success of resource rooms to meet the needs of students is this communication factor. Without communication, regular educators and special education teachers are not aware of what the other is doing with a particular child. This could lead to confusion, and the end result could be lowered achievement rather than improved achievement.

Another important role for the resource room teacher is to communicate and work closely with students' parents. Parent involvement can greatly enhance the success of students with disabilities; special education teachers need to encourage, facilitate, and reinforce this involvement. When students with mild disabilities are integrated into classes with their peers, it may be easy for parents to forget that their child is receiving specially designed instruction. When consistent and objective lines of coordinated communication are provided among regular teachers, special education personnel, and parents, fewer problems are likely to develop that can be attributed to a lack of information.

Regular Classrooms

Most students who are diagnosed with some type of mild disability will probably receive a majority of their services in regular classrooms. This started with the movement to integrate students with disabilities into "normalized" environments. It was a direct result of the passage of Public Law 94–142. One of the requirements of the legislation was for states to implement plans to train regular and special education teachers in how to implement the law. As regular teacher preparation programs continue to include content on managing the student with special needs in the classroom and as new materials are developed, the regular classroom teacher will be even better prepared to meet the needs of these students.

CHARACTERISTICS OF REGULAR CLASSROOMS

Students with mild disabilities receiving services in the regular classroom often participate in instruction designed for their nondisabled peers and from curricular components contained in their IEPs. The provision of specialized instruction can be through the regular classroom teacher (with support from special education and related personnel), a resource program, or through an itinerant teacher.

As a result of many students with disabilities spending more and more of their time in regular classrooms, the overall nature of these environments becomes more important for special educators. Elementary classrooms and secondary classrooms differ significantly. They differ in the orientation of the teacher to students, curricula, grading requirements, and horizontal arrangements (Smith, 1990). Table 3–7 provides a general description of regular classrooms at the elementary and secondary levels.

ADVANTAGES OF REGULAR CLASSROOMS FOR PLACEMENT OF STUDENTS WITH MILD DISABILITIES

The obvious advantage of placing students with mild disabilities in regular classrooms is that this is the "most normal" of the organizational arrangements and allows for maximum integration of these students with their nondisabled peers. Succinctly stated, it is the least restrictive environment possible. Students in secondary programs have the added advantage of benefiting from a variety of instructors teaching in the regular curricula as opposed to just one or two in a more restrictive environment. This approach is also extremely useful in rural settings where a wide variety of educational specialists may not be readily available.

By placing students with mild disabilities into regular classrooms, they assimilate more easily into the real world. Serving students in special education settings, even in resource rooms for part of the school day, does not reflect reality. Students in these settings are somewhat protected from the realities of regular classrooms. While this separation may be required for some students in order to help them develop specific academic and social skills, eventually they will have to be integrated into the nondisabled world. Regular classroom placements provide them with this opportunity during the school years. It also provides nondisabled role models for students to emulate; this can be very important.

TABLE 3-7 General Description of Regular Classrooms

ELEMENTARY SCHOOLS

- Lower grades are generally self-contained.
- Teachers certified as elementary teachers are responsible for the majority of students' programs.
- Curricula focus on basic skills.
- Instruction is generally large and small group.
- Schools are organized on a graded system with minimum age entry requirements.
- Upper elementary grades often become departmentalized.
- Role of elementary special education teacher focuses on helping students develop basic skills.

SECONDARY SCHOOLS

- Teachers focus on teaching specific subjects, such as history.
- Students generally receive instruction from 4–7 teachers daily.
- Curricula focus on state-approved curricula targeting college preparation, vocational preparation, or general academic.
- Basic skills instruction is extremely limited.
- Schools are organized on a graded system with a maximum age requirement.
- Role of secondary special education teachers focuses on remediating basic skills, helping students achieve success in mainstream classes, and facilitating socialization.

Source: Smith (1990). *Introduction to education,* 2nd Ed.

DISADVANTAGES OF REGULAR CLASSROOMS FOR PLACEMENT OF STUDENTS WITH MILD DISABILITIES

Along with advantages come disadvantages. Perhaps the greatest disadvantage of regular class placements for children with mild disabilities is the possible inability of the regular classroom teacher to address the unique learning and social needs of these students. Legal mandates may require placement in the least restrictive environment, but they do not necessarily ensure that a student will receive appropriate services.

Another disadvantage may be negative attitudes expressed by regular classroom teachers (Smith *et al.,* 1986). As our commitment to move children from special, segregated settings to the regular class becomes more of a reality, it may be an unsettling idea to some regular educators. With today's regular teachers "under the gun" to get results, they may become alarmed at the extra "burden" of students with disabilities in their classrooms. They may comment, "In addition to my thirty students, you want me to provide adapted instructions and materials to a kid from special ed.? Why doesn't the special ed. teacher handle that? I've only had one college class in special education and that content ranged from gifted to profound!"

An associated disadvantage is the relative novelty of having a special education teacher serve as a consultant. While inservice training may be provided to enable the special educator assume this new responsibility, some teachers prefer to maintain their own territory and want to teach in their own "space." For example, Mrs. Engert, a self-contained special education teacher of fifteen years, may feel a bit uncomfortable switching to the role of a consultant. Likewise, Mr. Dupont, a relatively new teacher, may feel the same uneasiness when asked to consult with teachers of considerable experience.

Thus, administrators of special education programs and teacher-educators need to be aware of the constantly changing inservice training needs of regular educators and special educators. Those concerns must be provided in very real, sensitive, and practical ways.

Community Settings

Educators of the very near future of secondary-aged students will probably find their work environment more closely aligned with the "real world" work settings their students move into after graduation. Instead of a resource room for students with mild disabilities, some teachers may be described as job coaches, transition specialists, or as educators within non-public school settings. Some of these nonschool agencies include programs offered by Associations for Retarded Citizens (ARCs) or a local office for the state Vocational Rehabilitation office. The ability to identify student strengths, weaknesses, and community options will all be critical skills for teachers of secondary students in the near future. A critical skill for those pursuing careers with older students who have mild disabilities will be their ability to work and collaborate with groups of individuals outside the traditional education setting.

Collaboration/Consultation Model for Students with Mild Disabilities

A relatively new option for supporting children with mild disabilities in the regular classroom is the collaborative /consultation model. This model emerged due to the stigma children were assigned due to their participation in "special class" work and from the lack of opportunities to generalize skills in the regular class (Weidmeyer & Lehman, 1991). The issue of collaboration has also been of great interest to professional organizations, and in particular, the Council for Exceptional Children (CEC). In an attempt to define, describe, and then train teachers to function effectively in the role of a collaborator, the following definition was developed.

> Collaboration is a generic (umbrella) term which is used to describe a style of interacting in which persons with diverse backgrounds/expertise voluntarily agree to work together to generate creative solutions to mutually defined problems. It is characterized by mutual trust and respect, open communication, and parity of contributions. The goal of collaboration is to more effectively meet the unique educational needs of exceptional students (Council for Exceptional Children, 1991).

The collaboration model is frequently used with children who have learning disabilities and mild mental retardation. This approach is often referred to as a "plug-in" model, since special educators work directly with students within the context of the regular class. In a less direct fashion, special educators also serve to determine the nature a student's learning problem and then work with the student and regular teacher to identify effective intervention strategies. Special educators/consultants also assist in monitoring the child's performance. These teacher consultants may also be helpful by identifying appropriate materials and supplementary teaching aids.

Phillips and McCullough (1990) suggest the following as general tenets of the collaborative approach.

1. Joint responsibility for problems (i.e., all professionals share responsibility and concern for all students).

2. Joint accountability and recognition for problem resolution.

3. Belief that pooling talents and resources is mutually advantageous, with the following benefits:

   a. Increased range of solutions generated.

   b. Diversity of expertise and resources available to engage problem;

   c. Superiority and originality of solutions generated.

4. Belief that teacher or student problem resolution merits expenditure of time, energy, and resources.

5. Belief that correlates of collaboration are important and desirable (i.e., group morale, group cohesion, increased knowledge of problem-solving processes and specific alternative classroom interventions) (p. 295).

The basic rationale for the collaboration/consultation model, therefore, is to encourage the involvement of numerous professionals, both regular education and special education, in the appropriate education of students with disabilities.

CLASSROOM ARRANGEMENTS

Regardless of the specific model used to provide special education and related services to students with disabilities, the physical arrangement of the classroom is important. Many students with mild disabilities have experienced significant failures, especially during their school years. Therefore, the physical arrangement of the classroom is important not only for the obvious reasons of preventing distractibility, facilitating teacher-student interactions, and promoting student collaborations, but to provide a sense of security for the student.

There are an infinite number of ways to physically arrange the classroom. In a special education classroom, whether the room is a resource room or special classroom, teachers need to consider the following student characteristics:

- general insecurity;

- poor social skills;

- short attention span;

- distractibility;

- behavior control problems;

- hyperactivity;

- need for audio-visual aids.

Teachers need to take advantage of the space they have available to promote learning and social interactions. Although it may seem that since there are fewer students in a resource room or special class room than in regular classes, less space is required. However, because of the need for learning centers, places for individual and small group instruction, and ways to eliminate distractions, the size of special education classrooms needs to be at least as large as regular classrooms.

Figure 3–3 provides an example of a floor plan for a resource room. Keep in mind that this is just a sample. Teachers should try different physical arrangements to determine which organization best meets their students' needs. For self-contained classrooms, teachers can modify the resource room sample to accommodate for more students at any one time. Some additional considerations within the resource room include:

- the proximity of students' desks to one another;

- a place or time of day/period for quiet activities;

- an area of the room designated for displaying student work;

- access to materials/supplies.

In designing classroom space, it is critical that a teacher is able to scan activities of all students from a variety of places within the class. Students will quickly learn areas that are difficult for teachers to observe and can thus open opportunities for students to kindle less-than-desired behaviors.

The Regular Education Initiative (REI)

The classroom options listed above subscribe to a dichotomous education system: one for children with disabilities and another for children who do not have disabilities. This separatist philosophy has become an issue of heated debate during the late 1980s (Will, 1986; Lilly, 1988; Wang & Walberg, 1988; Davis 1989). One reason for this controversy is the reported failure of the dual system to meet the needs of students with disabilities. Especially students with disabilities who exited the public school system only to encounter significant problems (Polloway, Patton, Epstein, & Smith, 1990; Zigmond, 1990). Davis (1989) noted that the current dual system is an illogical, discriminatory, and cost inefficient method of serving children with disabilities.

FIGURE 3-3 Example of Floor Plan for a Resource Room

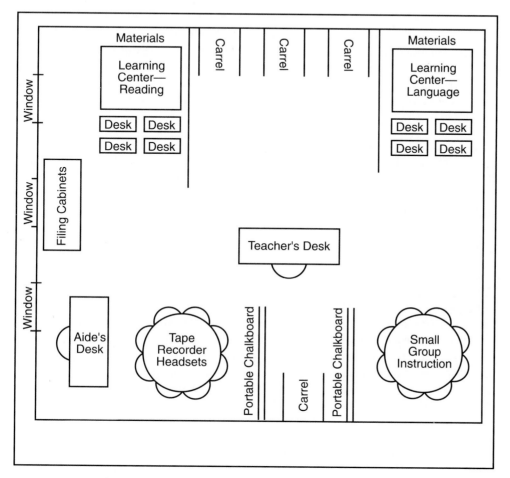

Source: Westling & Koorland (1988).

In a report published by the U.S. Office of Special Education and Rehabilitation Services (OSERS), Madeline Will (1986) reported on several important failures of the special education system. First, large numbers of students in special education programs were not learning successfully. Second, the use of the pull-out model of service delivery (where students are taken out of one class in order to receive specialized services somewhere else) was failing miserably. These concerns resulted in some professionals calling for the abolishment of the current dual model to one that would be more proactive and preventive in nature. Her final comment related to financial matters and the need to conserve scarce resources and to act as efficient as possible.

DEFINITION OF THE REGULAR EDUCATION INITIATIVE

Termed the **Regular Education Initiative (REI)** or, as some have termed it, the **General Education Initiative (GEI)**, this movement calls for a restructuring of how children with disabilities would receive services. It suggests that "the general education system assume unequivocal, primary responsibility for all students in our public schools—including identified handicapped students as well as those students who have special needs of some type" (Davis, 1989, p. 440). While it does not call for complete dissolution of special education as it exists, it does suggest the need for general and special educators to work more collaboratively at the school-building level. Ideally, all children who have mild disabilities would be served in the regular classroom.

This change would mean reorganizing the structure of services and massive retraining efforts of personnel. For example, proponents of this approach suggest that regular educators should take more of a responsibility for educating children with mild to moderate disabilities and have special educators serve more as consultants to regular educators than as teachers of children. This change alone would require substantial overhauling of teacher education programs, both for regular and special education teachers.

PROS AND CONS OF THE REGULAR EDUCATION INITIATIVE

The end product of REI would be a unified educational system for children, one where all children would benefit, not just children with disabilities. As such, this measure would also include a group of children who previously had been excluded from special assistance—children who are economically or socially disadvantaged and children who are bilingual.

On the other hand, critics of this approach argue that this plan was drafted by special educators, but it has a greater impact on the roles of the regular educators; regular educators have had little input into the plan. Commenting on the proposed REI, Lieberman (1985) notes, "it's similar to a wedding, in which we, as special educators, have forgotten to invite the bride (regular educators)" (p. 513).

Additionally, little is known about how the plan would actually work financially or administratively. Few people are willing to relinquish an old plan, be it as it may, with little information regarding the impact of one that is marketed as "new and improved." Before this plan can be implemented, educators from both sides will need to carefully review the feasibility of such an endeavor prior to taking a leap of faith.

IMPACT OF THE REGULAR EDUCATION INITIATIVE ON SERVING STUDENTS WITH MILD DISABILITIES

One can only speculate on the effects of an educational system where all children are educated together, separated perhaps, only by age. Research studies are available to suggest that education in the mainstream has a positive impact on both the academic and social abilities of children who have diagnosed disabilities, and on their peers, who do not. However, Davis notes that the REI debate "is focusing, in part, on quality-of-life issues—basic human needs issues that are much more global and significant than simply PL 94–142 compliance issues" (p. 445).

After gaining a lot of national attention when it was first introduced, the REI has more recently seemed to lose some support. Critics who have underlined the fact that major changes in the current special education system should not be made without an empirical basis for the change have seemingly captured the attention of policy makers. However, at this point it is definitely too early to tell how much of an impact the regular education initiative will have on special and regular education.

SUMMARY

This chapter provided information about the instructional setting used in special education for students with mild disabilities. The first section of the chapter provided information about the importance of the instructional setting. It was pointed out that where the services are provided is directly linked to the success of the services. The next major section of the chapter focused on the concept of least restrictive setting, as required by Public Law 94–142. Least restrictive setting was defined, and different models were presented to help describe the concept.

Special classes, as a setting for students with mild disabilities, were discussed. Characteristics of special classes, as well as advantages and disadvantages of special classes for students with mild disabilities were presented. The fact that special classes for this population are not used as often as in the past was noted. Finally, the role of teachers and other school support personnel was discussed.

The next major section presented information on the resource room. It was noted that resource rooms are currently the most widely used special education setting for students with mild disabilities. Types of resource rooms, and their current use were discussed. A discussion on the advantages and disadvantages of the resource room model was also presented.

The final section of the chapter dealt with regular classrooms and the regular education initiative. Regular classrooms were described, along with how they are used to serve students with mild disabilities. Advantages, disadvantages, and current use of regular classrooms to serve students in special education were presented. The regular education initiative was described, along with why many schools are moving to implement this newest service delivery model for students with mild disabilities.

REFERENCES

Bauwens, J., Gerber, S., Reisberg, L., & Robinson, S. (1991). *Academy for professional collaboration.* Reston, VA: Council for Exceptional Children.

Cegelka, P.T., & Prehm, H.J. (1982). *Mental retardation: From categories to people.* Columbus, OH: Merrill.

Council for Exceptional Children. (1991). Code of ethics of the Council for Exceptional Children. *Teaching Exceptional Children, 23*(2).

Cruickshank, W.M. (1977). Guest editorial. *Journal of Learning Disabilities, 10,* 193–194.

Danielson, L.C., & Bellamy, G.T. (1989). State variation in placement of children with handicaps in segregated environments. *Exceptional Children, 55*(5), 448–455.

Davis, W.E. (1989). The regular education initiative debate: Its promises and problems. *Exceptional Children, 55*(5), 440–446.

Deno, E. (1970). Special education as development capital. *Exceptional Children, 37,* p. 236.

Dunn, L.M. (1968). Special education for the mildly retarded: Is much of it justified? *Exceptional Children, 35,* 5–22.

Forness, S.R. & Kavale, K.A. (1984). Education of the mentally retarded: A note on policy. *Education and Training of the Mentally Retarded, 19,* 239–245.

Hallahan, D.P., & Kauffman, J.M. (1991). *Exceptional Children* 5th Ed. Englewood Cliffs, NJ: Prentice Hall.

Infant Health and Development Program. (1990). Enhancing the outcomes of low birth weight, premature infants: A multisite randomized trial. *Journal of the American Medical Association, 263,* 3035–3042.

Jenkins, J.R., & Heinen, A. (1989). Students' preferences for service delivery: Pull-out, in-class, or integrated models. *Exceptional Children, 55*(6), 516–523.

Lieberman, L.M. (1985). Special education and regular education: A merger made in heaven? *Exceptional Children, 55,* 513–516.

Lilly, M.S. (1970). Special education: A tempest in a teapot. *Exceptional Children, 37,* 42–49.

Lilly, M.S. (1988). The regular education initiative: A force for change in general and special education. *Education and Training in Mental Retardation, 23*(4), 253–260.

Martin, S.L., Ramey, C.T., & Ramey, S.L. (1990). The prevention of intellectual impairment in children of impoverished families: Findings of a randomized trial of educational daycare. *American Journal of Public Health, 80,* 844–847.

Meyen, E.L., & Skrtic, T.M. (Eds.) (1988). *Exceptional children and youth: An introduction* 3rd Ed. Denver: Love.

Morse, W.C. (1984). Personal perspective. In B. Blatt & R. Morris (Eds.), *Perspectives in special education: Personal orientations.* Glenview, IL: Scott Foresman.

Peterson, R.L., Zabel, R.H., Smith, C.R., & Smith, M.A. (1983). Cascade of services model and emotionally disabled students. *Exceptional Children, 49,* 404–410. In T.E.C. Smith, B.J. Price, & G.E. Marsh (Eds.), *Mildly handicapped children and adults.* St. Paul: West.

Phillips, V., & McCullough, L. (1990). Consultation-based programming: Instituting the collaborative ethic in schools. *Exceptional Children, 56,* 291–304.

Podemski, R., Price, B.J., Smith, T.E.C., & Marsh, G.E. (1984). *Comprehensive administration of special education.* Rockville, MD: Aspen Systems Corp.

Polloway, E.A., Patton, J.R., Epstein, M.H., & Smith, T.E.C. (1990). Comprehensive curriculum for students with mild handicaps. *Focus on Exceptional Children, 21,* 1–12.

Public Law 94–142. The Education of All Handicapped Children Act, 20 USC 1401; 34 Part 300.

Reid, D.K., & Hresko, W.P. (1981). *A cognitive approach to learning disabilities.* New York: McGraw-Hill.

Reynolds, M.C. (1973). Changing Roles of Special Education Personnel. Paper presented to UCEA. In T.E.C. Smith, B.J. Price, & G.E. Marsh (Eds.), *Mildly handicapped children and adults.* St. Paul: West.

Roberts, C., Pratt, C., & Leach, D. (1991). Classroom and playground interaction of students with and without disabilities. *Exceptional Children, 57*(3), 212–224.

Rich, H.L., & Ross, S.M. (1989). Students' time on learning tasks in special education. *Exceptional Children, 55*(6), 508–515.

Sabornie, E.J., Marshall, K.L., & Ellis, E.S. (1990). Restructuring of mainstream sociometry with learning disabled and nonhandicapped students. *Exceptional Children, 56*(4), 314–323.

Skeels, H.M., & Dye, H.B. (1939). A study of the effects of differential stimulation on mentally retarded children. *Convention Proceedings: American Association on Mental Deficiency, 44,* 114–136.

Smith, T.E.C., Price, B.J., & Marsh, G.E. (1986). *Mildly handicapped children and adults.* St. Paul: West.

Stainback, W.C., & Stainback, S.B. (1984). A rationale for the merger of special and regular education. *Exceptional Children, 51,* 102–111.

Stainback, S.B., & Stainback, W.C. (1989). Classroom organization for diversity among students. *National Social Studies of Education Yearbook, 88*, Part 2, 195–207.

U.S. Department of Education (1989). *Eleventh Annual Report to Congress on the Implementation of the Education of the Handicapped Act*. Washington, D.C.

Vergason, G.A. & Anderegg, M.L. (1991). Beyond the regular education initiative and the resource room controversy. *Focus on Exceptional Children, 23*, 1–10.

Yoshida, R.K. (1984). Perspectives on research. p. 56–72. In E.L. Meyen (Ed.), *Mental retardation: Topics of today—issues of tomorrow*. Lancaster, PA: Lancaster Press.

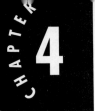

The Instructional Process

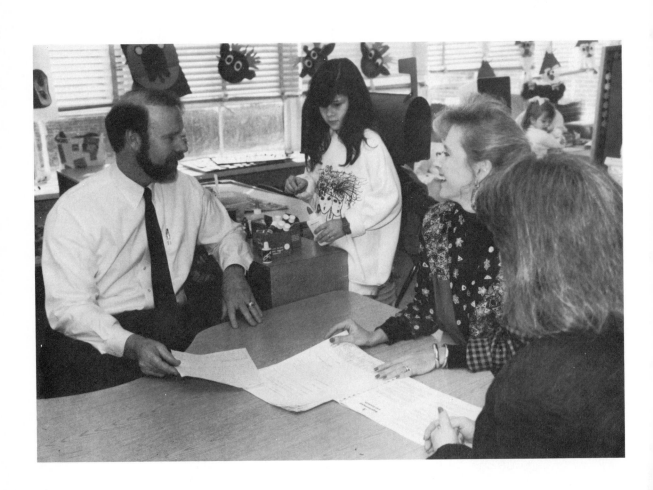

Outline

OBJECTIVES

After reading this chapter, you will be able to:

- describe the philosophical underpinnings of why our teaching of students with mild disabilities should be different

- understand the legal mandates and guidelines for making those instructional modifications

- describe the concept of "least restrictive environment"

- describe the components of an IEP

- specify the steps in the instructional process from Child Find to Program Evaluation

- list (and use) strategies to modify instruction for children who have mild disabilities

Introduction

The instructional process for children in special education incorporates a variety of activities that actually begin long before they enter a special education classroom. In a very general sense, that process includes 1. carefully designed methods for screening children who may benefit from specialized instruction; 2. objectively based assessment activities to determine the specific nature of the disability; and 3. curricular and teaching strategies that will enable those children to maximize their strengths and perhaps compensate for their weaknesses. An often overlooked but critically important step in this process is to evaluate that entire process to determine what has been effective and which components should be added, modified, or discontinued. What follows below is a description of the specific elements of the instructional process critical to providing appropriate services to children with disabilities.

DEFINING THE INSTRUCTIONAL PROCESS

The term "special education" implies that the instruction and materials that are provided to children with disabilities are somehow different than what is provided to children who do not have disabilities. That idea is the cornerstone that supports the notion that these children have the right to a free and appropriate public education. Yet, how do educators modify instructional methods and materials to address the unique needs of children with particular learning needs so that they are better prepared to meet the demands required of life in the mainstream? Much of what is "special" in special education is the consistent application of "good teaching" procedures that have demonstrated over time that they usually result in the acquisition of enhanced skills in a particular area. Yet, those components of "good teaching" are most successful when they are imbedded in a framework of specific steps that ultimately function to successfully integrate these children into the mainstream of their community.

The purpose of this chapter is to respond to the question of how special education is different, to offer suggestions that will facilitate making education for children with disabilities "special," and to describe the process components that not only meet the letter of the law (i.e., Public Law 94–142) but that lead to greater student/teacher success.

Early Efforts

One of the earliest efforts to modify instruction for people who "learn differently" was attempted by Jean-Marc-Gaspard Itard (1775–1838). Itard, a French physician, was given charge of a wild young boy, Victor, who displayed a variety of unusual learning characteristics. For five years, this ambitious doctor tried a variety of remediation and training strategies in an effort to change the developmental outcomes for this young lad, only to surmise that his efforts were unsuccessful. This failure is often regarded by historians as the first special education program (Haring, 1990).

In the absence of federal or local laws, previous research, established assessment procedures or curricular, Itard attempted to answer a variety of intriguing questions relative to the anticipated development of Victor. Two of the questions Itard addressed at the turn of the nineteenth century are still valid questions for today's contemporary educator as we approach the twenty-first century: 1. "To what extent can education compensate for delayed development . . . ?" and 2. "What are the critical features of effective training methods?" (Lane, 1976 p. 321). While educators may not be able to predict to what extent compensations in instructional methods can have on children who have delayed or impaired development, they are beginning to understand a few of the critical features that comprise effective training methods.

Ysseldyke and Algozzine (1990) provide five critical elements that help to answer the original question, "What makes special education so special?" These five elements include the objectives of instruction, individual education programs, content areas, instructional techniques, and instructional adaptations. Public Law 94–142, The Education of All Handicapped Children Act of 1975 (EHA), provides a mandated framework from which these modifications can be constructed.

The primary purpose of Public Law 94–142 is to:

> . . . assure that all handicapped children have available to them . . . a free appropriate public education which emphasizes special education and related services designed to meet their unique needs, to assure that the rights of handicapped children and their parents or guardians are protected, to assist States and localities to provide for the education of all handicapped children, and to assess and assure the effectiveness of efforts to educate handicapped children. (Public Law 94–142, sec. 601c)

Public Law 94–142 provides the legal framework for providing a free, appropriate public education (FAPE) to children between the ages of six and twenty-one years of age who have identified special needs.

More recently, the enactment of Public Law 99–457, the Education of the Handicapped Act Amendments of 1986, demonstrates a renewed commitment to this nations's preschool children who have special needs (Smith, 1990). Often described as a downward extension of Public Law 94–142, these amendments now insure that all students with disabilities between the ages of three and twenty-one are provided with a free, appropriate public education. Thus, this population is now considered to be a part of the definition of school-aged students identified under regulations within Public Law 94–142 (Strickland & Turnbull, 1990).

While many of the service provision features of Public Law 94–142 are maintained for younger children who have disabilities, perhaps the most notable difference between Public Law 94–142 and Public Law 99–457 is that Public Law 99–457 places a stronger emphasis on family involvement. Public Law 99–457 recognizes that young children are an inseparable part of a total family system and that early intervention efforts can only be successful when the family is actively involved as participants.

Additionally, while Public Law 94–142 provided incentives for serving preschool children (three to five years of age) prior to the mandates of Public Law 99–457, Part H of this new amendment provides financial incentives for states to also serve the youngest segment of our population, infants and toddlers (birth to two years of age).

MAJOR COMPONENTS OF PUBLIC LAW 94–142 RELATED TO THE INSTRUCTIONAL PROCESS

Any document, such as Public Law 94–142, that attempts to ensure that the diverse educational needs of children with disabilities are adequately provided can be difficult to understand

and even more complicated to implement. In an effort to simplify the major thrusts contained in Public Law 94–142, Strickland and Turnbull (1990) have summarized six broad service principles. These principles include:

- inclusion in a program of appropriate service;
- nondiscriminatory assessment;
- individualized education program;
- least restrictive environment;
- procedural safeguards; and
- parent participation.

Inclusion

As mentioned earlier, the notion of inclusion refers to the right that all children between the ages of three and twenty-one must be provided with a free and appropriate public education. Often referred to as the "zero reject" provision (Lilly, 1970), this component means that public school systems must serve all children within that age range who reside in their geographical area. Further, this notion encourages educators to examine all instructional options within the parameters of the regular class setting. Public Law 94–142 provides clear definitions for children identified as handicapped. Chapter 2 provides a listing of the thirteen specific categorical handicapping conditions covered under Public Law 94–142 and more recent amendments. These children, defined by federal statute, must be included in public school programs.

Nondiscriminatory Assessment

Prior to placement in a special education program, students must receive a comprehensive evaluation. A child must be assessed in all areas related to the suspected disability including (where appropriate):

- health;
- vision;
- hearing;
- social and emotional status;
- general intelligence;
- academic performance;
- communication status; and
- motor abilities.

The purpose of this evaluation is to substantiate the need for special education services; provide a basis for program planning; and establish a baseline for measuring progress (Meyen, 1988). Measuring the discrete skills of children with disabilities, however, can be a difficult task.

Optometrists, ophthalmologists, and audiologists are often able to measure visual and auditory abilities with a certain degree of accuracy since their diagnoses are based on objective and calibrated measurements. However, the ability to measure the less accessible abilities of cognition, learning potential, and related behaviors in children who have handicapping conditions are often less precise and subject to error (Sattler, 1988).

Of particular interest here are children from minority backgrounds. Cartwright, Cartwright, and Ward (1981) list four major minority groups in the United States. These groups include blacks (African descent), Hispanic (the second-largest, fastest-growing, and largest bilingual group), Asians/Pacific Islanders, and Native Americans. Native Americans include American Indians and Alaskans. This last group is represented by almost three hundred different languages and dialects.

By the year 2000, blacks, Hispanics, and other racially diverse groups will comprise one-third of the total population of the United States. Aramburo (1989) provides interesting statistics relative to today's educational population. For example, she notes that minorities comprise at least twenty-five percent of the total public school population in thirteen states and thirty-six percent in six states. Children from minority backgrounds are in the majority in the twenty-five largest school districts in America. Minority students in the state of California make up an estimated 50.8 percent of the 4.6 million students within that states' system. This problem becomes even more complex when considered within the context of special education services. Table 4–1 (on page 100) provides a recent analysis of where culturally diverse students fit into the special education system.

Problems often occur when children from culturally diverse environments enter an educational system that frequently is at odds with the way these children think and behave. Many of the evaluation instruments available have been found to be inherently discriminatory for children from minority backgrounds (Smith, Price, & Marsh, 1986). As a result, Public Law 94–142 recognizes the need to insure fair evaluations. Provisions of the law state that the practices used with population must be fair—without racial or cultural bias.

> Procedures to assure that testing and evaluation materials and procedures utilized for the purpose of evaluation and placement of handicapped children will be selected and administered so as not to be racially or culturally discriminatory. Such materials or procedures shall be provided and administered in the child's native language or mode of communication, unless it is clearly not feasible to do so, and no single procedure shall be the sole criterion for determining an appropriate educational program for a child. (Section 615-5C)

Even when examiners are sensitive and cautious regarding this issue, testing children from diverse cultural backgrounds can be particularly problematic for a number of reasons. First, tests are often designed to be used with large groups of children and must of the test information and test questions typically relate to the majority of the population and not minority groups. Second, tests frequently demand a linguistic style that may be culturally different from the minority student (Sattler, 1986).

Further, many of the norms used to compare childrens' performances are largely based on white, middle-socio-economic-class samples. Children raised in homes that are significantly different by cultural and economic measures should not be expected to compare favorably to this group. In addition, children from minority backgrounds may be hesitant to demonstrate their optimum capabilities to someone from a different culture (Sattler, 1988). Finally, there may be subtle cognitive differences in children from minority groups.

The literature is replete with situations where children from minority groups, the disadvantaged, or those who have multiple disabilities have ben subject to negative test bias (Mercer, 1976; Banks, 1977; Garcia, 1978; Sattler, 1988). In an attempt to rectify this situation,

TABLE 4-1 Participation of Racial and Ethnic Groups in Special Education

	RACIAL/ETHNIC GROUP				
	White	Black	Hispanic	Asian	Indian
Learning Disabled (LD):					
Percent LD	4.20	4.50	4.50	1.60	5.20
Percent of LD	71.24	17.35	9.77	0.96	1.14
Percent of general population	71.20	16.20	9.10	2.50	0.90
Mentally Retarded (MR):					
Percent MR	1.20	3.50	1.50	0.50	1.70
Percent of MR	56.99	37.79	9.12	0.84	1.04
Percent of general population	71.20	16.20	9.10	2.50	0.90
Emotionally Disturbed (ED):					
Percent of ED	0.60	0.80	0.40	0.10	0.50
Percent of ED	71.24	21.59	6.08	0.42	0.77
Percent of general population	71.20	16.20	9.10	2.50	0.90
Speech Impaired (SI):					
Percent SI	2.70	2.40	2.00	1.70	2.50
Percent of SI	76.94	15.55	7.30	1.71	0.92
Percent of general population	71.20	16.20	9.10	2.50	0.90
Gifted and Talented (GT):					
Percent GT	4.70	2.20	2.10	8.30	2.00
Percent of GT	79.92	8.48	4.56	4.98	0.44
Percent of general population	71.20	16.20	9.10	2.50	0.90

Source: Derived from information provided in J.D. Stern & M.O. Chandler (1987). *The condition of education: A statistical report.* Washington, D.C.: Office of Educational Research and Improvement, Center for Educational Statistics, pp. 64, 66.

the courts have been very clear in insuring that children are not excluded from an appropriate special education program (or included in one) due to discriminatory assessment procedures or violations of due process (*Diana v. State Board of Education*, 1970; *Larry P. v. Riles*, 1972).

In attempt to limit the negative effects of culturally determined test bias, Public Law 94–142, and subsequent amendments, state that evaluations must be appropriate for the child's cultural and linguistic background. That testing must be provided by personnel who are trained in that particular instrument with that particular population. Additionally, those tests should have sound psychometric properties (valid and reliable). Educational evaluations should be composed of several assessment measures and must be repeated at least every three years. One such test that addresses the needs of students from diverse racial and cultural backgrounds is the *System of Multicultural Pluralistic Assessment*

(SOMPA) (Mercer & Lewis, 1978). The SOMPA considers information from nine measures to assist in the development of a comprehensive assessment for educational and placement decisions. While critics of the SOMPA may argue that administration of this particular tool is too lengthy (five hours), it nonetheless permits personnel to capture an accurate picture of a child's abilities that is free from cultural or racial bias.

Individualized Education Program (IEP)

The core of providing "special" education to students with disabilities is the Individualized Education Program (IEP). The purpose of an IEP is to ensure that educational programs are designed to meet the specific needs of the exceptional learner. Eight major components compose the IEP.

1. A statement of the child's present level of educational performance, including academic achievement, social adaptation, prevocational and vocational skills, psychomotor skills, and self-help skills.

2. A statement of annual goals that describes the educational performance to be achieved by the end of the school year under the child's educational program.

3. A statement of short-term instructional objectives, which must be measurable intermediate steps between the present level of educational performance and the annual goals.

4. A statement of specific educational services needed by the child, (determined without regard to the availability of those services) including a description of:

   a. all special education and related services that are needed to meet the unique needs of the child, including the type of physical education program in which the child will participate, and

   b. any special instructional media and materials that are needed.

5. The date when those services will begin and the length of time the services will be given.

6. A description of the extent to which the child will participate in regular education programs.

7. A justification for the type of educational placement that the child will have.

8. A list of the individuals who are responsible for implementation of the individualized education program.

9. Objective criteria, evaluation procedures, and schedules for determining, on at least an annual basis, whether the short-term instructional objectives are being achieved (Federal Register, 1977).

When reviewing a child's present level of functioning, a variety of educational needs may emerge. It may not be appropriate or possible to deal with each of those identified concerns in a single IEP year (Lewis & Doorlag, 1987). Therefore, in concert with parents or significant caregivers, school personnel should prioritize which goals should be addressed first and focus on providing appropriate services to meet those goals.

Least Restrictive Environment

Public Law 94–142 specifies that children with disabilities are to be educated, to the maximum extent possible, with their peers who do not have disabilities. No longer do we question whether or not these children should be integrated with their peers and natural environments. The question that is often asked is *how* can instructional programs be designed for these children within the context of existing and often massive educational systems.

Research consistently demonstrates that when children with disabilities and children without disabilities are educated in integrated settings, positive outcomes are achieved by both groups (Hamre-Nietupski, Nietupski, Stainbach, & Stainbach, 1984). These positive outcomes include gains in academic skills, improvements in social relationships, and benefits to self-concepts. Additionally, when heterogenous groupings are used, it is often easier and cheaper to provide ancillary services (i.e., physical, occupational, and speech therapies).

Procedural Safeguards

A primary provision of Public Law 94–142 (and Public Law 99–457) is the establishment of procedural safeguards for children with disabilities and their parents. The exact interpretation of this provision has been difficult over the last two decades, but is, nonetheless, a very basic constitutional right guaranteed by the Fourteenth Amendment. In a proactive sense, these procedural safeguards were included to bring parents into the system to help them understand and question what was happening to their child. These provisions afford parents with a decision-making voice regarding educational opportunities that will be provided to their child. Often referred to as due process rights, these important provisions help to insure that all parties (school and families) have a method of assuring programmatic quality.

School districts must establish due process requirements in accordance with state and federal laws *and* make those procedures known to parents. When parents have questions regarding the program designed for their child or how that program is being implemented, the law provides parents with several rights, including the right to examine their child's records and the right to independent evaluations. This law also states that schools must notify parents in writing (in their native language, if possible) prior to changing the identification, evaluation, or placement of their child.

When a decision is made regarding an element of a child's special education program that is unacceptable to either the school or the parents, an impartial due process hearing may be requested. At this point parents have the right to counsel and experts in special education; the right to present evidence, cross examine, and compel the attendance of witnesses; and the right to a written or taped record of the hearing. If the findings of that hearing are still unsatisfactory to the parents, appeals can often be made to the state education agency (SEA) and then to the civil courts (Smith, 1981).

Parental Participation

A critical component in the development of a useful IEP is the notion of parent participation. Parents should be considered as an initial point of reference in the development of a tailor-made education plan rather than someone who comes to school only to sign an IEP form that has already been completed. Professionals should remember that parents (or other family members) may have little information regarding the IEP process and may be intimidated by the presence of several highly trained professionals who are asking for input.

Gress and Carroll (1985) offer several useful suggestions to facilitate the development of a healthy parent-professional partnership. It has been estimated that almost sixty percent of children who attend public schools today are from single-parent families. Add to that scenario the increasing levels of responsibility and stress that many of these single parents face in attempting to balance a career and child rearing tasks only increases the problem of parental involvement. Many sensitive educators look beyond the typical school hours (or days) to convene an IEP meeting. This action facilitates parental participation in the IEP process.

Another suggestion to enhance the quality of the parent-professional partnership is to consider the location of the IEP meeting. For a variety of reasons, some parents may have had negative experiences with a particular school or its personnel and may be hesitant to attend *any* meeting at *that* school. A lack of transportation to the IEP meeting may also be a major barrier to full participation for many parents. Holding the meeting at a neutral site (public library, church, or community activity center) may provide for a more positive, psychologically neutral interaction.

Professionals should also consider the importance of the actual setting where the IEP meetings are to take place, especially if this is the first IEP meeting for the parents. That meeting may bring to bear their worst fears. . . mental retardation?. . . a learning disability?. . . maybe "just" a mild bilateral hearing loss? To help these parents feel more relaxed, make sure the waiting area is clean and comfortable. The actual conference area (tables and chairs) should be arranged in such a way that it enhances communication and does not reflect an authority role by where someone sits. Remember, when meetings are held at the child's school, a territorial barrier can be created which may inhibit candid exchanges between parents and teachers.

When the meeting begins, it's often a good idea to restate the purpose of the meeting, what the expected outcomes are, and how much time is allotted (parents often have tight schedules, too). Realizing that parents may be somewhat hesitant to express their true feelings about the outcome of events in an IEP meeting ("Do I really want my child placed in that class?"), it's a good idea to follow-up that IEP meeting with a phone call from an IEP team member. This simple validation call gives the parents an opportunity to express their concerns and reiterates the staffs' desire for parental input and satisfaction.

All parents are eventually asked to sign the IEP document. That signature should indicate that individual's agreement with the information, goals, objectives, and methodologies contained in the document. However, as part of their due process rights, parents may refuse to sign the IEP and request further action in pursuit of appropriate educational services for their child.

The IEP Process

IEP: PRODUCT OR PROCESS?

An IEP is a statement of a child's present educational level, future educational goals, the educational services to be provided, and the extent to which the child will be able to participate in regular educational programs (Data Research, Inc., 1990). More simply, the philosophy behind the IEP is to guide decision making and formulate instruction.

The major steps in the IEP process include child find activities, the referral, screening and assessment of the student's strengths and weaknesses, placement in the least restrictive environment (see Figure 4–6) and the actual delivery of services. Public Law 94–142 is implicit about these key actions and events so that all implementation regulations are fulfilled (Smith, Price, & Marsh, 1983). Before examining the discrete steps in the development of an IEP, it is important to discuss two perspectives: the IEP as a product, and the IEP as a process.

The IEP as a Product

Many activities performed by school districts relative to IEP in the late 1970s and early 1980s focused on determining how to provide services to children that comply with the intent of the law (EHA). Now that many of those legal and logistical hurdles have been addressed, a number of school districts today focus on how to construct and implement the IEP document in an efficient, often computerized fashion (Ryan, & Rucker, 1986; Jenkins, 1987). However, when too much focus is placed on completing the product or IEP form, a number of issues often emerge (Marsh & Price, 1980). These include:

- Content area teachers complain about having handicapped students in the regular classroom.

- Special education teachers complain about the lack of cooperation they receive from regular teachers.

- Teachers resist input from specialists, asserting that they offer impractical suggestions that are not appropriate for the regular classroom.

- Parents express concern about what is happening to their child in the regular classroom.

- Monitoring personnel question the relationship between daily instructional activities and the comprehensive plan found in the files.

- All parties complain about the amount of time required to complete the IEP process.

Why do these kinds of problems occur? The answer may lie in the fact that each of the above mentioned groups of people attempted to address the letter of the law in completing the IEP form with little thought regarding what interactions would ensue that also involve other parties. Did the IEP team consider what consequences might result when Andy (who has a specific learning disability in the areas of math computation and reading comprehension) is placed in Mrs. Greene's fourth grade class? In her busy class (assume Mrs. Greene has thirty students) when will Mrs. Greene be able to learn how to implement those "curricular modifications" and how will she access those materials that have been "specially adapted for the special education student?" The question is not whether Andy belongs in Mrs. Greene's class with his playmates, but rather, how can the team help Mrs. Greene modify her schedule and the curricula for Andy.

Administrators and special education supervisors can be particularly helpful in this situation if they recognize and correct common misconceptions about IEP development. Podemski, Price, Smith, and Marsh (1984) have identified a few of those misconceptions, which include:

- The IEP is simply a form to be completed.
- Special educators are responsible for developing the IEP.
- The IEP is prepared as a legal precautionary document with little consequence on daily instruction.
- Persons most important in the development of an IEP are those who are most frequently associated with assessment (i.e., psychometrists, psychologists, etc.).

The IEP as a Process

When IEP is viewed as an active verb instead of just a noun, there are qualitative outcomes for both the student and staff. First, it is more likely that the student will receive services that are more comprehensive and appropriate when a process method is employed. Second, ownership in the IEP is more diverse and the roles of participants tend to encompass a more holistic view of the educational process. The student is set up to be more successful and professionals share in the joy of that success. Several authors (Podemski *et al.*, 1984) have noted that this process tends to be cyclical and usually involves three stages.

1. The initial stage concerned with child find and referral.
2. The intermediate stage devoted to evaluation and placement and completion of the IEP form.
3. The final stage involving daily programming and evaluation.

IEP team members also realize benefits in knowing about the types of services and expertise available within their system. This knowledge leads to better coordination of services, which reduces duplicate or redundant services.

Developing Components of the Instructional Process

A variety of strategies have been suggested for defining components of the instructional process (Maher, 1983; Smith, Price, & Marsh, 1983; Alter & Goldstein, 1986; Lewis & Doorlag, 1987; Strickland & Turnbull, 1990). Common to all of these approaches is a sequence of steps that insures not only a plan that meets the intent of the law, but one that provides for adequate development of appropriate educational experiences that lead to the child's maximizing future opportunities. Figure 4–1 identifies the major steps in this process.

CHILD FIND

The initial step in serving children who have handicapping conditions is to find them. This step is called Child Find and is a mandated requirement of Public Law 94–142. These activities are the direct responsibility of state and local education agencies who are charged with locating, identifying, and evaluating all children in their area who are in need of special education (Podemski *et al.*, 1984). Once children are identified within specific age and disability categories, they are identified to the state education agency (SEA) and to the U.S. Office of Education. This process then allows the local education agency (LEA) to be eligible to receive federal funds based on the number of children they have identified (Strickland & Turnbull, 1990). Local and state education agencies may request federal funds for up to twelve percent of the total school-age population. If the actual number of students who have been determined eligible for special education services exceeds twelve percent, the fiscal responsibility for serving those children is up to the local and state education agencies.

One of the first Child Find activities school districts employ is a public awareness campaign. These are usually informational posters or programs that describe the types of services that are available and how to access those services. Target sites for these campaigns may include supermarkets, churches, public health centers, and medical and related health offices.

Interagency cooperation is also valuable in identifying children who may be eligible for special education services. Agencies such as public welfare offices, after-school care centers, and municipally sponsored programs that serve children may be important links to segments of the population who may not realize that help is available.

REFERRAL

When a child has trouble meeting the demands in the family, school, or community, referrals are often made for special education services. Making a referral is a process of requesting information to decide if a student is eligible for those services. It is the initial step in accessing services. Referrals may be initiated by parents, teachers, or agency representatives serving the child. The two most common referral sources, however, are parents and regular classroom teachers. When children have mild disabilities (mental retardation, learning disabilities, or behavior disorders), parents unfamiliar with school routines or services or the exact nature of their childs' performance may not make a timely referral. As Wood (1984) notes, the child who has mild disabilities usually begins the educational process in a regular classroom. Unless the regular classroom teacher is able to identify these children quickly and modify their instruction, these students begin to fail academically and their self-concepts begin to deteriorate. Once children are identified as being eligible for special education services, they tend to adapt to changes in their curricula fairly well. But damage to a child's self-concept by school failure, peer isolation, or even ridicule because they are somehow "different" can be difficult to repair. Thus, it is critically important that regular classroom teachers understand the process for making appropriate

FIGURE 4-1 Steps in the IEP Process

1. Child Find Activities
2. Screening
3. Assessment of Strength/Needs
4. Design Educational Program (IEP)
5. Placement Decision
6. Implement IEP
7. Evaluate Program

referrals in their school system to decrease the risk of both academic failure and the development of poor self-concepts.

Classroom teachers should receive information on how children are referred to special education and what services are available. This information is often provided in an in-service manner and is termed "prereferral activities." Marsh, Price, and Smith (1983) have outlined three stages that are important in understanding the types of information that need to be shared at this point. This type of guidance should be provided throughout the referral process. These are 1. the exploratory stage, 2. the decision-making stage, and 3. the descriptive stage.

The exploratory stage helps to identify the existence of a problem. At this point, teachers should examine current examples of student work, attempt to modify their curricular approach and the environment, and determine how the student responds to those changes. Depending on the age of the student, it is also a good idea to talk to the student directly about your concerns. Previous teachers may also be a good source of information from a different perspective.

The second stage, decision making, is usually done in tandem with a school principal or other professional. Anecdotal records and information obtained in the exploratory stage is collated to determine if a referral for further testing is warranted. This step is important since it helps to validate early concerns. Deciding to make a referral for special education services is not easy. Often parents have a difficult time accepting the need for the action. Professionals should gather as much information as possible in order to make a good case for an actual referral.

The final step in this phase, description, involves the actual completion of the Referral Form. At this point parents must be advised that their child is being referred for a more complete evaluation.

SCREENING

Screening is an important step in determining if a child is eligible for special education. It is a process of obtaining objective information to determine if more intensive testing is necessary. By using standardized screening tests, teachers can quickly compare the performance of one child to how other children from a similar chronological age should be functioning in various areas. Screenings are often conducted in large groups, such as when children enter kindergarten or first grade. Screening may also be conducted throughout the school year with students in regular education programs to ascertain their progress. When a child's performance is below an expected range for children his age, teachers should begin to determine if additional, more indepth assessments should be conducted.

ASSESSMENT

Salvia and Ysseldyke (1988) define assessment as the process of collecting information that is used to make decisions about students. Children referred for special education services represent a wide variety of needs that generally cluster into one of four categories: physical needs, academic needs, classroom behavior needs, and social needs. Regardless of the primary referral reason, federal and state regulations may require that the following areas of development be considered in the course of developing appropriate programs and materials.

- Vision and hearing screenings.

- Speech/language evaluation.

- Intellectual assessment.

- Behavior/social rating measurement.

- Individual educational achievement and diagnostic tests.

- A review of the child's environmental, cultural, and economic disadvantage (often for diagnosis of a specific learning disability).

- A measurement of the child's classroom behaviors.

Thus, the areas that may have to be examined in any one child can be complex; involving the skills of a variety of professionals. This effort is often coordinated by the Eligibility Determination Committee (EDC). Those team members are responsible for organizing an appropriate assessment team, gathering assessment data, analyzing the results, and then synthesizing those results into a coherent and functional individualized education program.

IEP DEVELOPMENT

A basic consideration in the development of an IEP is that these comprehensive, detailed documents for guiding a students' curricula for a given year must be developed using a team approach. That team includes professionals, parents, and, when appropriate, the student. Recent amendments to Public Law 94–142 now insure a free and appropriate public education to thirteen different categories of exceptionality. These categories include children who are:

- deaf,
- deaf-blind,
- hard of hearing,
- mentally retarded,
- multi-handicapped,
- orthopedically impaired,
- other health impaired,
- seriously emotionally disturbed,
- have a specific learning disability (eg., autism),
- or have sustained a traumatic brain injury (U.S. Department of Education, 1990).

Because of this wide range, the nature of professionals who work and teach these children is tremendous. In addition to administrators, supervisors, transportation specialists, and building principals, the cadre of professionals working with this population include:

- special education teachers and consultants,
- nurses,
- psychologists/psychometrists,
- physical/occupational therapists,
- speech/language pathologists,
- nutritionists,
- audiologists,
- adaptive physical educators,
- medical personnel (physicians, surgeons, ophthalmologists, etc.), and
- regular education teachers.

The efforts of all these professionals are often augmented through the use of paraprofessionals—(Certified Occupational Therapists (C.O.T.A.s), Physical Therapy Assistants (P.T.A.s), and teaching assistants or aides. The ability to work in concert with one another, however, remains to be one of the greatest challenges in providing what these children need. Issues related to reponsibility, liability, and efficacy are still unresolved for many service delivery teams.

IEP Team Arrangements

Public Law 94–142 specifies that the development of an individualized education plan be developed from a multidisciplinary perspective. Figure 4–2 (on page 110) displays a variety of diagnostic and intervention team processes that have been utilized in the development of individualized education programs. Each approach or model has its own distinct advantages and disadvantages.

FIGURE 4-2 Advantages and Disadvantages of Selected Team Models

Type of Approach	Description	Advantages	Disadvantages
Multidisciplinary	Involves a cluster of professionals. Evaluations are independent. Results sent to central person or location.	Easy to schedule and useful when specific problems are presented. Useful when funds are limited and services are geographically diverse.	Isolated observations. Places a tremendous burden on team coordinator to interpret findings and generate programmatic recommendations.
Interdisciplinary	Evaluations may still be independent, but results and programmatic suggestions are discussed across disciplines.	Intervention options tend to be more compatible across disciplines. Focuses more on the "whole" child. Often a more stimulating work environment for team members.	Requires experienced administrative and planning skills. Greater time demands on team members. Risk turf protection issues.
Transdisciplinary	Cooperative working arrangement. The "Role Release" notion provides that team members educate each other in the skills of their "home" discipline.	Parents and students related to one person instead of many. Communication is less complicated. Easier to deliver diverse services especially in rural areas. Enhances professional skills of all team members.	Tremendous responsibility on other team members to master skills from other disciplines. Requires additional time for planning, coordination and training. Notion of role release may be a difficult transition for some members. State licensing may prohibit aspects of this model.

The development of an IEP can involve a variety of persons, but at a minimum should include a representative of the local school district—other than the child's teacher who is qualified to provide or supervise the provision of special education, the child's teacher, one or both of the child's parents or legal guardians, and the child, where appropriate.

Types of Teams

The multidisciplinary team approach evolved from a medical orientation whereby various specialists have expertise about specific parts or domains of the body (Peterson, 1981). This approach can be described as a method of obtaining discipline-specific information regarding various aspects of a child's development status.

In this model, children are usually seen in a one-on-one fashion by various professionals and assessment results are then compiled into an aggregate summary, often by a single team member. As shown in Figure 4–2, the primary advantage for using this approach over other team approaches is that the multidisciplinary team approach is most useful when team members are scattered across a large service delivery area. Since many of the school districts in the United States today are still described as rural (Helge, 1984), this model is particularly effective from a scheduling and coordination perspective.

The negative trade-off that does exists, however, is that observations and evaluations are conducted in isolation and team members rarely have an opportunity to share their insights, ideas, or hypotheses with one another. Consequently, the assimilation of programmatic recommendations can be difficult or even contradictory. Additionally, when team members work apart from one another, this isolation can lead to frustration and burnout.

Perhaps the most frequently used model in the development of an IEP is the interdisciplinary approach. In this model, team members may still conduct their evaluations independent of other professionals, but have the opportunity to come together and share their findings before a diagnostic label is assigned. The group dynamics available in this situation help facilitate goals and objectives that are more practical and realistic than is possible with a multidisciplinary approach. This model also helps when a clearcut definition or diagnostic category of a particular disability is not as apparent as when the child is considered in isolation. Perhaps the greatest disadvantage of this model is the requirement that all team members have to be gathered in a common location to formulate goals, objectives, activities, and evaluation criterion. This team approach requires a certain degree of planning and administrative skill that may be difficult in some school districts.

Take for example a school district that serves 300 children with disabilities who also require physical therapy services. It is not uncommon with many of today's service delivery schedules for those children to be served by a single therapist or by a therapist who is employed on a consultant basis. The demands on that single physical therapist or consultant to actively participate in all of the IEP meetings for the children they serve is extremely time intensive.

Perhaps the newest service delivery approach that has emerged over the last several years is the transdisciplinary approach. In this model, assessments may still be conducted in isolation by various team members, but the implementation of a child's educational program may be provided by only a few professionals.

This approach also emerged from a medically oriented service approach that was designed to serve infants in high risk, neonatal nurseries (Hutchinson, 1978). Since many of those children have diverse medical needs, the original purpose of this model was to decrease the number of different people who had contact with the child. This integrated service model reduced the risk for contamination to these fragile infants and increased the knowledge base and skills of primary service providers (nurses and parents). Thus, as Lyon and Lyon (1980) note, the transdisciplinary approach can be characterized as a joint team approach that promotes staff development and adds a new dimension to the team functioning—the concept of role release.

The notion of role release enables team members to share information among each other and can provide opportunities for cross-training in other discipline areas that might have been previously exclusive. For example, a physical therapist might train a regular classroom teacher how to address the physical needs (positioning, transferring, or handling) of a child with cerebral palsy who is mainstreamed into a regular seventh-grade science class.

Bricker (1976) characterizes teachers in this model as "educational synthesizers"—they assimilate assessment findings and recommendations and accomodate that information to the child's needs. With this added responsibility, teachers seek information and training from various support members, and then develop and implement those strategies in the classroom.

The greatest strength of this model is that it allows for greater team participation. This level of collaboration facilitates the development of a more accurate picture of the child's abilities and the subsequent formation of appropriate and functional goals and objectives. The least favorable component of this model is the amount of administrative energy that must be expended to allow team members to interact with and train each other.

Roles for Team Members

To meet the needs of students requiring special education services, a variety of related special education personnel may participate in the IEP process at the discretion of the parents or the local school district. The particular needs of each child will dictate the kinds of educational personnel that will need to be involved in the planning and implementation of an appropriate education plan. As mentioned earlier, some of these related personnel include physical and occupational therapists, adaptive physical education/recreation therapy specialists, social workers, speech/language pathologists, school psychologists/educational diagnosticians, vocational education teachers, job coaches, transition specialists, guidance counselors, reading specialists, paraprofessionals, and school administrators.

Each of these professionals adds their own expertise in such a way as to complement the activities and strengths of other team members. Yet, perhaps the most important team members are the child's parents. As previously discussed, parents have specific rights in the development of their child's IEP. Parents should be able to serve as equal partners on the team. This proactive approach toward parental involvement lays the foundation for building a strong partnership among all team members. Further, it assists parents (and often other family members) in developing a sense of ownership in the educational direction for their child. When parents sense that they are truly perceived as individuals with valid and useful information about the education of their child, they will be more likely to act in ways that professionals perceive as helpful and positive.

Of particular interest is the role the regular classroom teacher plays in the education of children who have mild disabilities. As noted earlier, a majority of the children who require special education services are mainstreamed into regular classes for at least a portion of the day. While the benefits of placing these children in classes with their peers strongly outweighs a segregationist argument (Stainback & Stainback, 1989), the success of this type of placement only occurs when the teacher prepares and mediates the learning environment and experiences so that children with mild disabilities can be successful.

Children who are provided with this type of placement often spend a majority of their day in the regular class and receive few, if any, direct special education services (Lewis &

Doorlag, 1987). The services that are provided are often through consultations between the special educator, related service personnel and the regular classroom teacher. Suggestions are made that may help the regular classroom teacher modify instructional strategies and alter the environment. This model of indirect services benefits students who have special needs, those who may not yet be identified (but who could benefit from special instruction), and the regular student.

Given the wide range of possible related special education personnel that may be needed to assist students achieve their maximum potential, consultation services may be provided in a variety of ways. For example, in the role of a consultant, the special educator may be able to suggest methods of insuring that the child with disabilities is provided with a number of teacher-mediated activities in the regular fourth-grade class that will increase the number of opportunities a child with disabilities has for meaningful interaction with their peers. A psychologist may be consulted to assist in the design of a behavior management program, and a special education teacher with expertise in the area of learning disabilities may be able to provide a number of strategies to help the regular classroom teacher adapt a reading program to fit a child's learning style.

An important (and often overlooked) member of the consultation model team is the regular classroom teacher. Input from these professionals is critical when designing a modification to an existing curricula that the regular classroom teacher is probably most familiar with. Additionally, the regular classroom teacher is the one team player who must maintain an accurate image of the "big picture" (i.e., the environment where the student with special needs will be expected to function as well as the peers that student will be interacting with on a day-to-day basis). Failure to engage the regular classroom teacher as a vital planner and implementer of special education services not only places a student's learning opportunities and potential at risk, but also jeopardizes harmonious team functioning.

Placement

One of the most critical decisions regarding the provision of appropriate services to children with disabilities is type of classroom placement(s) that is provided to the student. With the assumption that the regular classroom is perhaps the optimum placement option for children with mild disabilities, the regulations within Public Law 94–142 concerning this issue are fairly clear.

> . . . That special classes, separate schooling or other removal of handicapped children from the regular educational environment occurs only when the nature or severity of the handicap is such that the use of supplemental aids and services cannot be achieved satisfactorily (Federal Register, 1977b).

The implication (and actually, the mandate) here is that teachers will have attempted to modify the instruction and materials prior to referring a child for special education services. Yet, according to the findings of several authors, few substantial modifications are attempted prior to that initial referral (Strickland & Turnbull, 1990). Further, once a student is referred for an evaluation, it is highly likely that the student referred will be assessed (ninety-two percent) and finally enrolled in a special education program (seventy-three percent) (Algozzine, Christenson, & Ysseldyke, 1982).

Prereferral Activities

As suggested by its name, prereferral activities include a variety of strategies to modify both the teaching process and materials for children suspected of having a disability prior to a referral for special education services. Often referred to as prereferral intervention, this process is viewed as "an attempt to gain additional information to guide instruction in the regular classroom or to obtain compensatory education assistance within the regular program" (Strickland & Turnbull, 1990, p. 60). Yet, as mentioned earlier, few children are actually afforded the opportunity to demonstrate competence in the regular classroom when modifications are provided.

Strickland and Turnbull (1990) have identified several reasons why these prereferral activities often fail to take place. First, very few school districts have formal procedures for teachers to follow that enable them to modify instruction in the regular classroom. When those procedures do exist, it is often perfunctory in nature and is more likely used for documentation purposes rather than for substantive changes in curricular approaches.

Second, when policies and procedures are in place for teachers to make referrals, those policies often lack adequate criteria to make appropriate referral decisions or to assist the placement committee in making referral decisions or to assist the placement committee in making referrals that differentiate students in need of special education services and those who require remedial or second-language programs. The third reason that prereferral activities are often lacking in the standard protocol for many of today's public school children is the incorrect notion that special education services are the sole responsibility of the special education teacher. Often, the regular classroom teacher feels that he does not possess the specialized skills, resources, or time to address the academic needs of students in need of specialized instruction. For many children who have mild disabilities, the provisions contained in Public Law 94–142 for children with special learning needs were designed to avoid a separatist philosophy and to enhance the regular classroom environment and the activities therein so that those children could be maintained in the least restrictive environment.

In addition to meeting the mandates within Public Law 94–142, the use of a clearly defined and implemented prereferral program has a variety of positive benefits for students, teachers, and the educational system as a whole. When a functional array of prereferral activities are constructed, the first benefit many districts realize is that when referrals to special education are made, the nature of the information obtained during the prereferral phase is extremely helpful in determining the actual nature of the problem and usually results in more appropriate referrals.

Second, prereferral activities tend to result in programs that are often more cost-effective than programs that do not utilize prereferral intervention strategies (Affleck, Madge, Adams, & Lowenbraun, 1988). By combining existing resources within the school district many prereferral activities result in a decrease of resources that include time, personnel, and material costs that are typically involved in making referrals. Further, these activities tend to prevent fragmentation of services between regular education and special education services.

Figure 4–3 provides a suggested sequence of steps that are helpful to the regular classroom teacher in making appropriate referral-making decisions.

When teachers implement prereferral activities as suggested in Figure 4–3, the learning characteristics of the student in question are carefully considered and should result in either an individualized "regular classroom" placement or a sound base from which to refer

FIGURE 4-3 Suggested Sequence of Prereferral Activities/Intervention

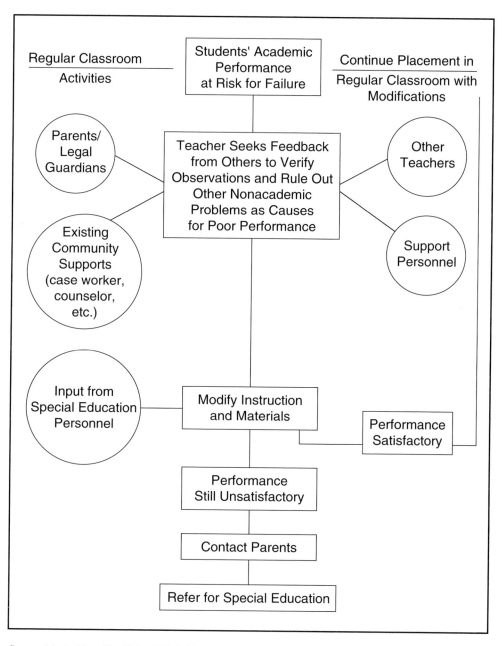

Source: Adapted from Ysseldyke, J. E. & Algozzine, B. (1990). *Introduction to special education,* 2nd Ed. Boston: Houghton Mifflin

the child for further testing. The use of a well-organized prereferral program also benefits other students in the class as well. Consider the accommodations suggested in Figure 4–4 for modifying instruction in the regular classroom. The skills a teacher gains by using some of those strategies may also be beneficial to other students who may not be experiencing significant difficulties but may demonstrate gains in their own educational competence.

After the teacher has followed a sequence of prereferral activities (gathered additional information about the student, modified the instruction and materials for the student), and the performance of that student is still unsatisfactory, then a referral for special education services should be made (see Figure 4–5 on page 118). Since the referral process for school districts can vary tremendously, be sure to include parents or legal guardians in the referral process. Failure to do so not only violates the rights of both students and parents, but can also create a less-than-favorable working situation among all parties. School personnel have sixty days from the date the referral is accepted by the Screening Committee until the Eligibility Determination Committee must make a placement decision.

As noted in Figure 4–5, the final decision to place a child in special education rests with the Eligibility Determination Committee (EDC). This committee can be the same as the Screening Committee. Parents have the right to appeal any decisions made by this committee as guaranteed by the Due Process regulations contained in Public Law 94–142.

Once the decision has been made to place a student in special education, a variety of placement options must be considered. The basic premise underpinning the placement decision is the notion of the Least Restrictive Environment (LRE). This concept insures that students with disabilities should have the optimal access to their chronological peers in an integrated setting. This concept "considers the student's educational needs in determining which of the placement alternatives facilitates (or least restricts) the student's opportunity for learning (Strickland & Turnbull, 1990, p. 20). Figure 4–6 (see page 119) provides an array, or "cascade," of the typical placement options available to students with disabilities. Note that placement options are ranked from least restrictive to most restrictive. Additionally, the width of each service option should correlate with the number of students who actually require that type of placement. Thus, a majority of students who have mild disabilities should probably be receiving services in the regular classroom with (or without) specialized services. When support services are provided to augment activities in the regular classroom it is often through the use of a resource room.

IMPLEMENTING INDIVIDUALIZED EDUCATION PROGRAMS

Writing IEPs

After the evaluation data have been analyzed and a decision to place a child in special education has been made, the next step is to design an appropriate intervention plan for all personnel involved in the education of the child. School personnel now have thirty days to design and implement the IEP.

The IEP has been described as a management tool that insures that the educational objectives are appropriate, and that those services are actually delivered and monitored (Torres, 1977). As such, teachers and related personnel should view the IEP document as a tool to be used in a proactive sense, to support the existing skills of the teacher rather than a rigid, inflexible form that negates creativity and spontaneity. It should be noted, however, that any changes to the IEP must be approved by the parents, local education

FIGURE 4-4 Prereferral Accommodations

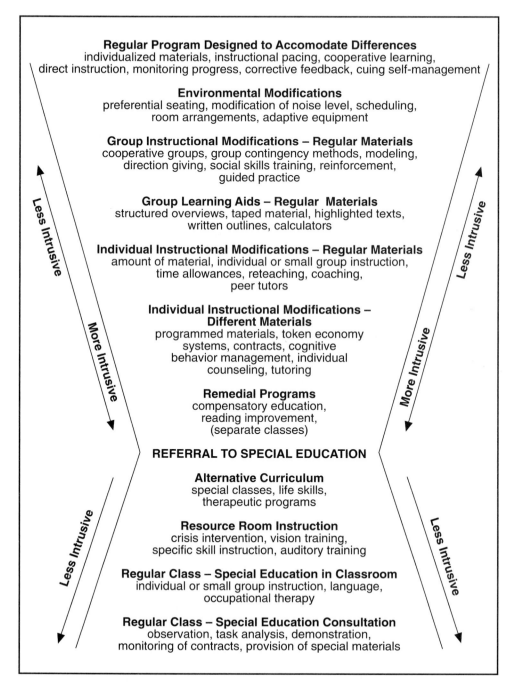

Regular Program Designed to Accomodate Differences
individualized materials, instructional pacing, cooperative learning,
direct instruction, monitoring progress, corrective feedback, cuing self-management

Environmental Modifications
preferential seating, modification of noise level, scheduling,
room arrangements, adaptive equipment

Group Instructional Modifications – Regular Materials
cooperative groups, group contingency methods, modeling,
direction giving, social skills training, reinforcement,
guided practice

Group Learning Aids – Regular Materials
structured overviews, taped material, highlighted texts,
written outlines, calculators

Individual Instructional Modifications – Regular Materials
amount of material, individual or small group instruction,
time allowances, reteaching, coaching,
peer tutors

**Individual Instructional Modifications –
Different Materials**
programmed materials, token economy
systems, contracts, cognitive
behavior management, individual
counseling, tutoring

Remedial Programs
compensatory education,
reading improvement,
(separate classes)

REFERRAL TO SPECIAL EDUCATION

Alternative Curriculum
special classes, life skills,
therapeutic programs

Resource Room Instruction
crisis intervention, vision training,
specific skill instruction, auditory training

Regular Class – Special Education in Classroom
individual or small group instruction, language,
occupational therapy

Regular Class – Special Education Consultation
observation, task analysis, demonstration,
monitoring of contracts, provision of special materials

Less Intrusive
More Intrusive
Less Intrusive

Source: Strickland, B. B., & Turnbull, A.P. (1990). *Developing and Implementing Individualized Education Programs,* 3rd Ed. Columbus, OH: Merrill, p. 69.

FIGURE 4-5 Steps in the Referral Process

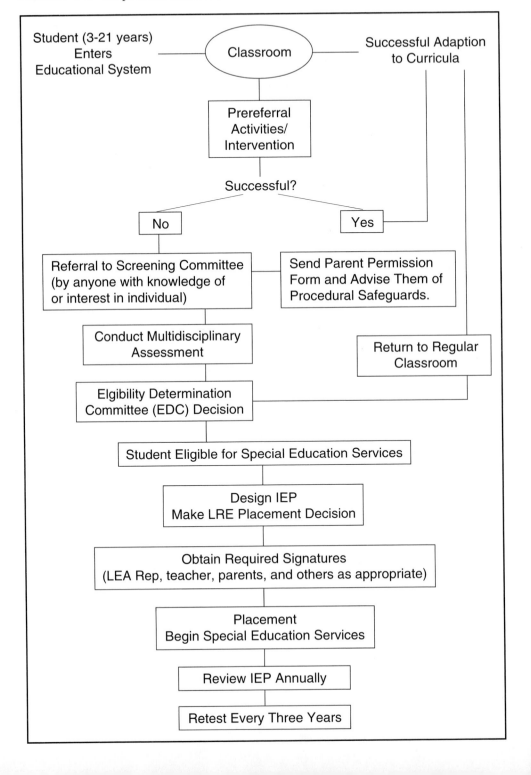

FIGURE 4-6 Placement Options along Continuum

Most Restrictive	Instruction in institution/hospital
	Instruction in home setting
	Instruction in special school apart from regular school building
	Instruction in special classroom in regular school building for the entire school day
	Instruction in resource room part of the school day
	Instruction in regular classroom with direct special assistance
	Instruction in regular classroom with indirect assistance
Least Restrictive	Instruction in regular classroom without any assistance except accommodations made by regular classroom teacher

agency (LEA) representative, the child's teacher, and other personnel affected by those changes. A sample IEP is provided in Figure 4–7 .

Time Lines for Developing IEPs

After it has been determined that a student has a disability and requires special education and related services, education personnel have thirty days from the date the Eligibility Determination Committee makes their decision to hold the initial IEP meeting (Federal Register, 1977b). Students should begin receiving the services immediately after that meeting. Certain exceptions have been made to that deadline. Some of those exceptions include situations when the IEP meeting is held during the summer months or while logistical arrangements (such as transportation) are being made.

INTERVENTION STRATEGIES

Realizing the complexity of developing an IEP, the driving thought in many teachers' minds is often, "What am I supposed to teach?" or "How am I supposed to teach this?" Perhaps the child presents a long list of educational needs and the teacher is not sure

FIGURE 4–7 Sample Individualized Education Program

—— YOURTOWN PUBLIC SCHOOLS ——
307 South Decatur Street
Yourtown, AL 36109
205-369-5110

INDIVIDUALIZED EDUCATION PROGRAM

NAME: _Johnny   Student_
BIRTHDATE: _9/23/79_ GRADE: _2_
SCHOOL YEAR: _1988-89_

EXCEPTIONALITY:
PRIMARY: _EMR_
SECONDARY: _SI_
IEP FROM: _12/14/88_ TO: _5/31/89_

PRESENT LEVEL OF PERFORMANCE SUMMARY

DATE	ASSESSMENT INSTRUMENT & SCORES	STRENGTHS	WEAKNESSES
11/30/88	KTEA: Mathematics - SS = 65 Reading - SS = 66 Battery Composite - SS = 66		Mathematics Applications and Computations Reading Decoding and Comprehension Spelling
11/4/88	Vineland: Age Equivalent = 4-4 SS = 64	Communication	Daily Living Skills Socialization
11/30/88	TOLD-I: SLQ = 72, LiQ = 62, SpQ = 72, SeQ = 80, SyQ = 61	Semantics	Syntax Listening

REGULAR CLASS PARTICIPATION (____ HOURS/WEEK)

Checks indicate regular services (REG), classroom modifications (MOD)
needed for regular class participation, and special education services (SPED).

	REG	MOD	SPED		REG	MOD	SPED		REG	MOD	SPED
READING			✓	LANGUAGE ARTS			✓	HEALTH	✓		
ENGLISH				SOCIAL STUDIES	✓	✓A		ART	✓		
SPELLING	✓	✓C		VOCATIONAL ED				HOMEROOM	✓		
MATH				HISTORY				LUNCH	✓		
LIBRARY	✓			SCIENCE	✓	✓A,C					
MUSIC	✓			PHYSICAL EDUC	✓						

MODIFICATION DESCRIPTIONS

A. Modify presentation   B. Modify environment   C. Modify time demands
D. Modify materials   E. Use of groups & peers   F. Use of teacher aide
G. _____

FIGURE 4-7 continued

YOURTOWN PUBLIC SCHOOLS
307 South Decatur Street
Yourtown, AL 36109
205-369-5110

MULTIDISCIPLINARY ELIGIBILITY REPORT

STUDENT _Johnny B. Student_ SCHOOL _Yourtown Elem._ DATE _12/5/88_

BIRTHDATE _9/23/79_ MEETING SITE _School Library_ TIME _3:05p.m._

REFERRAL DATE _10/11/88_ PERMISSION TO TEST/ "STUDENT RIGHTS" DATE _10/18/88_

AREA	DATE	ASSESSMENT INSTRUMENT, SCORES AND RESULTS
VISION	10/24/88	Snellen Chart, Telebinocular passed screening; wears glasses
HEARING	10/24/88	Puretone Audiometry / Tympanometry passed screening
INTELLIGENCE	11/29/88	Wechsler Intelligence Scale for Children – Revised Verbal = 65, Performance = 65, Full Scale = 62
COGNITION		
BEHAVIOR		
ADAPTIVE BEHAVIOR	11/4/88	Vineland Adaptive Behavior Scale – Classroom Edition Age Equivalent = 4-4, SS = 64
FINE MOTOR		
GROSS MOTOR		

FIGURE 4–7 continued

Yourtown City Schools
Individualized Education Program   page _____

The student will have the opportunity to participate as appropriate
in nonacademic and extra-curricular activities unless the IEP states
otherwise.

TYPE OF DIPLOMA: ☐ Regular   ☐ Advanced   ☐ Graduation Certificate

TRANSITION GOAL (By End of Ninth Grade or Age Fifteen)

___ *Not Applicable* _____

_____

_____

RELATED SERVICES		
SERVICE	HR/WK	PERSON(S) RESPONSIBLE
NONE		

SPEECH/LANGUAGE SERVICES   *1½*   HR/WK

TRANSPORTATION: ☒ Regular   ☐ Special

FIGURE 4-7 continued

Yourtown City Schools
Individualized Education Program   page _____

STUDENT NAME: _Johnny_ _Student_ SCHOOL YEAR: _1988-89_
AREA: _Reading_

Goals and objectives developed to move student to a less restrictive environment.	TYPE OF EVALUATION	PROJECTED CHECK DATE	DATE/DEGREE OF MASTERY
ANNUAL GOAL: _Johnny will improve decoding skills in reading._			
OBJECTIVE: _Using a listening station, Johnny will correctly decode 15 to 20 selected words within a 15_	_Student Worksheet_	_3/89_	_____
OBJECTIVE: _minute session._	_____	_____	_____
OBJECTIVE:	_____	_____	_____
OBJECTIVE:	_____	_____	_____

AREA: _Math_

Goals and objectives developed to move student to a less restrictive environment.	TYPE OF EVALUATION	PROJECTED CHECK DATE	DATE/DEGREE OF MASTERY
ANNUAL GOAL: _Johnny will improve math application skills._			
OBJECTIVE: _Using a computer software program calendar skills, Johnny will recognize the days of the week_	_Key Math_	_1/89_	_____
OBJECTIVE: _with 100% accuracy._	_____	_____	_____
OBJECTIVE:	_____	_____	_____
OBJECTIVE:	_____	_____	_____

FIGURE 4–7 continued

Yourtown City Schools
Individualized Education Program   page _____

STUDENT NAME: _Johnny_ _____ _Student_ ____ SCHOOL YEAR: _1988-89_

AREA: _Speech / Language_ _____

Goals and objectives developed to move student to a less restrictive environment.	TYPE OF EVALUATION	PROJECTED CHECK DATE	DATE/DEGREE OF MASTERY

ANNUAL GOAL: _Johnny will improve processing and production of selected syntactical structures._

OBJECTIVE: _Johnny will describe pictures or actions representing the targeted syntactical structures (subject/_

OBJECTIVE: _verb agreement, irregular plurals/ verb agreement) with 90% accuracy._

OBJECTIVE:			

SLP Tally — 4/89

OBJECTIVE: _____

OBJECTIVE: _____

AREA: _____

Goals and objectives developed to move student to a less restrictive environment.	TYPE OF EVALUATION	PROJECTED CHECK DATE	DATE/DEGREE OF MASTERY

ANNUAL GOAL: _____

OBJECTIVE: _____

OBJECTIVE: _____

OBJECTIVE: _____

OBJECTIVE: _____

FIGURE 4-7 continued

Yourtown City Schools
Individualized Education Program   page _____

STUDENT NAME: *Johnny*   *Student*   SCHOOL YEAR: *1988-89*
AREA: *Language Arts*

Goals and objectives developed to move student   TYPE OF   PROJECTED   DATE/DEGREE
to a less restrictive environment.   EVALUATION   CHECK DATE   OF MASTERY

ANNUAL GOAL: *Johnny will improve his*
punctuation skills.

OBJECTIVE: *When given a written assignment,*   *Teacher*   *2/89*   _____
Johnny will use a period at the   *made*
end of a statement and a question   *test*

OBJECTIVE: *mark where appropriate with*   _____   _____   _____
80% accuracy.

OBJECTIVE: _____   _____   _____   _____
_____
_____

OBJECTIVE: _____   _____   _____   _____
_____
_____

AREA: *Adaptive Behavior*

Goals and objectives developed to move student   TYPE OF   PROJECTED   DATE/DEGREE
to a less restrictive environment.   EVALUATION   CHECK DATE   OF MASTERY

ANNUAL GOAL: *Johnny will know and follow*
school rules.

OBJECTIVE: *Johnny will demonstrate*   *Teacher-*   *3/89*   _____
knowledge of defined classroom   *made*
rules by complying with these   *Progress Chart*

OBJECTIVE: *rules during class time 80%*   _____   _____   _____
of the time.

OBJECTIVE: _____   _____   _____   _____
_____
_____

OBJECTIVE: _____   _____   _____   _____
_____
_____

FIGURE 4-7 continued

Yourtown City Schools
Individualized Education Program   page _____

LEAST RESTRICTIVE ENVIRONMENT

Check the environment determined by the IEP committee:

☐ Regular Class   ☐ Sp. Ed./Part-Time Reg. Cl.   ☐ Public Residential
☐ Indirect Service   ☐ Self-Contained Sp. Ed. Cl.   ☐ Private Residential
☐ Direct Service   ☐ Public Day School   ☐ Homebound
☑ Resource Room   ☐ Private Day School   ☐ Hospital

A less restrictive placement was not selected for the following reasons:

In order to be successful in math and reading, Johnny Student requires a differentiated cirriculum, one-to-one instruction, and fewer distractions.

The following persons attended and participated in the development of this IEP on
_____.

IEP COMMITTEE MEMBERS
SIGNATURE   POSITION

Tom Student, Sr.   _____ PARENT _____
Peter Paddler   _____ LEA REP Principal
Susie Special   Sp. Ed. TEACHER _____
Jane Teacher   Second grade teacher
Tonya Talker   Speech/Language Pathologist

_____   _____
_____   _____
_____   _____
_____   _____

FIGURE 4-7 continued

Yourtown City Schools
Individualized Education Program   page _____

MODIFICATIONS FOR REGULAR CLASSES

Name: _Johnny_____ _Student_____ School Year: _1988-89_

It is necessary that modifications be made in your classroom for students because P.L. 94-142 provides that "...all handicapped students, including those in public or private institutions or other care facilities, are educated with children who are not handicapped, and that special classes, separate schooling, or other removal of handicapped children from the regular education environment occurs only when the nature or severity of the handicap is such that an education in regular classes with the use of supplementary aids and services cannot be achieved satisfactorily." 1300.550(b)(2)1

DIRECTIONS: Check ☑ each modification made.

Name of Course	Regular Teacher
1 _Spelling_	_Jane Teacher_
2 _Social Studies_	_Jane Teacher_
3 _Science_	_Mary Smith_

COURSES

1 2 3   **A. Modifying the presentation of the Material**

☐ ☐ ☐   1. Break assignment into segments of shorter tasks.

☐ ☐ ☐   2. When content mastery is questionable, investigate the use of concrete concepts BEFORE teaching abstract.

☐ ☑ ☑   3. Relate information to student's experiential base.

☐ ☐ ☐   4. Reduce the number of concepts introduced at any one time.

☐ ☐ ☐   5. Provide student with an overview of the lesson BEFORE beginning the lesson. (Tell student what student should expect to learn and why.)

☐ ☐ ☑   6. Monitor the level of language you use to communicate ideas. (Are you using vocabulary and complex sentence structures that are too advanced?)

☐ ☐ ☐   7. Schedule frequent, short conferences with student to check for comprehension.

☐ ☐ ☐   8. Provide consistent review of any lesson BEFORE introducing new information.

☐ ☐ ☐   9. Allow student to obtain and report information utilizing:
     ☐ cassette/tape recorders ☐ films   ☐ typewriters
     ☐ computers   ☐ dictation   ☐ calculators
     ☐ projects   ☐ interviews/oral reports

☐ ☑ ☐ 10. Highlight important concepts to be learned in text or material (color code key points; outline; study guides).

☐ ☐ ☐ 11. Space practice and drill sessions over time.

☐ ☐ ☐ 12. Monitor the rate in which you present material. (Do you talk too fast or give too much material at one time?)

☐ ☐ ☐ 13. Give additional presentations.
☐ ☐ ☐   a. Repeat original presentation.
☐ ☐ ☑   b. Provide simpler, more complete explanation.
☐ ☐ ☐   c. Give additional examples.
☐ ☐ ☐   d. Model skills in several ways.

☐ ☐ ☐ 14. Provide additional guided practice.
☐ ☐ ☐   a. Require more responses.
☐ ☐ ☐   b. Lengthen practice sessions.
☐ ☐ ☐   c. Schedule extra practice sessions.

FIGURE 4-7 continued

Yourtown City Schools
Individualized Education Program   page _____

1   2   3
☐ ☐ ☐   15. Make consequences more attractive.
☐ ☐ ☐   a. Increase feedback.
☐ ☐ ☐   b. Provide knowledge of results.
☐ ☐ ☐   c. Chart performance.
☐ ☐ ☐   d. Reward approximations.
☐ ☐ ☐   e. Give incentives to begin and to complete.
☐ ☑ ☐   16. Recognize and give credit for student's oral participation in class.
☐ ☐ ☐   17. Make arrangements for homework assignments to reach home with
                  clear, concise directions.
☐ ☐ ☐   18. Assign tasks at the appropriate level (lower reading/difficulty level).
☐ ☐ ☐   19. Give tests orally.
☐ ☐ ☐   20. Other: _____
☐ ☐ ☐   21. Other: _____

1   2   3   **B. Modifying the Environment**
☐ ☐ ☐   1. Use study carrels.
☐ ☐ ☐   2. Use proximity seating.
☐ ☐ ☐   3. Seat student in area free from distractions.
☐ ☐ ☐   4. Let student select the place which is best for student to study.
☐ ☐ ☐   5. Help keep student's space free of unnecessary materials.
☐ ☐ ☐   6. Use checklists to help student get organized.
☑ ☐ ☐   7. Use notebook for organized assignments, materials, and homework.
☐ ☐ ☐   8. Provide opportunities for movement.
☐ ☐ ☐   9. Other: _____
☐ ☐ ☐   10. Other: _____

1   2   3   **C. Modifying Time Demands**
☑ ☐ ☑   1. Increase amount of time allowed to complete assignments/tests.
                  (Contract with student concerning time allotment.)
☑ ☐ ☑   2. Reduce amount of work or length of tests (as opposed to allowing
                  more time).
☐ ☐ ☐   3. Teach time management skills (use of checklists, prioritizing time,
                  prioritizing assignments).
☐ ☐ ☐   4. Space short work periods with breaks or change of task.
☐ ☐ ☐   5. Set up a specific routine and stick with it.
☐ ☐ ☐   6. Alternate quiet and active time (short periods of each).
☐ ☐ ☑   7. Give student a specific task to perform within specific time limits.
☐ ☐ ☐   8. Other: _____
☐ ☐ ☐   9. Other: _____

            D. Modifying the Environment
1   2   3   1. Visual Motor Integration
☐ ☐ ☐   a. Avoid large amounts of written work (both in class and homework).
☐ ☐ ☐   b. Encourage student to select the method of writing which is most
                  comfortable (cursive or manuscript).
☐ ☐ ☐   c. Set realistic and mutually agreed upon expectations for neatness.
☐ ☐ ☐   d. Let student type, record, or give answers orally instead of writing.

FIGURE 4-7 continued

Yourtown City Schools
Individualized Education Program   page _____

1   2   3
☐ ☐ ☐   e. Avoid pressures of speed and accuracy.
☐ ☐ ☐   f. Provide student with carbon copy of lecture notes produced by
             teacher or peer.
☐ ☐ ☐   g. Reduce amounts of boardwork copying and textbook copying;
             provide student with written information.
☐ ☐ ☐   h. Other: _____
☐ ☐ ☐   i. Other: _____

1   2   3   2. Visual Processing
☐ ☐ ☐   a. Highlight information to be learned (color coding, underlining, etc.).
☐ ☐ ☐   b. Keep written assignments and work space free from extraneous/
             irrelevant distractors.
☐ ☐ ☐   c. Avoid purple dittos.
☐ ☐ ☐   d. Worksheets should be clear and well-defined.
☐ ☐ ☐   e. Go over visual task with student and make sure student has a clear
             understanding of all parts of the assignment BEFORE beginning.
☐ ☐ ☐   f. Avoid having student copy from the board. (Provide student with a
             written copy of the material. May copy teacher's manual or lecture
             notes.)
☐ ☐ ☐   g. Other: _____
☐ ☐ ☐   h. Other: _____

1   2   3   3. Language Processing
☐ ☐ ☐   a. Give written directions to supplement verbal directions.
☐ ☐ ☐   b. Slow the rate of presentation.
☐ ☐ ☐   c. Paraphrase material using similar language.
☐ ☐ ☐   d. Keep statements short and to the point.
☐ ☐ ☐   e. Avoid use of abstract language (metaphors, idioms, puns, etc.)
☐ ☐ ☐   f. Keep sentence structures simple; gradually introduce more complex
             sentences as student masters the ability to comprehend them.
☐ ☐ ☐   g. Encourage feedback from student to check for understanding. (Have
             student restate what you have said in student's own words.)
☐ ☐ ☐   h. Familiarize student with any new vocabulary BEFORE the lesson.
             (Make sure student can use this vocabulary not just recognize it.)
☐ ☐ ☐   i. Reduce amount of extraneous noise such as conversations, TV,
             radio, noises from outside, etc.
☐ ☐ ☐   j. Alert student's attention to key points with such phrases as, "This is
             important. Listen carefully."
☐ ☐ ☐   k. Ensure the readability levels of the textbooks used in class are
             commensurate with student's language level.
☐ ☐ ☐   l. Utilize visual aids to supplement verbal information. (Charts,
             graphics, pictures, etc., can be used to illustrate written and spoken
             information.)
☐ ☐ ☐   m.Utilize manipulative, hands-on activities whenever possible;
             establish the concrete experience base BEFORE teaching more
             abstract concepts.

FIGURE 4-7 continued

Yourtown City Schools
Individualized Education Program   page _____

1 2 3
☐ ☐ ☐   n. ALWAYS demonstrate to student how the new material relates to
            material student has previously learned.
☐ ☐ ☐   o. Other: _____
☐ ☐ ☐   p. Other: _____

1 2 3   4. Organizational
☐ ☐ ☐   a. Establish a daily routine and attempt to maintain it.
☐ ☐ ☐   b. Make clear rules and be consistent enforcing them.
☐ ☐ ☐   c. Contract with student, using a reward for completion of the contract.
☐ ☐ ☐   d. Provide notebook with organized sections such as:
                ☐ assignments due   ☐ calendar   ☐ homework
                ☐ time management schedules ☐ prioritized to-do lists
                ☐ study guides   ☐ class notes
☐ ☐ ☐   e. Avoid cluttered, crowded worksheets by utilizing techniques such as:
                blocking - block assignments into smaller segments.
                cutting - cut worksheets and give segments to students, segment by
                   segment.
                folding - fold worksheets into fourths, sixths, or eighths and place one
                   problem in each square.
                color coding, highlighting, or underlining - important information on which
                   student needs to focus.
☐ ☐ ☐   f. Hand out written assignments with expected dates of completion
            typed or written on one corner.
☐ ☐ ☐   g. To prevent misplaced assignments, provide student with file folders,
            notebooks or trays in which he can immediately place his work.
☐ ☐ ☐   h. Set aside a specific time for cleaning desks, lockers, organizing note-
            books, etc.
☐ ☐ ☐   i. Teach goal-setting skills.
☐ ☐ ☐   j. Teach decision-making/prioritizing skills.
☐ ☐ ☐   k. Teach time management skills.
☐ ☐ ☐   l. Other: _____
☐ ☐ ☐   m. Other: _____

1 2 3   **E. Use of Groups and Peers**
☐ ☐ ☐   1. Utilize cooperative learning strategies when appropriate.
☐ ☐ ☐   2. Assign a peer helper to:
☐ ☐ ☐   a. Check understanding of directions.
☐ ☐ ☐   b. Read important directions and essential material.
☐ ☐ ☐   c. Take carbon copies of lecture notes.
☐ ☐ ☐   d. Drill work.
☐ ☐ ☐   e. Summarize important textbook passages (on tape or in person).
☐ ☐ ☐   f. Record material dictated by student.
☐ ☐ ☐   g. Model appropriate responses.
☐ ☐ ☐   3. Other: _____
☐ ☐ ☐   4. Other: _____

FIGURE 4–7 continued

Yourtown City Schools
Individualized Education Program   page _____

1 2 3   **F. Use of Teacher Aide**
☐ ☐ ☐   1. _____
☐ ☐ ☐   2. _____
☐ ☐ ☐   3. _____
☐ ☐ ☐   4. _____
☐ ☐ ☐   5. _____

1 2 3   **G. Other (Specify)**
☐ ☐ ☐   1. Other: _____
☐ ☐ ☐   2. Other: _____
☐ ☐ ☐   3. Other: _____
☐ ☐ ☐   4. Other: _____
☐ ☐ ☐   5. Other: _____
☐ ☐ ☐   6. Other: _____
☐ ☐ ☐   7. Other: _____
☐ ☐ ☐   8. Other: _____
☐ ☐ ☐   9. Other: _____
☐ ☐ ☐ 10. Other: _____

Source: Alabama State Department of Education (1988). *Mastering the maze: The special education process.* Montgomery, AL: Program for Exceptional Children and Youth.

where to begin. On the other hand, a classroom teacher may have felt somewhat successful over the last ten years in her ability to teach basic sight words. And yet, Wayne, a student with a reading disability, is not progressing the way she had hoped he would. "Where do I begin?," she might ask. Figure 4–8 presents a variety of learning principles that may also facilitate learning and the motivation to learn. Those strategies have been found to be most helpful in assisting all students (with and without disabilities) achieve academic success. Those strategies are based on established and successful teaching practices and are rela-

FIGURE 4–8 Learning Principles

Factor	Principle
Appropriate Practice	A student is more likely to learn and retain that information if they have multiple opportunities to practice that skill in an appropriate setting with appropriate materials.
Distributing Practice	A student is more likely to learn if teaching is provided in short intervals.
Fading	A student is more likely to learn if physical and verbal supports/prompts are gradually removed.
Functional	A student will be able to learn more efficiently if objectives relate to real needs and wants.
Meaningfulness	A student is more likely to learn if learning tasks are meaningful to him or her.
Modeling	A student is more likely to learn if provided with a model of the expected outcome so that he or she can watch and then imitate.
Novelty	A student is more likely to learn if materials are novel or, in other ways, stimulate his or her interest.
Open Communication	A student is more likely to learn if comfortable with the lines of communication between him/herself and the instructor.
Pleasant Environment	A student is more likely to learn if the environment is pleasant and comfortable.
Prerequisites	A student is more likely to learn something new if he or she has mastered prerequisite skills.

tively simple to incorporate into all teaching/learning situations. Other chapters in this text will be helpful in teaching specific skills (math, reading, language arts, and so forth). Yet, there are three concepts that are common to all successful teaching approaches, regardless of the content. These concepts are involvement, generalization, and specificity.

Involvement

The first step is to involve the family and student (where applicable) in developing appropriate goals and intervention strategies. An IEP is not a document that is developed by "the professionals" that is then signed by parents. Parents may be helpful in identifying the concepts the student is most interested in learning and may be able to prioritize the tasks to be taught.

Generalization

Related to the idea of involvement is another component that will increase your likelihood of successful teaching—the concept of generalization. According to Haring (1985), skill generalization is when the student is able to respond appropriately in the absence of programmed training procedures. In much the same way that we act or perform differently in various situations (at work versus home versus church), students may be able to identify the word *restaurant* when it is printed in boldface, block letters on a flash card, but may not be able to find the word when it is printed in a different fashion in a phone book or on a marquee in a shopping mall. Skills that are attempted to be taught in isolation from other individuals or in contrived settings, often result in failure.

Consider the case of Chris, a seventeen-year-old student at Monmouth High, who has a specific learning disability in the area of mathematical calculations. A goal on his IEP states that Chris will be able balance his checkbook within $.05 on a monthly basis when provided with a bank statement, a check register, and a calculator. While Chris' teacher provides him with appropriate, commercially available materials and practice, Chris may never realize the importance of being able to balance his checkbook if Mom is always there to double check his "homework" and does not allow him to open a checking account in a real bank prior to graduation. It will be a sad awakening after Chris is graduated from high school, only to realize that he cannot deal with a basic skill required of independent living.

When students who have mild disabilities graduate from school (or otherwise leave) they are often living and working in the real world independently often with families of their own. If we truly believe that the mainstream of society is their ultimate environment, then we should provide multiple opportunities for them to practice their IEP objectives in the mainstream while we are still there to mediate when they err and celebrate when they succeed.

Specificity

Once you have determined what to teach, the next step is to develop the means to present it to the student and evaluate the success of your efforts. Behavioral objectives are written to guide instructional efforts and to insure consistency. Behavioral objectives are observable and measurable. That is you should be able to see what the student does and be able to measure it in some way. The simplest way to develop behavioral objectives is to ask yourself four questions:

...WHO is to perform the task?

...WHAT do you want them to do? (the outcome you expect)

...WHEN do you want them to do it? (remember generalization!)

and

...HOW WELL do you want them to do it?

For example:

...Willie

...will be able to recite his name and phone number

...when asked by his teacher and the school crossing guard

...with 100 percent accuracy

The accuracy to which a student completes a given objective is determined by the consequence of failure. Being able to name five colors, or tie shoelaces with minimal physical assistance is not as critical as, say, the ability to cross the street or dial 911 in an emergency. For other examples of IEP goals and objectives, see the sample IEP provided in Figure 4–7.

MATERIALS SELECTION

An important part of teaching is the materials that are selected for students to use. Depending on your particular classroom arrangement and the availability of funds, the materials selected to teach targeted goals and objectives can make the difference between an activity that children perform in a rote fashion or one that actively engages both the student and the teacher. The list of questions provided in Figure 4–9 will help you make a better decision when selecting materials. Making decision in this fashion initially takes time. However, when you systematically review materials according to the needs of your students, these questions should become second nature.

EVALUATION

In order to demonstrate that special education does make a difference, it is imperative that members of the special education team participate in a thorough evaluation of the teaching/learning process on an annual basis. This step is critical for several reasons. The most

FIGURE 4–9 Questions to Ask When Selecting Materials

- Cost?
- Are the materials on the students' level (chronological, developmental)?
- Is it consumable? How often will it (or parts) need to be replaced?
- In this computer age . . . how about parts? (availability and service)
- Is it durable?
- Are the materials colorful and attractive?
- Would your students enjoy using it?
- Are the materials consistent with your program theory/model?
- Do you need training to use it?
- Are the materials functional in nature? (Are you buying plastic fruit to teach nutritional concepts?)
- Can it be used for a variety of tasks or is its use limited to a few applications?
- Are the materials similar to products in the real world?

important reason is to verify that the student did, in fact, benefit from special education. Further, evaluating individualized education programs are essential to school district compliance with Public Law 94–142 and Public Law 99–457 and to the improvement of the delivery of special education services. This component of the IEP process can also provide a method for determining whether or not the expenditure of time, resources, and money were well spent. This process is often headed by the special education supervisor or a designated supervisor. When team members review the IEP and student performance characteristics, Smith, Price, and Marsh (1983) suggest that the following outcomes may be warranted:

- revise stated objectives;

- alter the service delivery process;

- change or modify personnel responsible for services;

- modify the roles that team members play in the students' program;

- alter the instructional procedures used; or

- terminate services (p. 148).

When team members are able to demonstrate positive gains for students in special education, there is another important, yet perhaps more subtle benefit—they made a difference. When special educators are asked why they chose their given profession, a common answer is, "because I wanted to help children who were disabled." The day-to-day professional life of a special educator is often richly rewarding and many parents are grateful for just about anything that is provided to their child.

While these reinforcers can be powerful, they often fail to sustain over the long run. Many teachers actually leave the profession. Bardo (1979) notes that salaries, benefits, and security in teaching is improving. However, as Walsh (1979) has found, teacher burnout is not uncommon and can lead to high absenteeism, alcohol abuse, and, ultimately, leaving the profession. Perhaps teachers leave the profession because they have not be able to see either the benefits of their efforts or ways to improve those efforts.

When school districts insure that IEPs are evaluated systematically, not only do they meet the minimum requirements of federal law, there are also benefits to the student, parents, special educators, and related personnel. In this context, teachers are able to see that their efforts to teach children with special needs have been successful. In those situations where the teaching was not successful, an effective evaluation process will enable team members to identify problems and perhaps indicate areas where the program can be improved to the benefit of both the student and teacher.

SUMMARY

Chapter four focused on how students with mild disabilities are taught. The primary organization of the chapter was around the assessment/IEP process. The introductory section of the chapter included a definition of the instructional process, as well as a brief description of early instructional efforts for students with mild disabilities. Components required by Public Law 94–142 that related to instruction were described. These included inclusion, nondiscrimination, individualized education program, least restrictive environment, procedural safeguards, and parental participation.

The next section of the chapter discussed the IEP process. The differences between using the IEP as a product and as a process were presented, along with a strong rationale to view the IEP as a process for instructional purposes. Developing the numerous components included in the instructional process was the next major section of the chapter. Specific steps, beginning with child find activities and culminating with IEP development and implementation were presented. Specific intervention strategies were also discussed in the chapter. This section not only included teaching techniques, but how to select and use various instructional materials.

REFERENCES

Algozzine, B., Christenson, S., & Ysseldyke, J. (1982). Probabilities associated with the referral to placement process. *Teacher Education and Special Education, 5,* 19–23.

Aramburo, D. J. (1989). Cultural pluralism—The numbers are still growing. *Exceptional Times.* Premier Edition. Reston, VA: Council for Exceptional Children.

Affleck, J.Q., Madge, S., Adams, A., & Lowenbraun, S. (1988). Integrated classroom versus resource model: Academic viability and effectiveness. *Exceptional Children, 54,* 339–348.

Alter, M., & Goldstein, M.T. (1986). The "6-S" paradigm: A tool for IEP implementation. *Teaching Exceptional Children, 18*(2), 135–138.

Banks, J.A. (1977). *Multiethnic education: Practices and promises* (Phi Delta Kappa, Fastback No. 87). Bloomington, IN: Phi Delta Kappa Educational Foundation.

Bardo, P. (1979). The pain of teacher burnout: A case history. *Phi Delta Kappan, 64*(4), 252–253. In T.E.C. Smith (Ed.), *Introduction to education,* 1990, St. Paul, MN: West.

Bricker, D. (1976). Educational synthesizer. In M.A. Thomas (Ed.) *Hey, don't forget about me! Education's investment in the severely, profoundly, and multiply handicapped.* Reston, VA: Council for Exceptional Children.

Data Research, Inc. (1990). *Handicapped students and special education,* Rosemount, MN: Author.

Cartwright, G.P., Cartwright, C.A., & Ward, M.E. (1981). *Educating special learners.* Belmont, CA: Wadsworth Publishing.

Federal Register. (1977a). *41,* Washington, D.C.: U.S. Government Printing Office, p. 5692.

Federal Register. (1977b). *42,* Washington, D.C.: U.S. Government Printing Office, pp. 42474–42515.

Garcia, R.L. (1978). *Fostering a pluralistic society through multi-ethnic education* (Phi Delta Kappa Fastback No. 107). Bloomington, IN: Phi Delta Kappa Educational Foundation.

Gress, J.R., & Carroll, M.E. (1985). Parent-professional partnership—and the IEP. *Academic Therapy, 20*(40), 443–449.

Haring, N. (1985). *Investigating the problem of skill generalization,* 3rd Ed. Seattle: Washington Research Organization.

Haring, N. (1990). Overview of special education. In N.G. Haring & L. McCormick (Eds.), *Exceptional Children and Youth,* 5th Ed. 2–43. Columbus, OH: Merrill.

Helge, D. (Ed.) (1984). The state of the art of rural special education. *Exceptional Children, 50,* (4).

Hutchinson, D. J. (1978). The transdisciplinary approach. In J.B. Curry & K.K. Peppe (Eds.), *Mental Retardation: Nursing approaches to care.* pp. 87–102. St Louis, MO: C.V. Mosby Co.

Jenkins, M.W. (1987). Effect of a computerized individual education plan (IEP) writer on time savings and quality. *Journal of Special Education Technology, 8*(3), 55–66.

Lane, H. (1976). *The wild boy of Averyon.* Cambridge, MA: Harvard University Press.

Lewis, R.B., & Doorlag, D.H. (1987). The mainstreaming team. In R.B. Lewis & D.H. Doorlag, *Teaching special students in the mainstream,* 2nd Ed. (pp. 19–39). Columbus, OH: Merrill.

Lilly, M.S. (1970). Special education: A tempest in a teapot. *Exceptional Children, 37,* 43–49.

Lyon, S., & Lyon, G. (1980). Team functioning and staff development: A role release approach to providing integrated educational services for severely handicapped students. *Journal of the Association for the Severely Handicapped, 3*(3), 250–256.

Maher, C.A. (1983). Development and implementation of effective individual education programs (IEPs): Evaluation of tow team approaches. *Journal of School Psychology, 21*(2), 143–152.

Maher, C.A. (1984). An approach to implementing IEP evaluation in the public Schools. *School Psychology Review, 13*(4), 519–525.

Marsh, G.E., II, & Price, B.J. (1980). *Methods for teaching the mildly handicapped adolescent.* St. Louis, MO: C.V. Mosby.

Marsh, G.E., II, Price, B.J., & Smith, T.E.C. (1983). *Teaching mildly handicapped children: Materials and methods.* St. Louis, MO: C.V. Mosby.

Mercer, J.R. (1976). Pluralistic diagnosis in the evaluation of Black and Chicano children: A procedure for taking sociocultural variables into account in clinical assessment. In C.A. Hernandez, M. J. Haug, & N.N. Wagner (Eds.), *Chicanos: Social and psychological perspectives* (2nd Ed.), (pp. 183–195). St. Louis: Mosby.

Mercer, J.R., & Lewis, J.F. (1978). *System of multicultural pluralistic assessment.* San Antonio, TX: The Psychological Corp.

Meyen, E.L. (1988). A commentary on special education. In E.L. Meyen & T.M. Skrtic (Eds.), *Exceptional children and youth.* Denver: Love.

Podemski, R.S., Price, B. J., Smith, T.E.C., & Marsh, G.E. II. (1984). *Comprehensive administration of special education.* pp. 1–48, Rockville, MD: Aspen.

Public Law 94–142. The Education of All Handicapped Children Act, 20 USC 1401; 34 Part 300.

Public Law 99–457. The Amendments to the Education of the Handicapped Act of 1986, Section 619, Parts B & H.

Ryan, L.B., & Rucker, C.N. (1986). Computerized *v.* noncomputerized individual education programs: Teachers' attitudes, time, and cost. *Journal of Special Education Technology, 8*(1), 5–12.

Slavia, J., & Ysseldyke, J.E. (1988). *Assessment in special and remedial education,* 4th Ed. Boston: Houghton Mifflin.

Sattler, J.M. (1988). Assessment of ethnic minority children. In J.M. Sattler, *Assessment of children,* 3rd Ed. (pp. 563–596). San Diego: Sattler.

Smith, T.E.C. (1990). *Introduction to education.* St. Paul, MN: West.

Smith, T.E.C., Price, B. J., & Marsh, G.E. (1986). *Mildly handicapped children and adults.* St. Paul: West.

Stainback, S.B. & Stainback, W.C. (1989). Classroom organization for diversity among students. *National Social Studies of Education Yearbook,* Part II, *88*, 195–207.

Strickland, B.B. & Turnbull, A.P. (1990). *Developing and implementing individual education programs,* 3rd Ed. Columbus, OH: Merrill.

Torres, S. (Ed.) (1977). *A primer on individualized education programs for handicapped children.* Reston, VA: The Foundation for Exceptional Children.

U.S. Department of Education (1981). *Assistance to states for educating handicapped children: Interpretation of the individualized education program (IEP).* Washington, D.C.: U.S. Government Printing Office.

U.S. Department of Education (1990). Definition Amendments to Public Law 94–142.

Walsh, D. (1979). Classroom stress and teacher burnout. *Phi Delta Kappan, 61*(4), 252. In T.E.C. Smith, *Introduction to education*, 1990, St. Paul, MN: West.

Wood, J.W. (1984). *Adapting instruction for the mainstream.* Columbus, OH: Merrill.

Ysseldyke, J.E., & Algozzine, B. (1990). *Introduction to special education*, 2nd Ed. Boston: Houghton Mifflin Co.

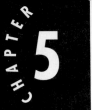

Receptive Language: Teaching Reading and Listening Skills

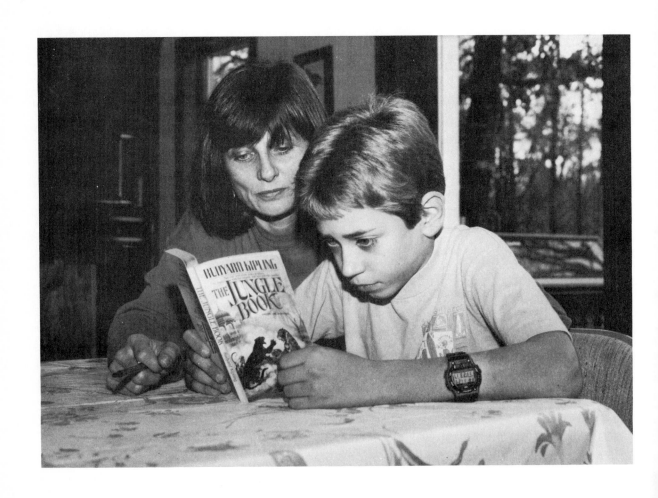

Outline

OBJECTIVES

After reading this chapter, you will be able to:

- discuss the importance and status of reading in our society;

- define reading;

- describe the five generalizations about reading;

- discuss reading problems and students with disabilities;

- describe the major approaches to teaching reading;

- describe the major remedial reading approaches;

- define listening;

- describe how to assess listening skills;

- discuss approaches to teach listening skills.

Introduction

Receptive language skills are critical for individuals to effectively communicate and learn. Indeed, being able to listen and understand what someone is saying and to read and comprehend printed materials helps set humans apart from other animal species. Some individuals have deficits in receptive language and find themselves at a major disadvantage in our language-dependent society. Without the ability to receive information in oral and written forms, people have problems getting and holding jobs, communicating with peers, and understanding what teachers say (Polloway & Smith, 1992).

Information is received in two ways: listening to auditory information and reading visual information. Limitations in either of these skills greatly reduces the cognitive abilities of children and adults. Children routinely need to be able to obtain information from listening and reading in school. Teachers generally "tell" students things, either facts to be learned or directions to be followed, or have students read to obtain information. Deficits in either of these skills means a significant reduction in the ability of the student to process incoming information. Imagine not being able to read well enough to understand facts presented in a history or biology textbook or not being able to attend to the teacher during an important lecture. How can students learn if they are not capable of acquiring information through reading or listening (Polloway & Smith, 1992).

Social interactions among children also require the ability to receive information. Listening and responding accordingly are very important for social activities. Children frequently shy away from their peers who are different in any way; the inability to listen and therefore participate in verbal interactions, would likely result in such rejection (Smith, Price, & Marsh, 1986). Think about being in a social setting and not being able to interact because of limited listening skills. Our likely behavior would be similar to that of many children—escape from the situation.

Adults must also have abilities in listening and reading. Success in most jobs requires these abilities (Peters & Lloyd, 1987). Listening to directions and instructions from supervisors or reading information is critical. Can you think of any job that does not, at least from time to time, require the ability to receive information through listening or reading? Even jobs that do not require listening and reading skills directly frequently require individuals to be able to receive and process information through one of these channels.

Adults in social interactions also need to be able to listen and read. Listening is more likely needed in social settings. Without the ability to listen and then participate in verbal exchanges, individuals are at a major social disadvantage. While reading may not be directly related to social interactions, people often discuss things that they have read. Also, adults may find themselves in social settings where they have to read something, such as a menu or program.

Problems in listening or reading can result in major problems for students and adults. Trying to get along in our society, which is so dominated by language, is very difficult when experiencing receptive language problems. This chapter will present information concerning receptive language problems and their impact on school-age children. Ways to assess these deficiencies as well as remediate the problems will be provided.

Teaching Reading

NATURE OF READING

Reading is an extremely important skill for school-aged individuals. Not only is reading a key element in the curriculum of elementary schools (Smith, 1990), but it is required as a means of acquiring information for all courses (Polloway & Smith, 1992). Reading deficiencies in the elementary school can result in poor grades, lowered self-concept, and social rejection. Reading weaknesses in higher grades can negatively affect academic success in history, literature, science, or any other subject area that requires students to process information from written materials. Reading is probably the single most important skill students learn in elementary grades. With good reading, students have an advantage in acquiring information in other courses; deficits in reading result in a major disadvantage for students. For example, students who can read a chapter in history and comprehend the content well enough to pass a test have a strong advantage over students who have to read the chapter over and over and who still may not be able to remember and later retrieve facts.

Reading is a complex process that can be defined in many different ways. Guerin and Maier (1983) note that reading is:

- recognizing letters that make words;

- sounding out a sequence of sounds to make words;

- recognizing symbols that have meaning;

- recognizing words that, put together, make sentences that convey ideas;

- identifying words and understanding what they mean; and

- understanding what the author is trying to say (pp. 237–238).

Luftig (1989) defined reading as "the conversion of print into auditory equivalents and the subsequent interpretation of those equivalents into meanings based on previously learned language" (p. 287).

The Commission on Reading noted five generalizations about reading (Anderson *et al.*, 1985). The first generalization is that reading must be a constructive process. This means that the art of reading requires more than simply calling words. It requires the reader to use personal experiences and background knowledge to adequately interpret what is read. Background knowledge about a particular topic helps children understand what they read (Rowe & Rayford, 1987).

A second generalization noted by the commission is that reading must be fluent (Anderson, 1985). Readers who have to take time to decode many of the words they are reading are at a disadvantage compared to others who can read "effortlessly." Excessive decoding can interrupt the flow of reading and make it more awkward and less efficient (Hargis, Terhaar-Yonders, Williams, & Reed, 1988; Samuels, 1988). The commission cited the strategic nature of reading as the third generalization. This means the understanding of the different levels of reading (Anderson, 1985). For example, reading a newspaper requires less attention to detail than reading a chapter in a textbook for an exam. Good readers adjust their reading effort and style according to the content of the material and purpose for the reading.

The fourth generalization relates to the importance of motivation to reading (Anderson *et al.*, 1985). If students are not motivated to learn to read initially or to improve reading skills later, they reading will be less than optimal. Just like any curricular area, if readers do not see the relevance in reading, they are less inclined to make a strong effort to improve their reading skills (Madden, 1988). A primary task for teachers, therefore, is to motivate students to read. Making reading fun and rewarding should be a key component in the curriculum of every elementary school.

The final generalization noted by the commission relates to the continuous development of reading (Anderson *et al.*, 1985). While many students learn to read early in their elementary years, reading skills should continue to improve throughout the school years with practice (Blair & Rupley, 1988; Hargis *et al.*, 1988). Adults who continue to read and practice their reading improve their reading skills (Dowhower, 1987). There are many people who rarely use their reading skills except for functional reading, such as for road signs or menus. Other adults use their reading a great deal, either for pleasure or work-related activities. It is likely that those adults who read extensively are better readers than those who rarely read.

Teachers who are involved in reading instruction should consider all five generalizations noted by the Commission on Reading (Anderson *et al.*, 1985). They should consider whether each generalization is a possibility within their existing reading programs. For example, students need to be able to read a passage without spending a great deal of time decoding words that should be familiar and be able to use contextual clues to comprehend the reading materials. Weaknesses in these areas should be addressed by teachers. By evaluating reading programs in light of the five generalizations, teachers can determine weaknesses in the reading program and steps to improve the program.

READING PROCESS

The reading process involves visual motor skills, perceptual skills, and an interpretation of symbols by the brain. It is generally broken down into two major components: "reading" the words, or decoding, and understanding what is read, or comprehension (Cooper, Warncke, & Shipman, 1988; Samuels, 1988). Although there are many subskills involved in the reading process, they can all be grouped within the decoding or comprehension categories.

Decoding is the process of making sounds out of letters and letter groups, and blending these sounds together to form words (Luftig, 1989). Decoding can be oral, when an individual reads the word out loud, or silent, when the word is decoded, or "read" without actually saying the word. In either case, the letters that form a word are matched with sounds that result in a word.

Simply decoding, or "reading" words does not automatically mean that the words read are understood. Comprehension refers to the understanding of what is read (Samuels, 1988; Luftig, 1989). Without comprehension, the reading process is virtually useless. It does not do you any good to be able to read something if you do not understand what it means. The major purpose of reading is to understand something (Luftig, 1989). Many students appear to be good readers because they can read orally or silently very easily. However, this fluent decoding may not be followed by comprehension of the material.

Although reading programs differ in how various reading skills are sequenced, there is a general sequence of skills that are usually included. Table 5–1 describes the reading

TABLE 5–1 General Sequence of Reading Skills

GRADE	SKILLS ACQUIRED
Kindergarten	Identify sounds and pictures Express ideas in complete verbal sentences Understand meaning of words such as *above* and *far* Understand concepts of size, small, etc. Recognize and identify colors Organize objects into groups Match forms Understand beginning concepts of number
Grade 1	Recognize letters of alphabet; can write and give sound Auditory and visual perception and discrimination of initial and final consonants Observe left to right progression Recall what has been read Aware of medial consonants, consonants blends, digraphs Recognize long sound of vowels; roots words; plural forms; verb endings *-s, -ed, -ing*; opposites; pronouns *he, she* Understand concept of synonyms, homonymns, antonyms Understand simple compound words Copy simple sentences, fill-ins
Grade 2	Comprehension and analysis of what has been read Identify vowel digraphs Understand varient sounds of *y* Identify medial vowels Identify diphthongs Understand influence of *r* on preceding vowel Identify three-letter blends Understand use of Suffix *-er* Understand verb endings (for example, *stop, stopped*)
Grade 3	Recognize multiple sounds of long a in *ei, ay, ey* Understand silent *e* in *-le* endings Understand use of suffix *-est* Know how to change *y* to *i* before adding *er, est*

(continued)

TABLE 5-1 General Sequence of Reading Skills (cont'd.)

GRADE	SKILLS ACQUIRED
Grade 3 continued	Understand comparative and superlative forms of adjectives Understand possessive form using *s* Use contractions Identify syllabic breaks
Grade 4	Recognize main and subordinate parts Recognize unknown words using configuration and other words attack skills Identify various sounds of *ch* Recognize various phonetic values of *gh* Identify rounded *o* sound formed by *au, aw, al* Use and interpret diacritical markings Discriminate among multiple meaning of words
Grade 5	Read critically to evaluate Identify diagraphs *gn, mb, bt* Recognize that *augh* and *ough* may have round *o* sound Recognize and pronounce muted vowels in *el, al, le* Recognize secondary and primary accents Use of apostrophe Understand suffixes *-al, -hand, -ship, -ist, -ling, -an, -ian, -dom, -ern* Understand use of figures of speech; metaphor, simile Ability to paraphrase main idea Know ways to paragraphs and developed Outline using two or three main heads and subheadings Use graphic material
Grade 6	Develop ability for critical analysis Recognize and use Latin and Greek roots, such as *photo, tele, graph, geo, auto* Develop generalization that some suffixes can change part of speech, such as *-ure* changing an adjective to noun *(moist -moisture)* Understand meaning and pronunciation of homographs Develop awareness of shifting accents

Source: Guerin & Maier, 1983. *Informal assessment in education.* Palo Alto, CA: Mayfield Publishing Co., pp. 245–246. Used with permission.

skills that are likely taught at various grade levels. Special education teachers need to understand the general sequence of these skills in order to determine an approximate reading level for students as well as appropriate reading intervention program for implementation.

STATUS OF READING IN TODAY'S SCHOOLS

Since the reform reports were issued in the late 1970s and early 1980s, there has been a great deal of publicity about the quality of education in American schools. The most heralded report, *A Nation at Risk*, issued by the National Commission on Excellence in Education, reported several facts that greatly disturbed the American public. Among the findings:

- forty-two percent of students in high school completed a general curriculum as opposed to a college preparatory curriculum;

- homework for high school students has been decreasing;

- academic achievement in general has been decreasing;

- students in the United States spend significantly less time in school than students in other industrialized countries.

While these findings did not specifically relate to reading skills, they did express a general concern about the status of public education. In addition to *A Nation at Risk*, several other reports issued during the same era were highly critical of education. The *Action for Excellence* report, issued by the Commission of the States (1983), was more specific in recommendations related to corrective actions. This report called for the development and implementation of competencies in reading and other basic academic areas (Ornstein, 1985).

Reading abilities of students have also been evaluated through the analysis of nationally administered, standardized tests. The following summarizes much of the existing data that has been reported on the reading skills of students and adults in our society.

1. Functional illiteracy exists in approximately 23 million Americans (*A Nation at Risk*, 1983);

2. Functional illiteracy exists in approximately thirteen percent of all seventeen-year-olds (*A Nation at Risk*, 1983);

3. Scores on the Scholastic Aptitude Test (SAT) have declined during the years between 1963 and 1980 (*A Nation at Risk*, 1983);

4. Approximately 820,000 young adults (fifteen-to-eighteen year olds) are functionally illiterate (*Reading Report Card and Literacy: Profiles of America's Young Adults* (1985).

Although these figures reveal some startling facts, illiteracy outside the United States is even more staggering. Carceles (1990) reported that among the world population, approximately twenty-seven percent of individuals capable of reading are illiterate. Statistics that reveal the reading levels of students and adults with disabilities make it apparent that this group of individuals has significant problems in the area of reading (Smith, Price, & Marsh, 1986; Polloway & Smith, 1992).

READING AND STUDENTS WITH MILD DISABILITIES

As would be expected, students with mild disabilities frequently experience problems in reading (Smith, Price, & Marsh, 1986). The very nature of mental retardation results in below average achievement in all areas, and the literature includes many studies that reflect the below-average reading abilities of students in this category (Strichart & Gottlieb, 1982; Polloway *et al.*, 1987; Crews, 1988). One recent study found that students classified as mentally retarded scored significantly below their nonretarded peers on the Florida State Student Assessment Test. On the reading subtests of this exam, only 5.6 percent of students with mental retardation received a passing score (Crews, 1988).

Reading disabilities are also found in a large number of children with learning disabilities. In fact, problems in reading are the primary academic deficit found among students with this disability (Rivers, 1986; Snider & Tarver, 1987; Fessler, Rosenberg, & Rosenberg, 1991). In a study that investigated the performance of students with learning disabilities on the Florida State Student Assessment Test, it was found that these students scored well below their nondisabled peers in all areas of reading (Algozzine *et al.*, 1988). Table 5–2 compares the performance of students with learning disabilities and their nondisabled peers on the reading subtests. In another study, Rivers (1986) studied the characteristics of 200 elementary students with learning disabilities and found that the most prevalent academic deficit among the sample was reading; she found reading problems in 54.5 percent of the population studied. Still another recent study reported that 57 percent of students with learning disabilities experienced problems in reading, language, and math skills (Fessler *et al.*, 1991).

Reading problems among students with learning disabilities do not disappear after they leave high school. In a study that compared college students with learning disabilities

TABLE 5–2 Performance of LD and Non-LD Students on Reading Sub-Tests

SKILL AREA	LD STUDENTS MEAN SCORE	NON-LD STUDENTS MEAN SCORE
Who, What, When	3.76	4.74
Pictures, Maps, Signs	3.67	4.41
Identify Informed Sources	3.43	4.54
Indexes/Dictionary	3.39	4.46
Cause and Effect	3.31	4.55
Written Directions	3.31	4.55
Diagrams and Tables	3.19	4.16
Main Idea (implied)	3.06	4.48
Paragraph Conclusion	3.06	4.35
Main Idea (stated)	2.87	4.32
Facts and Opinion	2.78	4.32

Source: Algozzine, B., O'Shea, D.J., Stoddard, K., & Crews, W.B. (1988). Reading and writing competencies of adolescents with learning disabilities. *Journal of Learning Disabilities, 21*, 154–160.

to their nondisabled peers, results confirmed the significant lowered reading ability of the students with learning disabilities (Morris & Leuenberger, 1990). Older adults with learning disabilities also exhibit problems in the area of reading (Rogan & Hartman, 1990; Sitlington & Frank, 1990).

Students classified as emotionally disturbed or behaviorally disordered also experience problems in reading (Epstein & Cullinan, 1982). These students frequently score a year below their chronological age peers in most academic subjects, including reading (Kauffman, 1989; Fessler, Rosenberg, & Rosenberg, 1991). In one study, it was determined that fifty percent of students who had been classified as emotionally disturbed or behaviorally disordered who had learning problems experienced deficiencies in reading or language (Fessler *et al.*, 1991). After reviewing numerous studies concerning the characteristics of students with behavior disorders, Mastropieri, Jenkins, and Scruggs (1985) concluded that academic problems, including reading, were prevalent among this population of students.

Although the exact nature of reading problems experienced by students with disabilities will vary from individual to individual, there are some general reading characteristics of students classified as having disabilities. These include the following (Wallace, Cohen, & Polloway, 1987).

1. *Readiness skills*   Frequently students with disabilities lack reading readiness skills, such as visual and auditory discrimination, directionality, and memory.

2. *Word analysis and word recognition*   Often there are problems with word analysis and word recognition due to letter reversals, word reversals, and problems with phonetic skills.

3. *Comprehension abilities*   The heart of reading comprehension, is often the major weakness found in students with disabilities. Problems in all three levels of comprehension (literal, interpretive, and critical) are present.

4. *Study skills*   Students with disabilities often experience problems in study skills, such as adequate use of the table of contents in reading materials and note taking.

5. *Oral reading skills*   Mispronunciations and problems with word phrases are examples of the oral reading skills often deficient among students with disabilities.

6. *Literacy interests*   Many students with disabilities are not taught to enjoy literature and reading. Therefore, their appreciation for leisure reading time is likely minimal.

Students with mild disabilities, therefore, are likely to experience many different problems in the area of reading. These students will receive their reading instruction in a variety of settings. These could include regular classrooms and resource rooms. The exact setting will be determined by the individual education program (IEP) which takes into consideration the least restrictive environment requirement of federal and state legislation. Through special education programs and accomodations made in regular classrooms, regular and remedial reading activities should be implemented to reduce the impact of these problems.

METHODS TO TEACH READING

Teaching reading is a major activity in our schools, especially elementary schools (Smith, 1990). Most elementary classrooms have a daily reading period. For students with disabilities, reading instruction may also occur in secondary schools. There are numerous ways to teach reading; however, regardless of the methods used, teachers should consider several affective principles that relate to teaching students reading skills (Culyer, 1988).

1. Students must believe in their ability to learn to read.
2. Students must believe in the ability of their teachers to teach them to read.
3. Students must have teachers who believe in their ability to teach the students to read.
4. Students must experience consistent success and positive reinforcement in their efforts to learn to read.

These affective principles are important because of the need for students to believe in themselves. Students must believe that they are capable of learning. For many students with disabilities, failure has been a regular occurrence. The failure cycle must be broken, and students must develop a positive self concept in order to benefit from reading instruction. This is even more critical in reading because of its relationship with other academic areas.

There are several different ways to teach students to read. They are generally broken down into three major groups: phonics approaches, skills approaches, and whole language approaches. Some commercial as well as teacher-made programs use a variety of methods that may overlap. However, these three approaches form the basis for most reading programs.

Phonics Approaches

Phonetic reading approaches teach students how to decode words using a phonics approach. Instruction focuses on teaching students the relationships between certain letters and letter groups and sounds (Salend, 1990). Individuals learn to associate the approximately forty to forty-four sounds in the English alphabet, also called phonemes, with letters and groups of letters in the English language (Baumann, 1988). A basic understanding that students must develop in order to read effectively is phoneme-graphene associations and sound blending. For example, students must learn that the "t" sound, when blended with the "oo" sound makes the word *to*. These skills are mandatory, to some degree, regardless of the reading approach used. The goal of phonics instruction is for students to be able to "consistently use information about the relationship between letters and sounds and letters and meanings to assist in the identification of known words and to independently figure out unfamiliar words" (Anderson *et al.*, 1985, p. 43). Students who possess good phonics skills are able to "read" words they have never encountered through phonics analysis (Shuman, 1987). Remember how you "sounded out" words that were unfamiliar to you? This is an example of using phonics analysis.

There are two ways to use phonics instruction in reading programs, explicit phonics instruction and implicit phonics instruction. In explicit phonics instruction, sounds of letters are taught in isolation and then blended together to form words. Blending individual sounds into blended units is not an easy task. Many children are capable of relating sounds to letters, but have difficulty when attempting to blend the sounds into words. In the implicit phonics instruction, sounds are not taught in isolation, but are taught as part of words. Although most reading programs use the implicit phonics approach, some teachers continue to teach phonics explicitly (Anderson *et al.*, 1985).

There is a long-standing controversy regarding the use of a phonics reading approach. On the one hand, proponents of the phonics method believe that this model can facilitate reading for all students, especially those with reading disabilities. On the other hand, some professionals argue that phonics instruction results in students "plodding" through their reading by carefully analyzing each word; this often leads to sounding out words without comprehending the meaning of the passage (Wallace & McLoughlin, 1988) and limited skills in transferring rules for phonetic analysis to unknown words (McClure, 1985). A lack of perfect symmetry between letters and sounds also makes total phonics instruction difficult (Baumann, 1988). It should be kept in mind that phonics is only the first step in a long process that results in optimal reading for students (Anderson *et al.*, 1985).

Regardless of the problems associated with phonics approaches, there are a number of reading series that use phonics as the basis for the reading program. These include (Lerner, 1988):

- *Breaking the Code* (Open Court);

- *Building Reading Skills* (McCormick & Mathers);

- *Keys to Reading* (The Economy Company);

- *Learning About Words Series* (Teachers College Press);

- *New Phonics Skilltexts* (Charles E. Merrill);

- *Phonics We Use* (Riverside);

- *Phonovisual Program* (Phonovisual Products, Inc.);

- *Speech-to-Print Phonics* (Harcourt Brace Jovanovich);

- *Wordland Series* (Continental Press).

Whole Word Approaches

Another primary model to teach reading in our schools is the whole word approach. Students who are taught to read using this model are able to read words without decoding or applying phonetic analysis; the words are instantly recognized (Baumann, 1988). This "ability to automatically recognize words that are frequently used in basic reading material (the, you, said, in, etc.) is an important goal for all readers" (Wallace *et al.*, 1987, p. 175). Studies have revealed the whole word approach to be effective with students with disabilities (Barudin & Hourcade, 1990). An obvious advantage of the whole word approach is that students can read more quickly; they do not have to decode or phonetically analyze words. An obvious disadvantage: students may not be able to read words that are unfamiliar. In general, it was thought that children would learn to read more rapidly if they learned to recognize whole words (Anderson *et al.*, 1985).

TABLE 5-3 Format for Introducing Sight Words

TEACHER	STUDENTS

Teacher writes on board: sat, mud, fit, sad.

1. Teacher models.
    a. "You are going to read these words without saying the sounds out loud."
    b. "My turn. Watch my mouth. I'll say the sounds to myself, then I'll say the word." Teacher points to the first word, moving lips and whispering each sound as she points to each letter. After saying the sounds subvocally, she says "What word?", signals, and says the word "sat."
    c. Teacher models with one more word.

2. Teacher tests group on all the words.   *Students sound out words, whispering sounds. "Sssaaat."*
    a. "Your turn." Teacher points to left of first letter. "As I point to the letters, sound out this word to yourselves." Teacher loops from letter to letter touching under each continuous sound letter for about one second. "What word?" (Signal.)   *Students say word at normal rate. "Sat."*
    b. Teacher repeats step 2(a) with remaining words in list. Teacher presents the list until students correctly identify all words.

Source: Carnine, D., Silbert, J., & Kameenui, E.J. (1990). *Direct instruction reading,* 2nd Ed. Columbus, OH: Merrill, p. 116. Reprinted with permission.

When using a whole word approach, new words are taught either in an isolated manner or within a sentence or passage (Salend, 1990). When teaching new words within a sentence or passage, students are able to use context clues to help them determine the new word. Words are also taught in an introductory format and a practice format. Table 5–3 describes the format for introducing sight-reading words, while Table 5–4 provides an example of using the practice format. Note that the specific process involved requires a slightly different approach.

Whole Language Approaches

A newer technique to teach reading that is gaining popularity in some schools is the whole language model. Using this approach, reading is taught as part of the overall language process, which includes language, literacy, and content learning. When using the whole language model, basal readers and other books specifically designed to teach reading are not used. Rather, teachers use real books, both fiction and non-fiction, to teach basic reading

TEACHING READING **153**

TABLE 5–4 Practice Format for Sight-Reading Words in Lists

TEACHER	STUDENTS

Teacher writes on board: sad, not, fit, am, sun, fin.

1. "You're going to read these words the fast way. When I point to a word, sound it out to yourself. When I signal, say the word the fast way."
2. Students read words with a three-second pause.
3. a. Teacher points to left of the first word,   *"Sad."*
    pauses three seconds, then says, "What word?", and signals.
    b. The teacher continues the same procedure, as in step 2 (a), with the remaining words.
3. Students read entire word list again with a two second pause.
    a. Teacher has the students read words again with only a two-second pause.
4. Teacher gives individual turns.
    a. Teacher points to word, pauses two seconds, then calls on a student.
    b. Teacher repeats step 4 (a) with remaining words.

Source: Carnine, D., Silbert, J., & Kameenui, E.J. (1990). *Direct instruction reading,* 2nd Ed. Columbus, OH: Merrill, p. 117. Reprinted with permission.

skills and enable students to improve those skills (Polloway & Smith, 1992). Students are encouraged to read for meaning rather than through decoding activities (Salend, 1990).

Studies that have investigated the effectiveness of whole language reading instruction in the United States have had mixed results. When used by good teachers, the whole language methods seem to work extremely well; however, the method results in only average reading performance in the majority of cases (Anderson et al., 1985). Regardless of the effectiveness of the whole language model, teachers trying to implement this approach may encounter barriers. These could include limited resources, lack of professional development, simple misperceptions about whole language, and resistance to change from teachers (Ridley, 1990).

When using a whole language model, the selection of appropriate materials is still an important part of the program. Rhodes and Dudley-Marling (1988) suggest that teachers use the following questions to guide materials selection.

1. Were the materials written for authentic communicative purposes?
2. Do the materials use natural language?
3. Are the materials relevant to the background experience of students?

4. Do the materials invite lengthy engagement in reading?

5. Do the materials encourage divergent responses?

6. What can the student learn about the world as a result of using the materials?

7. Are the materials representative of out-of-school materials?

8. Are the materials predictable (p. 87)?

BASAL READING SERIES

Even though there are many models available for teachers to use in reading instruction, the majority continue to rely on a basal reading series approach (Hitchcock & Tompkins, 1987; Barr & Sadow, 1989). Basal reading programs are complete reading instruction packages that provide all the materials necessary to teach reading. Basal reading programs appear to be the driving force in reading instruction in this country (Anderson *et al.*, 1985). In one recent study, it was concluded that fully eighty-five percent of the school-aged children learn to read using a basal reading series (Barnard & Hetzel, 1989). An interesting note is that while the vast majority of schools continue to use a basal reading approach, the idea that "packaged" reading programs should be used has been challenged for many years. It seems that professionals "talk down" about basal reading series but use them anyway.

There are numerous basal reading series available for schools. While they differ in some respects, the majority include reading books for students sequenced on the basis of difficulty, a teacher's guide with instructions for daily reading activities, workbooks for students, and supplementary story books (Shuman, 1987). In addition, some have film strips, audio tapes, flash cards, and other supplementary instructional materials. "An entire basal reading program would make a stack of books and papers four feet high." (Anderson *et al.*, 1985, p. 35)

Using a basal reading series has both advantages and disadvantages. Probably the most important advantage is that a basal reading series enables all teachers to teach reading in a systematic manner. Teachers who are new or who have not had a great deal of preparation regarding reading instruction are able to implement an effective reading program with a basal reading series. This can be reassuring for new teachers who have strong doubts about their ability to teach children how to read. On the other hand, an important disadvantage of the basal model is that teachers are frequently limited in the activities they can implement in reading instruction. Although they are not bound only to the activities and sequence of the basal series, too often teachers rely strictly on the content of the commercial program. Having a structured set of activities available is tempting for teachers who may want to implement other instructional activities but are limited in their time for preparation and instruction.

READING PROBLEMS

Reading receives a great deal of attention in our entire educational system. However, even though this subject area is a principal focus in elementary schools, many students experience significant reading disabilities (McGill-Frazen, 1987). Reading problems are complex. They can result from socioeconomic factors, psychological factors, educational factors, or physical factors (Ekwall & Shanker, 1988). Table 5–5 describes some of the factors in each of these major categories that can cause reading problems.

TABLE 5-5 Factors Associated with Reading Disabilities

FACTOR	COMPONENTS
Physical Factors	eyes and seeing
	auditory difficulties
	laterality, mixed dominance, and
	directional confusion
	neurological problems
Psychological Factors	emotional problems
	intelligence
	self-concept
Socioeconomic Factors	ethnic factors
	socio-economic factors
	language factors
Educational Factors	teachers' personalities
	teaching methods for reading
	school policies
	materials used in reading
	class size
	time spent on reading instruction

Source: Ekwall, E.E., & Shanker, J.L. (1988). *Diagnosis and remediation of the disabled reader,* 3rd Ed. Boston: Allyn & Bacon.

Regardless of the factors related to the reading disability, there are several types of reading problems that are typically found among students. These include problems related to reading habits, word recognition errors, comprehension errors, and miscellaneous symptoms (Mercer, 1987). Smith (1983) lists several common problems experienced by some students who suffer from reading disabilities. These include 1. omitting letters, syllables, or words; 2. inserting extra letters, words, or sounds; 3. substituting words that look or sound similar; 4. mispronouncing words; 5. reversing words or syllables; 6. transposing letters or words; and 7. repeating words or using improper inflection during oral reading. Table 5–6 (on page 156) summarizes various behaviors associated with the major kinds of problems described by Mercer (1987).

ASSESSMENT OF READING PROBLEMS

Prior to developing and implementing intervention programs for students to improve reading, a comprehensive assessment of these reading skills should be completed. Assessment in the area of reading can be formal or informal. Many teachers use both types of assessment data to develop a comprehensive evaluation of the child in question.

TABLE 5-6 Behaviors Associated with Reading Problems

	CHARACTERISTICS
Reading Habits	tense movements, such as frowning, fidgeting losing reading place insecurity resulting in refusing to read or crying holding materials too close
Word Recognition Errors	omitting or inserting words substituting words reversing letters in words mispronouncing words hesitating between words for more than five seconds not recognizing known words
Comprehension Errors	poor recall regarding reading content
Miscellaneous Errors	jerky reading, inappropriate word grouping

Source: Mercer, C.D. (1987). *Students with learning disabilities.* Columbus, OH: Merrill.

Formal Reading Assessment

Formal assessment generally consists of standardized, norm-referenced tests that are designed to compare the student taking the test with a "typical" group of children similar in age and other characteristics. Results from these tests show a student's grade equivalent, age equivalent, percentile rank, or some other standard score.

Reading is one of the most tested areas in schools. There are three general areas assessed with reading tests: oral reading skills, decoding skills, and comprehension skills (Luftig, 1989). Because reading is evaluated so extensively, there are numerous formal assessment instruments available that focus on reading skills. Many norm-referenced, general achievement tests, such as the Peabody Individual Achievement Test-Revised (PIAT-R), Wide Range Achievement Test-Revised (WRAT-R), and Kaufman Test of Educational Achievement (K-TEA) include one or more reading subtests. These tests are often used to provide a general description of a student's reading ability levels (Salvia & Ysseldyke, 1991). While they do provide an overview of reading skills, these tests do not allow assessment of specific areas in reading and are therefore of limited value in determining appropriate intervention strategies for students.

To obtain more indepth assessment information about reading, tests specifically designed to test reading skills should be used. There are many such tests available for professionals to use. These range from comprehensive, individualized diagnostic reading tests, such as the Stanford Diagnostic Reading Test (Karlsen, Madden, & Gardner, 1985) to more specific reading tests that focus on particular areas, such as oral reading skills, like the Gray Oral Reading Test-Revised (Wiederholt & Bryant, 1986; Polloway & Smith, 1992). Table 5-7 describes the characteristics of several formal reading tests available. Users of

TABLE 5–7 Characteristics of Formal Reading Tests

TEST	GROUP (G) OR INDIVIDUAL (I)	GRADE LEVEL	READING AREAS ASSESSED
Test Batteries			
Diagnostic Reading Scales (Spache, 1981)	I	1–7	Three word recognition lists and twenty-two passages of increasing difficulty are used to assess word recognition, word analysis, and comprehension. Twelve supplementary phonics tests are also included to assess areas such as consonant and vowel sounds, blending, initial consonant substitution, and auditory discrimination.
Durrell Analysis of Reading Difficulty (Durrell & Catterson, 1980)	I	1–6	Oral reading passages and accompanying comprehension questions are included, as well as paragraphs for silent reading and listening comprehension. Specific subtests deal with oral reading, silent reading, listening comprehension, and word recognition and word analysis. Additional subtests are included in listening vocabulary, sounds in isolation, spelling, visual memory of words, identifying sounds in words, and prereading phonics abilities.
Gates-McKillop Reading Diagnostic Tests (Gates & McKillop, 1962)	I	2–6	The subtest areas include oral reading (with error analysis), flash presentation and untimed presentation of words, flash presentation of phrases, knowledge of word parts, recognition of visual forms representing sounds, and auditory blending. Supplementary tests assess spelling, oral vocabulary , syllabication, and auditory discrimination.
Stanford Diagnostic Reading Test (Karlsen, Madden, & Gardner, 1976)	G	1–12	The test measures specific reading skills in vocabulary (auditory vocabulary, word meaning, word parts);

(continued)

TABLE 5–7 Characteristics of Formal Reading Tests (cont'd.)

TEST	GROUP (G) OR INDIVIDUAL (I)	GRADE LEVEL	READING AREAS ASSESSED
Test Batteries			
Stanford Diagnostic Reading Test (Karlsen, Madden, & Gardner, 1976) continued			decoding (auditory discrimination, phonetic analysis, structural analysis); comprehension (word reading, reading comprehension– literal and inferential); rate (reading rate, fast reading, scanning, and skimming).
Woodcock Reading Mastery Tests-Revised (Woodcock, 1986)	I	K–college and adult	The test includes six subtest areas: visual auditory learning, letter identification, word identification, word attack, word comprehension (antonyms, synonyms, analogies), and passage comprehension.

Source: Mercer C.D. (1987). *Students with learning disabilities.* Columbus, OH: Merrill. p. 380-381. Reprinted with permission.

these tests should always consider the reliability and validity of the tests for specific groups of students, as well as the appropriateness of the sample used to standardize the test.

Informal Reading Assessment

While formal, norm-referenced reading tests can provide information that gives grade levels and age levels, informal measurement of reading skills often results in more useable assessment data for developing individual intervention programs. Wallace, Cohen, and Polloway (1987) describe five different methods for informally assessing reading skills. These include 1. observation, 2. interviews and oral questioning, 3. informal reading inventories, 4. cloze procedure, and 5. informal teacher-constructed tests.

Observations Observations provide an excellent source of assessment information concerning students' reading skills. Observations can be systematic or nonsystematic. Systematic observation is when the assessor sets out to observe specific behaviors. For example, if a teacher were interested in a student's oral reading skills, special attention would be given to the child during an oral reading activity. This would provide information about the student's specific strengths and weaknesses in oral reading. Nonsystematic observation is when the assessor observes a general classroom situation; there is no specific behavior targeted. While this form of observation may provide a great deal of information about the general nature of a student's reading skills, or the reading skills exhibited by a class, it will most likely not provide the in-depth observational information about a child's reading skills that could be obtained through systematic observation.

Regardless of the type of observation used, the following guidelines should be considered when collecting assessment information through observations.

1. Reading and writing should be observed over a period of time in a number of different contexts.

2. The setting, as well as students' reading and writing behaviors, must be thoroughly considered.

3. Teachers should also consider their own behavior as part of students' instructional settings.

4. Observations should be regularly summarized and recorded.

5. In many cases it's helpful if observations are supplemented with pictures, audiotapes, or videotapes.

6. Observations of students don't have to be unobtrusive.

7. There are times when it's useful to ask students questions to clarify what's been observed.

8. Observation need not be excessively time-consuming. (Rhodes & Dudley-Marling; 1988, pp. 37-38)

These guidelines ensure that useful data regarding reading skills are obtained through observations. Observing students without consideration for some of these points may result in the collection of information that is not helpful in developing and implementing remedial programs.

After collecting data through observations, teachers need to analyze the information to determine specific strengths and weaknesses of the child. Through an analysis of a student's reading skills, the following questions may be answered.

■ What word analysis skills does the child utilize?

■ Does the child depend on one analysis skill (e.g., sounding words out)?

■ How extensive is the child's sight vocabulary?

■ What consistent word analysis errors are made by the child?

■ Are particular words or parts of words consistently distorted or omitted?

■ Does the child read too fast, too slow, or word by word?

■ Are factual questions answered correctly?

■ Is the child able to answer comprehension questions requiring inferential and critical reading ability? (Wallace & McLoughlin, 1988, pp. 140–141)

Information obtained from these questions can result in specific actions by teachers. For example, if it is concluded that the student does not have word analysis skills sufficient to decode new words, steps can be taken to teach these skills. Likewise, if a student reads too slowly, instruction can focus on expanding eye gaze to increase reading rate.

An observational checklist may be used to collect information about students' reading skills. Checklists are beneficial to the observer because they provide some structure to the observation. This ensures that the observer attends to particular behaviors that have been determined to be important for the development of reading programs. Several of the diagnostic readings tests, such as the *Gates-McKillop-Horowitz Reading Diagnostic Tests* and the *Durrell Analysis of Reading Difficulty*, contain checklists, and many teachers develop their own checklists. In addition, some commercial reading programs may include checklists. Figure 5–1 provides an example of a reading diagnostic checklist.

Interviews and Oral Questioning   Interviewing and questioning students enables teachers to gather information regarding reading interests and attitudes, word analysis skills, word recognition skills, and reading comprehansion skills. Students can be encouraged to talk about their interests in reading and what they like and do not like about reading (Wallace *et al.*, 1987). Finally, interviewing students about what they have just read is an excellent method of assessing comprehension of their reading. In fact, Salvia and Ysseldyke (1991) believe that this is the best way to measure reading comprehension.

Informal Reading Inventory   Informal reading inventories (IRIs) consist of a series of graded reading passages and questions used to determine reading level and comprehension skills (Choate & Rakes, 1989). They range from the preprimer level to seventh or eighth grade levels. Students generally are required to read two passages, one orally and one silently. At the end of the passages, students are asked questions about the content of the passage. Through analysis of word recognition skills, noted during oral reading, teachers are able to determine a word recognition level. Likewise, the use of questions to determine comprehension of the content allows the teacher to determine general comprehension skills (Ekwall & Shanker, 1988).

Informal reading inventories can be useful for several purposes. These include:

- to determine proper placement of students in reading programs;

- to determine the independent, instructional, and frustration reading levels of students;

- to determine number and types of oral reading problems; and

- to determine comprehension skills of students (Ekwall & Shanker, 1988).

Teachers frequently develop their own informal reading inventories, often from the reading materials used in the classroom. Luftig (1989) provides a list of guidelines that teachers can use when creating informal reading inventories. These include the role of questions in the process, as well as general rules such as how questions should be asked. Table 5–8 (on page 162) summarizes these guidelines.

Cloze Procedure   The cloze procedure provides another method of informally assessing reading skills, both reading level and comprehension (Luftig, 1989). Using the cloze model, every *n*th word is left out of a reading passage and replaced with a blank. Students

FIGURE 5-1 Example of Reading Diagnostic Checklist

Rating	Area Reviewed

Oral Reading

1. Word-by-word reading
2. Incorrect phrasing
3. Poor pronunciation
4. Omission
5. Repetitions
6. Inversions or Reversals
7. Insertions
8. Substitutions
9. Basic sight words not known
10. Sight vocabulary not up to grade level
11. Guesses at words
12. Consonant sounds not known
13. Vowel sounds not known
14. Vowel parts and/or consonant clusters not known
15. Uses morphological skills
16. Uses context clues
17. Good comprehension

Oral/Silent

18. Good vocabulary
19. Adequate vacabulary

Study Skills

20. Unaided recall scanty
21. Well organized response
22. Locates information well
23. Skims materials well
24. Adjusts reading rate based on reading content
25. Reading rate good

Other Abilities

26. Good knowledge of alphabet
27. Good spelling ability
28. Good dictionary skills

Key: F – frequent; S – sometimes; N – never

Source: Ekwall, E.E. (1985). *Locating and correcting reading difficulties*, 4th Ed. Columbus, OH: Merrill.

TABLE 5-8 Guide for Making Questions for Informal Reading Inventory

1. Sequence questions in same order information is presented.

2. Main questions come before detailed questions.

3. Focus questions only on important material.

4. Check all questions to make sure that some questions cannot be answered based on previous questions.

5. Ensure that the same answer does not fit more than one question.

6. Do not use questions that can use more than one answer.

7. Do not use questions that can be answered correctly by individuals who have not read the passage.

8. Ensure that any pictures in the text do not provide clues for questions.

9. Keep questions short and simple.

10. Use who, what, when, where, how, or why questions.

11. Do not start questions with negative statements.

12. Do not include questions that require lists.

13. Use some questions that require word definitions.

14. Do not use questions that require opinions.

15. Avoid questions that only require yes/no or true/false answers.

Source: Luftig, R.L. (1989). *Assessment of learners with special needs.* Boston: Allyn & Bacon.

fill in the blank with a word that "makes sense" with the remainder of the sentence. Some general characteristics of the cloze procedures include:

- words can be deleted at various intervals, however, most research is based on deleting every 5th word;

- the first and last sentence are generally left intact;

- passages may vary in length, however, approximately 250 words is the average number;

- administration of the cloze method is similar to administering a group standard-ized reading test (Ekwall & Shanker, 1988).

The following passage presents an example of the cloze technique. Keep in mind that this method of assessment can be easily done with classroom reading materials.

Nick and Chris were twins. Tony was their 1. _____ friend. The three boys stood in front 2. _____ the big store. They could not stop 3. _____ at the red bike in the store 4. _____. (Guerin & Maier, 1983, p. 253)

Informal Teacher-Made Tests　Tests that are developed by teachers to informally as-sess students' reading skills are another excellent method for diagnosing reading problems (Wallace *et al.*, 1987). These tests are directly related to the reading curriculum used in the classroom, making a direct link between assssessment data and classroom intervention (Polloway & Smith, 1992). Teacher-made tests can be designed to measure any reading skill. Therefore, teachers who desire specific information about a child's reading ability are able to secure such information through the use of these tests.

When developing teacher-made tests, Guerin and Maier (1983) give the following recommendations.

1. Reduce instructional goals to a sequence of objectives that lead to each goal.

2. Construct items that measure performance that is directly related to the skill steps leading to an objective.

3. Establish criterion levels to reflect the degree of performance that ensures consistent success and provides the basic entry skill needed for subsequent objectives.

4. Include enough items (four to ten) to establish clearly that the results accurately represent the student's level of performance.

5. Create a pool of pretested items so that the same item does not need to be used in repeated testing.

6. Evaluate and redesign items so that they are clear and accurate measurements of a learning step. (p. 40)

Parents and Reading Assessment　The role of parents in reading assessment is very important. By informally observing children on a daily basis in the home environment, par-ents may be able to provide significant input into the assessment process. This information may prove extremely helpful in diagnosing reading problems. Ekwall and Shanker (1988) suggest that the following information can be obtained from parent interviews.

- Parental views of student's problem

- Emotional climate of the home

- Health factors

- Reading materials available at home

- Library habits and time spent reading

- Study habits and study environments

- Parental expectations

- Social adjustment

- Independence and self-concept

- Duties at home

- Sleep habits

- Successful practices with the student

- Previous tutoring and results

This kind of information might be helpful for teachers during the development and implementation of reading programs. Better understanding the home environment makes it easier for teachers to develop appropriate programs for students experiencing reading problems.

REMEDIAL READING APPROACHES

Students with mild disabilities frequently exhibit reading problems. As noted, these problems can relate to decoding, comprehension, or the many subskills associated with each. When the reading problems experienced by students are significant enough to warrant intervention, specific entries in the student's IEP should reflect goals, objectives, and intervention techniques that focus on reading (Smith, Graves, & Aldridge, in press). For these students, reading remediation may actually take place twice each day, once in the special education resource room and once in the regular classroom (O'Sullivan, Ysseldyke, Christenson, & Thurlow, 1990).

The exact location for the reading remediation will be determined by the content of the IEP. The overriding factor when providing reading remediation for students with disabilities is the same as providing other services to these students, the least-restrictive-environment mandate. Public Law 94-142 requires that students with disabilities be educated with nondisabled peers as much as possible. Therefore, remedial reading instruction for these students might be in regular classrooms, special education classrooms, or a combination of the two.

The important role of parents in reading remediation should not be overlooked. Public Law 94-142 mandates the involvement of parents in educational programs for students with disabilities. It has been previously noted that parents can play a very important role in assessing reading problems. They can also participate in effectively implementing remedial reading programs. By carrying out remedial activities at home, providing a conducive atmosphere for reading, and modeling reading behaviors, parents can increase the chances for progress in reading.

There are numerous reading remediation programs designed to improve the reading abilities of these students. These include commercial remedial reading programs, specific remedial models, and teacher-made activities. Often teachers use several different reading programs. Since there is no one particular reading program that is effective with all children, teachers need to be flexible in determining which program to use in their classrooms. Having an array of options available makes it more likely that an appropriate program can be developed for each child.

General Considerations in Reading Remediation

There are several general considerations when implementing reading remediation programming. Ekwall and Shanker (1988) make the following suggestions.

1. Review materials previously learned as often as possible until responses are automatic.

2. Illustrate new concepts with verbal explanations.

3. Limit directions for oral and written assignments. For example, divide a three-part assignment into three parts and give directions for each part separately. (As with all suggestions in this section, procedures used depend on the capabilities of the student.)

4. Provide a working environment that is as free of distractions as possible. Use study carrels or reading and study areas isolated from other students.

5. Introduce new or distracting words with color cues such as a green letter at the beginning of a word and a red letter at the end of a word.

6. Give the student sufficient time to respond to oral questions. One study showed that teachers allow on average about two to three seconds for a student to answer. Allow at least five to ten seconds if needed; in some cases half a minute may be more appropriate.

7. Encourage the student to verbalize the response when writing something new.

8. Encourage the student to use a finger, pencil, ruler, or piece of paper with a window cut in it when reading, if needed.

9. Many experts have suggested permitting students to give oral answers to tests in their regular classroom if unable to produce adequate written responses. However this reinforces an undesirable habit. It is usually better to modify the time allowed for completion or to provide questions that require short answers. (p. 360)

In addition to these general considerations, Ford and Ohlhausen (1988) add that teachers should focus on functional reading, use incentives, and arrange for cross-grade involvement in the reading process to take advantage of student-helpers. Also, teachers should provide reading instruction in an environment that is relatively free from distractions (Choate & Rakes, 1989).

Remedial Phonics Approaches

Some remedial reading programs focus on the use of phonics. While the specific sequence of phonics skills used to teach children may vary from child to child, there is a sequence of skills that are usually taught to students with disabilities when teaching reading. These include:

1. initial and final consonants;
2. consonant blends and digraphs;
3. short vowels;
4. long vowels;
5. silent letters;
6. vowel digraphs;
7. vowel dipthongs (Wallace, Cohen, & Polloway, 1987, p. 180)

A basic understanding that students must develop in order to read effectively is phoneme-grapheme associations and sound blending. These skills are mandatory, to some degree, regardless of the reading approach used. Fuchs and Fuchs (1984) describe a beginning reading remedial program that emphasizes the phoneme-grapheme associations. In this program, students are taught letter-sound associations and blending skills. Teaching letter-sound associations is accomplished using demonstration and prompting activities. For example, the teacher initially demonstrates the association between a letter and sound. A sound is presented, and the teacher shows which letter is associated with that sound as well as how the sound is produced.

In step two pictorial and verbal cues are initially provided for a prompt, but they are faded as quickly as possible to enable the student to learn the association. Figure 5–2 describes activities for some of these exercises. The final step in this process is practice. Students are expected to practice the grapheme-phoneme associations depicted on their letter cards at least twice each day. The criterion for completion of this activity is when fifty letter sounds are properly pronounced in a one minute period (Fuchs & Fuchs, 1984).

The second process in the model is teaching sound blending to produce words. Again, demonstration, prompts, and practice are the key elements of the instructional process. The teacher actually models blending of three letter cards into a consonant-vowel-consonant (CVC) word. This provides students with a real example of sound blending (Fuchs & Fuchs, 1984).

Gillingham-Stillman Approach

The Gillingham method is a multisensory approach that requires students to trace letters as they say them out loud (Gillingham & Stillman, 1970). The system relies a great deal on phonics and a systematic learning sequence (Lerner, 1988). Students are taught to recognize and say ten letters (a, b, f, h, i, j, k, m, p, t,) by learning the sound associated with each letter. Students "view the letter, hear the sounds they make, link the letters to their sounds, and write the letters." (Salend, 1990, p. 321) After learning these ten letters and their corresponding sounds, students begin blending the sounds together to form words.

Remedial Whole Word Approaches

Some remedial reading programs are based on teaching reading using the whole word model. When teaching students with disabilities how to read using a whole word approach,

FIGURE 5–2 Example of Grapheme-Phoneme Associations and Picture, Verbal, and Gestural Prompts

Associations Gra-pheme	Pho-neme	Prompts Pictorial	Verbal	Gestural
a	a		None	Move letter card to mouth as if to bite card.
c	k		"This is a *cute, kitty, cat*."	Move letter card to shoulder as if to hug the cat. As the teacher hugs the card, his/her head bends down and left arm curls up to form the shape of *c*.
h	h		"Sit in this chair quietly. Only say *h*."	Put finger to mouth as if to mimic "sh."
o	o		None	Point to lines of legs coming from *o*.
p	p		None	Move letter card down, as if falling.
x	ks		None	Make an *X* on chest.
y	y		"This says 'yummy'."	Point to spot on letter card where mouth says "yummy."

Source: Adapted from Fuchs, L.S., & Fuchs, D. (1984). Teaching beginning reading skills: A unique approach. *Teaching Exceptional Children, 17,* 48–53.

teachers should gradually introduce new words and provide a great deal of reinforcement and practice for students. The following presents some specific techniques for using the whole word approach with disabled students.

- Label objects around the classroom.

- Develop picture dictionaries using magazine photographs and illustrations.

- Use word games that emphasize common sight words.

- Have students listen to a tape recording of sight words while following a worksheet of the same words.

- Make flash cards for individual or group practice sessions.

- Always introduce sight words in a sentence.

- Point out unusual configurations of various sight words.

- Classify sight words by categories (people, things, animals, etc.). (Wallace *et al.*, 1987, p. 178)

When using a whole word approach, teachers need to focus initial attention on words that are frequently used in the English language. The *Dolch* word list is an example of words used frequently. Table 5–9 includes the 220 words on the *Dolch* list. Ensuring that students are able to read the words on the *Dolch* list is an excellent beginning for teaching students with disabilities how to read.

TABLE 5–9 Dolch Word List

PREPRIMER		PRIMER		FIRST		SECOND		THIRD	
1.	the	45.	when	89.	many	133.	know	177.	don't
2.	of	46.	who	90.	before	134.	while	178.	does
3.	and	47.	will	91.	must	135.	last	179.	got
4.	to	48.	more	92.	through	136.	might	180.	united
5.	a	49.	no	93.	back	137.	us	181.	left
6.	in	50.	if	94.	years	138.	great	182.	number
7.	that	51.	out	95.	where	139.	old	183.	course
8.	is	52.	so	96.	much	140.	year	184.	war
9.	was	53.	said	97.	your	141.	off	185.	until
10.	he	54.	what	98.	may	142.	come	186.	always
11.	for	55.	up	99.	well	143.	since	187.	away
12.	it	56.	its	100.	down	144.	against	188.	something
13.	with	57.	about	101.	should	145.	go	189.	fact
14.	as	58.	into	102.	because	146.	came	190.	through

(continued)

TABLE 5–9 Dolch Word List (cont'd.)

PREPRIMER	PRIMER	FIRST	SECOND	THIRD
15. his	59. than	103. each	147. right	191. water
16. on	60. them	104. just	148. used	192. less
17. be	61. can	105. those	149. take	193. public
18. at	62. only	106. people	150. three	194. put
19. by	63. other	107. Mr.	151. states	195. thing
20. I	64. new	108. how	152. himself	196. almost
21. this	65. some	109. too	153. few	197. hand
22. had	66. could	110. little	154. house	198. enough
23. not	67. time	111. state	155. use	199. far
24. are	68. these	112. good	156. during	200. took
25. but	69. two	113. very	157. without	201. head
26. from	70. may	114. make	158. again	202. yet
27. or	71. then	115. would	159. place	203. government
28. have	72. do	116. still	160. American	204. system
29. an	73. first	117. own	161. around	205. better
30. they	74. any	118. see	162. however	206. set
31. which	75. my	119. men	163. home	207. told
32. one	76. now	120. work	164. small	208. nothing
33. you	77. such	121. long	165. found	209. night
34. were	78. like	122. get	166. Mrs.	210. end
35. her	79. our	123. here	167. thought	211. why
36. all	80. over	124. between	168. went	212. called
37. she	81. man	125. both	169. say	213. didn't
38. there	82. me	126. life	170. part	214. eyes
39. would	83. even	127. being	171. once	215. find
40. their	84. most	128. under	172. general	216. going
41. we	85. made	129. never	173. high	217. look
42. him	86. after	130. day	174. upon	218. asked
43. been	87. also	131. same	175. school	219. later
44. has	88. did	132. another	176. every	220. knew

Source: Johnson, D.D. (1971). The Dolch list reexamined. *The Reading Teacher, 24,* 455–456. Reprinted with permission.

Functional reading follows along the line of teaching students to recognize words that are used often, as well as words that are critically important for independent functioning and safety. For example, individuals need to know that the word "poison" means that the contents should not be consumed. Likewise, the word "danger" should alert the individual that caution should be maintained. For students about to exit high school and enter the job market, the ability to read job application forms and other adult reading materials is critical.

There are numerous lists of "so-called" survival words. These words should be taught as soon as possible for all students. For students with disabilities whose reading skills may always be deficient, emphasis on teaching these words is even more critical. Table 5–10 provides an example of these kinds of words.

Regardless of the word list to be taught, Simms and Falcon (1987) suggest a method for using sight words in remedial reading. Using their approach, words are categorized into semantic categories. Examples include:

- action words (example: pick, put, buy)

- away words (example: away, down, there)

- connecting words (example: because, but)

- feeling words (example: hurt, laugh)

- little words (example: if, to, as)

- question words (example: who, where, what)

- sharing words (example: gave, get, help)

- life words (example: live, look, grow)

Once words are categorized into these kinds of groups, students are taught the words in groups using any method frequently used to teach sight words. This particular approach can be used with any sight word list.

TABLE 5–10 Survival Words

poison	explosives	blasting
danger	flammable	gentlemen
police	doctor	pull
emergency	go	down
stop	telephone	detour
hot	boys	gasoline
walk	contaminated	inflammable
caution	ladies	in
exit	dynamite	push
men	ambulance	nurse
women	girls	information
warning	open	lifeguard
entrance	out	listen
help	combustible	private
off	closed	quiet
on	condemned	look
up	wanted	

Source: Polloway, C.A., & Polloway, C.H. (1981). Validation of a survival vocabulary. *Academic Therapy, 16,* 446.

Edmark Reading Program   The *Edmark Reading Program* (Edmark Associates, 1972) is an example of a commercial reading program based on the whole word approach. Masters and Mori (1986 note that the goal of the *Edmark* program is for students to be able to recognize words and know their meaning. The program includes 227 lessons, each focusing on 1. recognizing words, 2. following directions, 3. picture-phrase matching, and 4. oral reading from storybooks (Wallace *et al.*, 1987). The original purpose of the program was to teach students with mental retardation a sight word vocabulary of 150 words (Wallace *et al.*, 1987).

There are several advantages of the *Edmark* program for students with mental retardation. These include:

- lessons are broken into small, teachable units;

- students are allowed to progress through the lessons at their own rate;

- positive reinforcements are an integral part of the program (Wallace *et al.*, 1987).

The program has been shown to be successful with students who are experiencing disabilities.

The Fernald Approach   Grace Fernald developed a remedial reading and spelling program in 1943 that has continued to be used more than forty years. While the model has been modified numerous times over the past several decades (Adelman & Taylor, 1989), the approach uses a multisensory format and requires students to use the visual, auditory, kinesthetic, and tactile senses (Lerner, 1988). Hence, the program has been called the VAKT model. The method basically uses a whole word approach, focusing on recognizing words rather than sounds associated with letters.

Salend (1990) describes the Fernald method as a four-step process. In step one, students trace a model of a word, saying each syllable of the word during the tracing movement. Students are encouraged to use the new word in a story. Activities in this step are repeated until the student can write the word from memory. In step two of the Fernald method, students try to write the new word after seeing the model and visualizing the word with their eyes closed; they do not trace the word first. The words are then compared to the model. In step three, students try to read the word, then write the word from print. Finally, in the final step of the Fernald method, students attempt to read new, unfamiliar words through comparisons with known words (Salend, 1990). Research suggests that the use of a multisensory, kinesthetic model, such as the Fernald model, is effective with disabled students (Barudin & Hourcade, 1990).

Whole Language Remedial Approaches

As the whole language reading model has become popular in regular elementary classrooms, it has also become a focus in reading remediation. Marino and Gerber (1990) describe an application of the whole language model to students with disabilities. The four steps of the approach are:

1. Teaching a list of sight words to students.

2. Having students write sentences using words from the sight word list previously mastered.

3. Using teacher-made books that include words from the mastered sight word list.

4. Reading in a commercial, reading series.

This application of the whole language approach takes advantage of basal series for application purposes without totally relying on the basal approach.

When using the whole language reading mode, an important step is conferencing. The reading conference is when the reader shares with someone (teacher, parent, volunteer, other student) what has been read. Many schools use adult volunteers to serve as the "teacher" role in the conferencing process. The person in this role listens to the student's story, without undue criticism. The key is for students to read their stories and gain confidence in their reading and writing skills. An important principle in the reading conference is that the student has ownership of the reading. That is to say that the student decides what to do with what has been read (Rhodes & Dudley-Marling, 1988).

Language Experience Approach

This reading approach incorporates students' experiences and language for instructional purposes. Students relate stories to teachers, who write the story. Students then learn to read their own stories. After learning how to write, students write their own stories (Gillespie-Silver, 1982). This approach to reading enables students to conceptualize written material as follows:

What I can think about, I can talk about.

What I can say, I can write (or someone can write for me).

What I can write, I can read.

I can read what others write for me to read." (Lerner, 1988, p. 376)

The language experience model is similar to the whole language reading method in several ways. A series of prewritten, reading books is not used, and students rely on their own subject content for reading materials.

Ekwall and Shanker (1988) suggest the following procedure for using the language experience model with disabled students.

1. Discuss some event of great interest. Afterward ask students if they would like to write a story about it.

2. As students dictate the story, write it on chart paper using the following methods:

    a. Use manuscript or cursive writing, whichever is common to the age-grade level of the group.

    b. Use a heavy writing instrument such as a felt-tip pen.

    c. Use the language of the students and do not attempt to alter it.

    d. Make sure students see the words as they are being written.

    e. Try to adhere to the one important event and follow a sequence of events.

    f. Use one-line sentences for severely disabled readers and gradually increase sentence length as improvement is noted.

    g.   In beginning each new sentence, emphasize the fact that you start on the left and proceed to the right.

    h.   Emphasize the return sweep from the end of one sentence to the beginning of the next.

3. After the story has been completed, reread it as a choral exercise. Either you or a child may point to each word as it is read. It is important that the word being read is the same one being pointed to.

4. Have individual children take turns rereading the story sentence by sentence.

5. Duplicate the story on a large piece of tagboard and have students cut it into sentence strips. These can then be put in a pocket chart to form the original story. Go back to the original chart when necessary. Also let students rearrange the sentences to form a different order of events.

6. After students have read the story over many times, you may wish to cut the tagboard sentences up into words and let students form the original sentences and new sentences.

7. As more stories are dictated and read and as students build a larger sight vocabulary, you may wish to duplicate stories on ditto paper and give each student a copy to be cut up into sentences and/or words for building varying story order and new sentences.

8. As students' reading ability grows, you should begin to let each student write and illustrate his or her own stories. These can be bound into booklets with attractive covers on them indicating the author of each book. Students should then begin to read each other's books.

9. A great deal of emphasis should always be placed on rereading materials that were written earlier, as children require a great many exposures to each word before it becomes a sight word. After sight vocabularies begin to grow considerably, students can begin to read library or trade books. (pp. 110–111).

Direct Instruction

A general teaching approach that has significance for remediating reading is direct instruction. This particular model emphasizes teacher-led group activities that focus on individual needs (Mandlebaum, 1989). Direct instruction in reading attempts to teach essential skills using the most efficient means available. A great deal of research data collected in large-scale studies has supported the direct instruction approach in teaching reading skills (Carnine *et al.*, 1990).

Direct instruction includes three critical components: organization of instruction, program design, and teacher presentation techniques. The first component, organization of instruction, deals with the way teachers organize their reading programs to take maximum advantage of the amount of time students spend on reading activities. In order to do this, teachers must schedule efficiently and have appropriate materials available. Students need to be engaged in reading activities as much as possible to optimize learning opportunities. Not scheduling students properly and not being prepared with appropriate materials only wastes time that could better be spent on reading activities (Carnine *et al.*, 1990).

Program design, the second component of direct instruction, is the teacher's ability to use appropriate programs to meet the specific needs of students. This could encompass using the right program for a particular child, or actually developing a program for a single student whose needs are not being met by other approaches. The final component of direct instruction is the way teachers present reading instruction. Being able to use different methods, such as small group instruction, oral reading, and monitoring, at appropriate times is a critical component of the direct reading program (Carnine *et al.*, 1990).

Teachers can adopt programs for direct instruction, or use commercially prepared programs that utilize the direct instruction approach. One such commercial program is Direct Instructional System for Teaching Arithmetic and Reading (DISTAR). The DISTAR reading system (Englemann & Bruner, 1984) is a very structured reading program that is based on directed instruction, drill, and repetition (Lerner, 1988). It was originally developed for use with disadvantaged and slow learning students, but it has since been revised to be used with students who experience reading disabilities (Wallace, Cohen, & Polloway, 1987).

DISTAR is used with small, homogeneous groups of students and is fast paced. An advantage of the DISTAR program for students with disabilities is that constant, positive reinforcement is provided during the reading program. This works well with disabled students who have experienced significant failure and who need constant reassurance of their success. The DISTAR program initially focuses on left-right and sequencing skills, then it encourages blending through a say-it-fast approach (Wallace *et al.*, 1987).

Other Remedial Programs

There are some remedial programs that do not specifically fit into one of the major groups previously described. These programs have been used with varying degrees of effectiveness with students who are experiencing reading problems.

Merrill Linguistic Reading Approach   The Merrill Linguistic Reading Program (Otto, Randolph, Smith, & Wilson, 1975) is a structural, linguistic model. The program is designed for students in first through sixth grades who need a structured format. A basic premise of the program is that most words and sentences used have many similarities; students need to be taught these similarities. The program includes reading books, skills books, a testing series, reinforcement materials, and practice kits (Gillespie-Silver, 1982).

SQ3R   There are several different strategies that can be used to help students develop comprehension skills. One method that has been used for several years is the SQ3R method. The SQ3R reading program includes five steps: survey, question, read, recite, and review. Developed in the early 1960s, this method is primarily designed to help students improve comprehension skills. Mercer (1987) describes the activities that occur in each step.

1. *Survey*   The initial step has the reader scanning the material to be read. Headings, introductory statements, summaries, margin notes, and graphic aids such as tables and charts are the primary focus during this step. The purpose is to give the reader an overview of the materials.

2. *Question*   Questions are developed by the reader based on the information acquired during the survey step. These questions will help focus the reader's attention on specific content during the reading stage.

3. *Read*   During this step in the SQ3R method, the reader reads the material and attempts to answer the questions previously developed. The reader may wish to take notes during this step.

4. *Recite*   After reading the materials, the reader attempts to recite the answers to the previously formulated questions. This is done without using the reading materials or any notes made during reading.

5. *Review*   The reader checks the answers to the questions to the content in the reading passage. Sections may be reread if the reader feels that additional clarification is needed.

High Interest-Low Vocabulary Materials   Elementary-aged students with reading problems generally have appropriate-level materials that represent their chronological-age interest. However, as students get older and their reading levels remain at lower elementary levels, finding age-appropriate materials that are on the appropriate reading level becomes a problem. There are some materials that have been developed that focus on high interest materials with a low reading level. Lerner (1988) provides us with a list of the programs with these characteristics.

- *Challenger* (New Readers Press) with one through six reading level;

- *Focus: Reading for Success* (Scott, Foresman) with a K through eight reading level;

- *High Action Reading Series* (Modern Curriculum Press), reading level two through six;

- *Key-Text* (The Economy Company), reading level pp through eight;

- *New Directions in Reading* (Houghton-Mifflin) with a two through seven level;

- *The New Open Highways Program* (Scott, Foresman), level one through eight;

- *Program de lectura en espanol* (Spanish) (Houghton-Mifflin), reading level K through eight;

- *Quest* (Scholastic) with a reading level of two through eight;

- *Rally* (Harcourt Brace Jovanovich), grade level two through eight;

- *The Reading Connection* (Open Court), with a reading level of second through eleventh grade, fifth month;

- *Reading for Today* (Steck-Vaughn), reading level one through five;

- *Scott, Foresman, Spanish Reading Program* (Scott, Foresman), one through five;

- *Spanish Reading Series* (The Economy Company), grade level one through five; and

- *Sprint Reading Skills Program* (Scholastic), with a grade level of one through five.

Teacher Made Materials and Activities

In addition to commercially prepared materials, teachers can develop their own age-appropriate, level-appropriate materials. A key in the development of these materials is the readability level of the materials. Even with stimulating content, students will have difficulty reading materials that are too difficult. Therefore, teachers must determine the readability of materials to ensure that the level meets the needs of students.

There are several ways to determine the readability of materials. The easiest way is to simply review the materials and make a judgment about the readability level. Teachers who have had a great deal of experience teaching students at various age levels can often make good readability estimates. New computer technology can also be used to determine readability (Ekwall & Shanker, 1988). There are also formulas that teachers can apply to reading materials to develop readability levels. Although these formulas vary, most contain some of the following (Carnine, 1990):

average length of words;

relative frequency of words;

length of sentences;

relative complexity of sentences.

Each readability formula will provide specific guidelines for using these criteria.

Teacher Activities   There are numerous activities that teachers can use to help students with reading problems. In fact, the creativity of the teacher is the only factor that limits reading remediation activities. One method teachers use to teach reading skills is modeling. Modeling can be defined as providing opportunities for students to observe appropriate reading behaviors (Slavin, 1988; Woolfolk, 1990). Teachers can model reading skills by reading to students or reading silently (Mandlebaum, 1989). Students without reading problems can also serve as reading role models for those experiencing problems. By giving students the opportunity to observe appropriate reading behaviors, teachers provide examples that could be followed by other students. The process of modeling "minimizes the guesswork in learning how reading works." (Duffy, Roehler, & Hermann, 1988, p. 762) Modeling can help students develop oral reading skills, silent reading skills, and comprehension skills (Roe, Stoodt, & Burns, 1987).

Associated with modeling is peer tutoring. Labbo and Teale (1990) describe a way to have cross-age helpers improve reading skills. In this approach, students with good reading skills read with students who have reading problems. The conclusion from the study suggested that "a cross-age program is a promising way of helping poor readers in the upper elementary grades to improve their reading." (p. 368)

Lipson and Wickizer (1989) describe a process where students' reading abilities are improved by making them more cognizant of their own reading abilities. For example, students are intentionally stopped during their reading to describe what they are doing. At this juncture, teachers should provide specific feedback concerning the child's reading activities. In order to provide specific feedback, teachers should 1. listen carefully to the child's description, 2. attent to the child, 3. describe the strategy the child is using, and 4. provide reinforcement to the child for using specific strategies.

Methods to Teach or Improve Comprehension

As previously stated, without comprehension skills reading is a relatively moot process. Individuals read in order to understand the written language presented. Comprehension is a major component of reading and is often a skill deficit for students with disabilities (Fowler & Davis, 1985; Sinatra, Berg, & Dunn, 1985; Graves, 1987). There are some students who can read orally with perfection without having any comprehension of the content.

There are several ways to help students improve their comprehension skills. The *SQ3R* method previously described, as well as storytelling, are excellent examples of ways to improve reading comprehension. Fowler and Davis (1985) present a method for improving the reading comprehension of students with mild mental retardation. This model, called the story frame approach, uses frames developed by the teacher that help focus the student's attention during the reading process. The frames can be reused in subsequent reading activities. Examples of frames that must be completed when using this model include 1. the problem in this story _____; 2. it started when _____; and 3. the story ends _____.

This method is actually a modified cloze process or advance organizer. Cudd and Roberts (1987) suggest that when using story frames, teachers focus their initial intervention on simple frames. After students successfully learn how to use these simple frames, more complex frames can be utilized. The success of story frames results in providing the reader prereading cues that help keep students focused on the story content (Fowler & Davis, 1985).

Another method for improving reading comprehension of students with disabilities is through semantic mapping (Sinatra *et al.*, 1985). Semantic mapping enables students to organize and categorize the information they obtain through reading. Students can be taught how to do this with graphic illustrations of the relationships among the different components in the reading passage. A semantic map is similar to a diagram of a sentence. Important parts of the reading passage are put into specific categories that make it easy for the student to remember what was read.

Graves (1987) described several methods for improving comprehension skills for students with disabilities. These methods include one that helps students find the main idea in a story by writing the main idea sentence for a reading passage. In this method, students first write the main idea of a story based on a group of sentences. After mastering this process, students select a main idea from a list of possible ideas based on a short reading section.

Other methods Graves (1987) suggests to build comprehension skills include ordering instruction developmentally and using learning strategies. In the first method, ordering instruction developmentally, students are taught how to locate factual information from a reading passage. Following this, they are given opportunities for drawing inferences from reading materials. The learning strategies approach teaches students to use various strategies to facilitate comprehension. For example, note taking during reading and understanding how to look for important facts, such as bold type and margin notes, help students focus on the important content.

Wallace *et al.*, (1987) suggest several general procedures for building and improving comprehension skills for students with disabilities.

- Have students answer *when, where, who, what,* and *why* questions as they read.

- Encourage students to predict what may happen in a story based upon what was already read.

- Have students ask comprehension questions of the teacher or other students.

- Allow at least five seconds after each question for the student to think of the response.

- Teach students to follow an author's organization by pointing out signals, markers, and headings.

- Have students retell a particular passage in their own words.

- Teach students to reread sections that they do not understand.

- Discuss pictures or illustrations in the text as a clue to comprehension.

- Practice the ability to read in phrases or "chunking" to process thought units within a sentence.

- Teach students to form a mental image of what they read about.

- Provide direct instructions on meanings of words in the reading passage.

- Have students locate nonsense material purposely placed in a passage. (pp. 187–188)

GROUPING FOR READING INSTRUCTION

A topic found in all reading textbooks is grouping students for reading instruction. We all remember reading groups; some students are in the bluebirds, some in the redbirds, and some in the blackbirds. Although the groups are never labeled with ability levels, students know which group is the top and which group is the bottom. In most every elementary classroom where instruction in reading is part of the curriculum, teachers put students into small groups to teach reading skills. The idea for homogeneous grouping is to allow the teacher to teach students at their optimal rate (Anderson *et al.*, 1985).

In the lower elementary grades, teachers generally have three or four reading groups. The reading group for students with the best reading skills should be the largest group, generally eight to twelve students. Only three or four students should be assigned to the group for students with the lowest reading skills. The key factor in assigning students to groups should be the number of letter-sound correspondences and words known by individual students (Carnine, Silbert, & Kameenui, 1990).

As students get older, teachers may need to change their group placement. A critical consideration for teachers is that placement in a reading group is always only temporary. Students should be able to move from group to group as their skills require. Grouping students for reading will be enhanced if several teachers group students among classrooms. The more teachers and students available for reading groups results in more appropriate groups. Grouping should start with students who have the fewest reading skills and culminate in grouping students with the best reading abilities (Carnine *et al.*, 1990).

While grouping students for reading instruction can be beneficial, teachers also need to be aware of some possible negative outcomes. These include:

- students in lower groups frequently get less silent reading time than students in higher groups (Anderson *et al.*, 1985);

- less is often expected of students in lower groups (Smith *et al.*, 1986);

- it may be difficult for students to move among groups (Anderson *et al.*, 1985); and

- students in lower groups do not have good reading models.

As a result of these and other problems, the Commission on Reading recommends that teachers use instructional arrangements other than simply relying on reading groups. Whole class instruction is an option, as well as grouping students for small-group purposes rather than grouping based on ability levels (Anderson *et al.*, 1985).

SENSORY TRAINING AND READING PROBLEMS

Over the years, there have been numerous professionals who have advocated the relationship between sensory perception and reading abilities. These individuals have promoted sensory perceptual remediation as a way of facilitating reading gains. Supporters of this notion were widespread during the 1960s; however, during recent years the credibility of this approach has been severely challenged (Smith *et al.*, 1986; Mercer, 1987; Lerner, 1988).

Research findings have consistently found limited or no relationships between sensory perception and reading skills (Smith *et al.*, 1986; Marsh, Price, & Smith, 1983). Certainly, the research has not supported the notion of remediating reading deficiencies through training in sensory perception. Unfortunately, "despite ample research refuting such claims, private sensory screening and training programs flourish in the U.S." (Casbergue & Greene, 1988, p. 197) Teachers need to be aware of the lack of empirical data supporting perceptual-motor training and be able to explain this limitation to parents who may wish to experiment with different intervention strategies.

TECHNOLOGY AND READING INSTRUCTION

Reading instruction, like many different academic areas, lends itself well to uses of instructional technology. The computer explosion of the 1980s had a tremendous impact on the uses of computers in education. For example, the number of computers in schools increased from 13,986 in 1982 to more than 30,000 in 1983, more than doubling in a single academic year (National Center for Education Statistics, 1984). In the 1986-1987 school year, there were more than two million computers in public schools (Goodspeed, 1988). With such widespread increase in the number of computers, computer applications have grown rapidly.

The most likely model for computer usage in instruction is through computer assisted instruction (CAI). CAI can be defined as a two-way communication and learning process between the learner and computer. When using CAI, learning is individual and focuses on the unique needs of the learner. CAI is primarily used in drill-and-practice, tutorial, and simulations (Lockard, Abrams, & Many, 1987).

Technology can be used in reading instruction in a variety of applications, but CAI is the primary mode. Drill-and-practice, information presentation through the use of tutorials, simulations, and problem solving activities are the predominant means of using CAI in reading (Wallace & McLoughlin, 1988). Drill-and-practice helps supplement more traditional reading instruction (Wallace *et al.*, 1987).

As with any teaching tool, the computer can be used improperly and result in "busy work" time for students. Simply allowing students to play games and perform redundant drill activities does not take advantage of the technology. Perkins (1988) suggests that, when using computer technology, teachers combine computers with other instructional materials, form small groups to work together on computer projects, provide direct teaching as well as student monitoring, and facilitate generalization of learned skills.

When selecting appropriate computer software for reading instruction, school personnel should be aware of the many different qualities that are necessary for effective materials. For example, software should be evaluated for sight vocabulary, word identification, comprehension, and study skills (Scott & Barker, 1987). Table 5–11 presents a checklist that might be helpful in selecting software for reading instructional activities.

Teaching Listening Skills

Just as reading is a critical skill for students in order to process information from written materials, listening is important for processing oral information. Without listening skills, students are at a major disadvantage in school settings. Think of all the information and instructions teachers provide students orally. As students get older, less and less information is presented visually in classrooms; teachers tend to rely on lectures and "telling" students information. In fact, lecturing is the most predominantly used instructional method used at the secondary level (Smith, 1990). Limited listening skills can result in a significant problem.

NATURE OF LISTENING

Listening is not a simple process where the ear transmits information to the brain; it involves many different components. Among the many parts of listening are auditory acuity, attention to auditory signals, sound discrimination, auditory memory, and listening comprehension (Polloway & Smith, 1992). The majority of children do not have any problems with listening. With the exception of simply not paying attention, listening is generally not problematic. However, for a small number of children, deficits in listening are significant enough to cause problems. These children may not "hear" the oral message and are therefore left out of what is going on around them. This could be the result of hearing problems, for example, being hard of hearing or deaf, or it could result from simply having listening problems.

TABLE 5–11 Checklist for Evaluating Reading Software

	RESPONSE		
QUESTION	Yes	No	Comments

1. Are appropriate hardware and peripherals available?

2. Are there back-up discs available?

3. Does software match the reading curriculum?

4. Can software be incorporated in lesson plans?

5. Is the software cost efficient?

6. Are there written materials that describe how the software should be used?

7. Does the software require a management system?

8. Is in-service training or staff development included in the program?

9. Is there an opportunity to preview the software?

10. Can the software be used as a self-paced program?

11. Are the graphics well done?

12. Do students like the software?

Source: D. Scott & J. Barker (1987). Guidelines for selecting and evaluating reading software: Improving the decision making process. *The Reading Teacher, 40,* 884–887.

ASSESSING LISTENING PROBLEMS

Just as reading skills need to be assessed before appropriate intervention techniques can be determined and implemented, listening skills also need to be determined to facilitate appropriate intervention programs. Formal or informal approaches are used to assess listening skills.

Formal Assessment of Listening Skills

Formal methods to evaluate listening skills generally use one of the following models (Burns & Richgels, 1988):

1. rote recall—ability to recall information presented orally;

2. following directions—ability to listen and follow directions given orally;

3. multiple-choice—ability to select correct response from a multiple-choice format after listening to information;

4. free recall—ability to retell a story that has been read orally; and

5. informal reading inventory—ability to respond orally to questions related to content read to the student in sequentially more difficult passages.

There are only a few formal tests available to assess listening skills. Most of these are in the form of subtests found in tests for language arts. The best advice when attempting to evaluate a student's listening skills is to use informal assessment practices. This will not only provide more flexibility in the potential ways to assess listening, but it will also afford more useable information.

Informal Assessment of Listening Skills

Teachers are in an excellent position to observe listening skills and assess their students ability to listen. Everyday oral communication between children and others provides an excellent opportunity for informally assessing listening skills in a natural language environment. Whereas formal tests of listening require students to "perform" certain tasks, often in contrived settings, informal assessment simply occurs as part of the student's routine communication process.

Just as with any area, teachers will likely do a better job of assessing listening skills if they have a structured format to follow. There are numerous checklists available to assess listening skills. Table 5–12 presents an example of a listening check list.

METHODS TO TEACH LISTENING SKILLS

Students who display listening deficits need assistance to develop skills to enable them to process auditory information. There are several assumptions that must be made about listening instruction before attempting to remediate listening deficits. These include:

1. Listening skills are teachable to some students.

2. Students cannot simply be made to listen; situations can be manipulated to facilitate the improvement of listening skills.

3. Listening must be active between the speaker and listener.

4. Listening is easily incorporated into any teaching activity.

5. There are different forms of listening and therefore different ways to teach listening (Wallace *et al.*, 1987).

TABLE 5-12 Checklist to Determine Listening Skills

	SETTINGS SKILLS USED			
LISTENING SKILLS	Informal	Academic	Small Group	Large Group
1. Pays attention				
2. Discriminates environmental sounds				
3. Recognizes environmental sounds				
4. Attends to important auditory stimuli				
5. Pronounces common words correctly				
6. Follows oral directions				
7. Recalls facts heard				
8. Remembers concepts heard				
9. Answers orally asked questions properly				
10. Participates in conversations and discussions				

Source: Wallace, G., Cohen, S.B., & Polloway, E.A. (1987). *Language Arts.* Austin, TX: PRO-ED. p. 81.

Storytelling

One of the oldest activities, and one that can be used effectively to help students develop listening skills is storytelling. Peck (1989) notes that storytelling is experiencing a "renaissance" in schools. Storytelling can help children develop a positive attitude about oral and written expression (Roney, 1989). One of the most important aspects of storytelling is the bond that can develop between the teller and listener (Nelson, 1989). Storytelling can occur in just about any setting. A school classroom is an excellent site for storytelling, as well as outside on the playground, on the school bus, or in the assembly room. Teachers often set aside specific times for storytelling. They may tell the stories, or they may rotate the story telling among students.

Advanced Listening Organizers

One of the primary components of a listening program is to ensure that students are attending to the auditory stimuli. Without attending to the auditory signal, students are not capable of comprehending the message. Therefore, teaching students to pay attention to auditory information is important. There are many different ways teachers can help students focus on auditory information. In one such model, Forster and Doyle (1989) describe a process that relies on taped news broadcast. Students listen to the broadcast and complete missing information included on an outline they are given. This activity helps students focus on the information and "listen" for certain facts.

The activity just described is a form of a listening advanced organizer. Listening advanced organizers provide cues about what to listen for. By providing students with an outline of the information they are about to hear, they are better able to attend to the auditory information and comprehend the material (Robinson, 1989). For example, if you are listening for directions on getting to a particular place, you pay more attention to the speaker when directions start to be given.

Teacher Listening Role Model

One excellent way to improve listening skills of students is for teachers to demonstrate good listening skills. Just as teachers can model appropriate reading skills, they can also model effective listening skills. Teachers need to attend to students who are trying to tell them something. Often teachers ignore students and do not pay attention to those who are desparately trying to get their attention. Other than those cases where teachers are using "planned ignoring" in an attempt to limit reinforcement for inappropriate behaviors, they should always try to be attentive to their students. By paying attention to students, teachers are setting a good example and are serving as good listening models for their students.

Because teachers often get caught up in the hectic activities of the classroom, they may not realize that they are not listening to some students. Teachers have a tendency to listen to certain students and inadvertently ignore others. Often the students who are not "heard" are those with mild disabilities. One way teachers can avoid this oversight is to keep a daily log and make notes by each student's name as that student is "listened to". Teachers might also set orchestrated interactions with each student to model proper listening.

Activities for Improving Listening Skills

Materials to teach listening skills are in our everyday environment. Teachers can have students listen to a variety of different auditory information as part of listening exercises. Wallace, Cohen, and Polloway (1987) list the following real-life listening activities that can help students become better listeners.

- Listening to the news, a comedy show, or movie.
- Talking to a friend.
- Taking notes in class.
- Arguing with a sibling.
- Learning new information.

- Following a parent's directions.

- Responding to instructional questions.

- Listening to a story.

- Hearing a lecture.

- Listening to records.

- Making arrangements.

- Using the telephone.

- Taking orders for materials/services.

- Interviewing for a job.

- Listening to a joke.

These activities are simple; they do not require expensive materials or elaborate instructions. They are simple, everyday activities that help students focus their auditory attention. The key is that teachers can use real life situations to teach the natural skill of listening.

Lerner (1988) describes several different ways to enhance listening skills of students. These include 1. activities to teach auditory awareness, 2. activities to facilitate understanding words, 3. ways to help students understand sentences, 4. activities to teach listening comprehension, and 5. teaching critical listening skills. Examples of activities in these areas include:

Teaching Auditory Awareness

Use real objects or pictures of objects to teach initial consonants.

Make up riddle rhymes to teach sounds.

Play bingo with consonant blends instead of numbers.

Facilitating Understanding Words

Use real objects to teach names of objects.

Teach verbs that can be illustrated, such as "jump."

Teach classes of objects, such as food and clothes.

Facilitating Understanding of Sentences

Have students follow directions given in sentences.

Have students identify the correct picture out of a series of pictures that best describe a story.

Have the students use the cloze technique to fill in a missing word from a sentence.

Teaching Auditory Memory Skills

Read a story and ask questions about specific details.

Read a story and have the student arrange a series of pictures in the same sequence as in the story.

Read a set of directions on how to make something; have students try to make the object after the reading.

Teaching Critical Listening Skills

Tell a story with parts that do not fit; have students identify those parts.

Have students listen to advertisements on a radio or television and describe how the seller is trying to convince the buyer.

Finally, Choate and Rakes (1989) suggest several strategies to help students develop listening skills. The following describes some of these methods.

1. Use instructional adaptations to facilitate listening, such as arranging seating to limit distractions and maximize use of visual aids.

2. Screen out auditory and visual distractors by having students sit without looking at doors and windows, and using background music to screen out auditory distractors.

3. Implement a cuing system so students will be aware when something important is going to be said.

4. Have students verbally sum up what was recently discussed.

5. Have students practice listening to audio tapes with the volume at different levels.

6. Have students retell stories.

7. Read a passage out loud and then ask questions that require more than simple answers.

8. Use a modified cloze method; read a story and leave out one important sentence. After reading the story, give students an option of three sentences, one of which fits into the story.

9. Read a story then ask questions that require students to make judgments.

10. Read a story and have students imagine sound effects that would fit. Then reread the story with students supplying the sound effects.

SUMMARY

This chapter has focused on receptive language. The beginning of the chapter noted the importance of receptive language for humans. Specifically, it was noted that without the ability to understand spoken language through listening and the ability to understand written language through reading, humans would not have achieved their successes. It was then noted that for some individuals, deficits in listening or reading create major problems in academic work, vocational settings, and social interactions.

Teaching reading was the next major section in the chapter. The nature of reading was discussed, with an emphasis on the fact that reading is a very complex process that includes decoding information as well as comprehending its content. Problems in decoding prevent comprehension; problems in comprehension make the decoding process fairly unimportant. Individuals need to have skills in both major areas. How to assess reading skills was discussed. It was noted that, although there are numerous norm-referenced tests available, informal assessment procedures, such as informal reading inventories and observations, provide extremely valuable information.

The primary methods of teaching reading, including phonics, whole word, and whole language methods, were discussed. It was noted that no one particular method has been adopted universally. In fact, there appears to be overlap among the major approaches. Regardless of the method used, the majority of schools continue to rely on basal reading programs as a core for reading instruction. These programs provide a scope and sequence of skills, as well as materials for students and teachers to follow.

A new method of teaching reading, the whole language model, has been gaining popularity over the past several years. This approach does not use reading textbooks, but relies on students learning to read using "real" reading materials. Students use their own writing, as well as novels and other documents, to develop reading skills.

For students with disabilities, problems in reading are common. In fact, it was noted that students with mild mental retardation, learning disabilities, and behavior disorders, frequently exhibit problems in reading. Reading remediation programs must be used to facilitate reading among these students. Ways to improve reading were discussed, including commercially prepared programs to teacher-made activities.

The final section of the chapter focused on teaching listening skills. It was noted that, like reading skills, deficits in listening result in major problems in academic, vocational, and social settings. Although most students listen very adequately, some students experience problems with listening. For these students, teachers need to develop intervention programs that will focus on improved listening.

The chapter included information about how to assess listening skills as well as ways to improve the listening skills of students with deficits. It was noted that informal assessment generally provides better information than formal assessment, and that teacher-developed activities can be created in the natural setting of the classroom. These activities can greatly help students with their listening skills.

REFERENCES

Adelman, H.S., & Taylor, L. (1989). The Fernald techniques from a motivational perspective. *Academic Therapy, 24,* 243–259.

Algozzine, B., O'Shea, D.J., Stoddard, K., & Crews, W.B. (1988). Reading and writing competencies of adolescents with learning disabilities. *Journal of Learning Disabilities, 21,* 154–160.

Anderson, R.C., Hiebert, E.H., Scott, J.A., & Wilkinson, I.A.G. (1985). *Becoming a nation of readers: The report of the commission on reading.* Washington, D.C.: The Center for the Study of Reading.

Barnard, D.P., & Hetzel, R.W. (1989). *Selecting a basal reading program.* Lancaster, Pennsylvania: Technomic Publishing Co.

Barudin, S.I., & Hourcade, J.J. (1990). Relative effectiveness of three methods of reading instruction in developing specific recall and transfer skills in learners with moderate and severe mental retardation. *Education and Training in Mental Retardation, 25,* 286–291.

Baumann, J.F. (1988). Direct instruction reconsidered. *Journal of Reading, 31,* 712–718.

Burns, J.M., & Richgels, D.J. (1988). A critical evaluation of listening tests. *Academic Therapy, 24,* 153–162.

Carnine, D., Silbert, J., & Kameenui, E.J. (1990). *Direct instruction reading,* 2nd Ed. Columbus, OH: Merrill.

Casbergue, R.M., & Greene, J.F. (1988). Persistent misconceptions about sensory perception and reading disability. *Journal of Reading, 32,* 196–203.

Choate, J.S., & Rakes, T.A. (1989). *Reading: Detecting and correcting special needs.* Boston: Allyn & Bacon.

Cooper, J.D., Warncke, E. W., & Shipman, D.A. (1988). *The what and how of reading instruction.* Columbus, OH: Merrill.

Cudd, E.T., & Roberts, L.L. (1987). Using story frames to develop reading comprehension in a 1st grade classroom. *The Reading Teacher, 41,* 74–79.

Culyer, R. (1988). Using single concept cards and sentences for affective and effective reading. *Academic Therapy, 24,* 143–152.

Duffy, G.G., Roehler, L.R., & Herrmann, B.A. (1988). Modeling mental processes helps poor readers become strategic readers. *The Reading Teacher, 41,* 762–767.

Ekwall, E.E., & Shanker, J.L. (1988). *Diagnosis and remediation of the disabled reader,* 3rd Ed. Boston: Allyn & Bacon.

Epstein, M.H., & Cullinan, D. (1982). Characteristics of mild behavioral disorders. In T.L. Miller & E.E. Davis (Eds.) *The mildly handicapped student.* New York: Grune & Stratton.

Fessler, M.A., Rosenberg, M.S., & Rosenberg, L.A. (1991). Concomitant learning disabilities and learning problems among students with behavioral/emotional disorders. *Behavioral Disorders, 16,* 97–106.

Fowler, G.L., & Davis, M. (1985). The story frame approach: A tool for improving comprehension of EMR children. *Teaching Exceptional Children, 17,* 296–298.

Fuchs, L.S., & Fuchs, D. (1984). Teaching beginning reading skills: A unique approach. *Teaching Exceptional Children, 17,* 48–53.

Gillespie-Silver, P. (1982). Meaning-seeking strategies and special reading programs. In T.L. Miller & E.E. Davis (Eds.) *The mildly handicapped student.* New York: Grune and Stratton.

Graves, A.W. (1987). Improving comprehension skills. *Teaching Exceptional Children, 19,* 63–65.

Guerin, G.R., & Maier, A.S. (1983). *Informal assessment in education.* Palo Alto, CA: Mayfield Publishing.

Hargis, C.H. Terhaar-Yonkers, M., Williams, P.C. & Reed, M.T. (1988). Repetition requirements for word recognition. *Journal of Reading, 31,* 320–327.

Labbo, L.D., & Teale, W.H. (1990). Cross-age reading: A strategy for helping poor readers. *The Reading Teacher, 43,* 362–369.

Lerner, J. (1988). *Learning disabilities,* 5th Ed. Boston: Houghton-Mifflin.

Lipson, M.Y., & Wickizer, E.A. (1989). Promoting self-control and active reading through dialogues. *Teaching Exceptional Children, 21,* 28–32.

Luftig, R.L. (1988). *Assessment of learners with special needs.* Boston: Allyn and Bacon.

McClure, A.A. (1985). Another way to teach reading to learning disabled children. *Teaching Exceptional Children, 17,* 267–273.

Madden, L. (1988). Improve reading attitudes of poor readers through cooperative reading teams. *The Reading Teacher, 42,* 194–199.

Mandelbaum, L.H. (1989). Reading. In G.A. Robinson, J.R. Patton, E.A. Polloway, and L.R. Sargent (Eds.) *Best practices in mild mental retardation.* Reston, VA: Division on Mental Retardation, Council for Exceptional Children.

Marsh, G.E., Price, B.J., & Smith, T.E.C. (1983). *Teaching children with mild disabilities.* St. Louis: C.V. Mosby.

Mastropieri, M.A., Jenkins, V., & Scruggs, T.E. (1985). Academic and intellectual characteristics of behaviorally disordered children and youth. In R.B. Rutherford (Ed.) *Monograph in behavioral disorders.* Tempe, AZ: Arizona State University.

Mercer, C.D. (1987). *Students with learning disabilities.* Columbus, OH: Merrill.

Morris, M., & Leuenberger, J. (1990). A report of cognitive, academic, and linguistic profiles for college students with and without learning disabilities. *Journal of Learning Disabilities, 23,* 355–361.

Peck, J. (1989). Using storytelling to promote language and literacy development. *The Reading Teacher, 43,* 138–141.

Peters, E., & Lloyd, J. (1987). Effective instruction in reading. *Teaching Exceptional Children, 19,* 58.

Polloway, E.A., & Smith, T.E.C. (1992). *Teaching language skills to exceptional learners,* 2nd Ed. Denver: Love Publishing.

Rhodes, L.K., & Dudley-Marling, C. (1988). *Readings and writers with a difference: A holistic approach to teaching learning disabled and remedial students.* Portsmouth, NH: Heinemann.

Ridley, L. (1990). Enacting change in elementary school programs: Implementing a whole language perspective. *The Reading Teacher, 43,* 640–646.

Roe, B.D., Stoodt, B.D., & Burns, P.C. (1987). *Secondary school reading instruction in the content areas,* 3rd Ed. Boston: Houghton-Mifflin.

Roney, R.C. (1989). Back to the basics with storytelling. *The Reading Teacher, 42,* 520–523.

Rowe, & Rayford, (1987).

Samuels, S.J. (1988). Information processing abilities and reading. *Journal of Learning Disabilities, 20,* 18–22.

Salend, S.J. (1990). *Effective mainstreaming.* New York: MacMillan.

Scott, D., & Barker, J. (1987). Guidelines for selecting and evaluating reading software: Improving the decision making process. *The Reading Teacher, 40,* 884–887.

Simms, R.B., & Falcon, S.C. (1987). Teaching sight words. *Teaching Exceptional Children, 20,* 30–33.

Sinatra, R.C., Berg, D., & Dunn, R. (1985). Semantic mapping improves reading comprehension of learning disabled students. *Teaching Exceptional Children, 17,* 310–314.

Smith, T.E.C. (1990). *Introduction to education,* 2nd Ed. St. Paul: West Publishing.

Smith, T.E.C., Price, B.J., & Marsh, G.E. (1986). *Mildly handicapped children and adults.* St. Paul: West Publishing.

Snider, V.E., & Tarver, S.G. (1987). The effect of early reading failure on acquisition of knowledge among students with learning disabilities. *Journal of Learning Disabilities, 20,* 351–356.

Strichart, S.S., & Gottlieb, J. (1982). Characteristics of mild mental retardation. In T.L. Miller and E.E. Davis (Eds.) *The mildly handicapped student.* New York: Grune & Stratton.

Wallace, G., Cohen, S.B., & Polloway, E.A. (1987). *Language arts.* Austin: PRO-ED.

Wallace, G., & McLoughlin, J.A. (1988). *Learning disabilities: Concepts and characteristics,* 3rd Ed. Columbus, OH: Merrill.

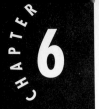

Expressive Language: Teaching Written and Oral Expressive Skills

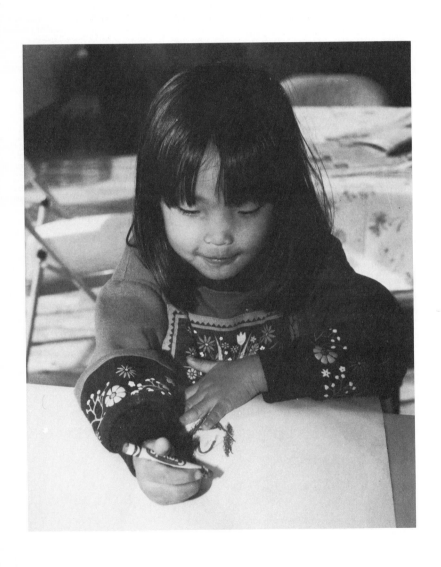

Outline

OBJECTIVES

After reading this chapter, you should be able to:

- describe the importance of expressive language;
- describe the major components of expressive language;
- describe how to assess expressive language skills;
- describe how to teach handwriting skills;
- discuss specific ways to improve spelling skills;
- describe how to assess written expression skills;
- describe some of the common methods to teach written expression;
- discuss the importance of oral expressive language;
- describe considerations in teaching oral expressive language.

Introduction

One of the most important skills that separate humans from other animal species is the ability to express themselves with language. While many other animal species are able to express themselves with various sounds, gestures, and movements, no species can match humans in the repertoire of expressive language skills. Their abilities to communicate, both orally and in written form, distinguish human beings from the rest of the animal kingdom. No doubt, these skills are partly responsible for the supremacy of humans over other animals.

Expressive language includes both written and oral language. Skills in both these areas are vitally important for individuals to function in our society. Being unable to speak or write severely limits our ability to communicate. The higher level of cognitive competence experienced by humans would be of limited benefit without expressive language abilities. Students who are unable to express themselves either in writing or orally are at a major disadvantage in school (Polloway & Smith, 1992). Think of the frustrations you would feel if you were unable to express your feelings to your friends or your needs to your parents or teachers. And how do limitations in oral expression affect a student in the third grade or limitations in written expression impact a student in the tenth grade? Obviously, a great deal of information flows from teachers to students, but the information flow from students to teachers is just as critical. Students express their feelings on topics orally and in writing, respond to questions orally and in writing, and complete assignments that require oral and written responses. Weaknesses in these areas result in frequent failures for students.

The consequences of not being proficient in oral or written language do not end when a student leaves school. Adults must be able to express themselves in vocational and social settings. Many jobs require workers to use oral or written expressive language. Individuals who have difficulties in these areas may not be eligible for certain jobs. For example, a telephone operator and a receptionist need to be able to express themselves orally. Likewise, newspaper reporters need to be able to use written expression. Even in jobs that do not require specific skills in oral and written expression, workers need to be able to express themselves in a general sense. Workers on an assembly line, for example, need to be able to indicate when the "line" needs to be stopped or slowed down, and when additional parts are needed to continue a particular job (Polloway & Smith, 1992).

Unfortunately, while the importance of oral and written expression is obvious, these skills are frequently not emphasized in the school's curriculum. Alexander (1983) noted the following regarding written expression.

- Composition is allocated less instructional time than reading in the elementary school, or than literature in the secondary school.

- The product receives greater attention than the process—composition instruction consists of assigning and evaluating.

- Composition consists of a set of skills that does not fit neatly into a scope and sequence schema.

■ Composition instruction suffers from several negative environmental factors: standardized tests focus on editing and correctness; commercial texts emphasize the product; and objectives of language arts instruction feature mechanics, usage, and punctuation. (p. 55)

While these concerns are related to instruction in written expression, similar problems exist in the area of oral communication. In fact, there is probably less time spent on oral expression skills in our schools than on written expression skills. Teachers rarely, except possibly in a class specifically designed for speech, focus on developing oral language skills.

It is impossible to determine which form of expression, written or oral, is more important. It is possible to state that deficiencies in either of these can have significant consequences for individuals at all age levels. Without the ability to express complicated messages, the human species moves much closer to other animal species down the ladder of sophisticated communication competence. Being able to receive and understand language, as well as build responses, are of little use without the ability to express the response. This chapter will describe problems experienced by students in written and oral expression and provide suggestions for remediating these problems.

A consideration when dealing with expressive language skills is multicultural concerns. As previously noted, the population in the United States continues to become more culturally diverse. Many students currently enrolled in public school programs are from minority cultural groups, and this cultural diversity is becoming more and more pronounced (Polloway & Smith, 1992). The language of many students from minority cultural homes often presents problems. For many students, English is a second language. The fact that English may not be the primary language spoken in the home environment often results in problems for students and the learning process.

Special education teachers must take into consideration different language patterns used by children from minority cultures. Assessment and intervention practices may need to be altered to appropriately serve this population of children. While professionals at one time considered the language used by these students to be deficient, the prevailing opinion is that the language is different, but not deficient (Polloway & Smith, 1992). These language differences present unique problems for school personnel who provide intervention services for students with disabilities from minority groups.

Written Language

Of all the different forms of communication, written language is the most complex. Indeed, it is considered by some to be the "highest achievement in language for all modern cultures" (Barenbaum, 1983, p. 12). Written language is not a simple skill, but a combination of myriad subskills, including 1. appropriate verbal concepts in receptive and expressive oral language, 2. the ability to read, 3. the ability to spell, 4. the ability to write legibly, and 5. the ability to transform ideas into logical, understandable information (Lutwig, 1989). The following sections describe some of the elements included in written language.

HANDWRITING

Handwriting is the mechanical component in written language. It is basically a perceptual motor skill that requires the person writing to know what is to be written, understand how to translate that information into letters and words, and then make those letters and words in such a manner that someone else can read and comprehend the information (Polloway & Smith, 1992). Handwriting is neither easily taught nor quickly learned; it can be characterized as a complex task that students learn over a period of several years (Bain, 1991).

In schools, both teachers and students use handwriting on a daily basis (Herbert, 1987). Teachers use handwriting to write on the board, write on students' papers when providing feedback, and making notes. They also use handwriting in written communications to parents concerning their child's performance and daily activities. Teachers with poor handwriting skills are inappropriate models for students. This is especially true at the elementary level where instruction in handwriting commonly occurs.

For students, the importance of good handwriting skills should be obvious; most assignments and tests are written, and teachers expect most written communications from students to be handwritten. If this handwritten communication is illegible or of significantly poor quality, teachers may develop a negative impression of the student that could carry over into other activities (Polloway & Smith, 1992). Students must also use handwriting to take notes in classes. If this handwriting is illegible, it may be of limited use at a later time when the student needs to study for a test or review notes for other purposes. For these, as well as other reasons, the handwriting skills of students are critical to their educational success (Phelps, Stempel, & Speck, 1985).

Although handwriting proficiency is very important to students, it is rarely considered a top priority in classrooms. Bain (1991) calls handwriting "the stepchild of written language." (p. 44) There are several reasons why instruction in handwriting has received such limited attention. These include:

- the process of handwriting instruction is tedious;

- improvement in handwriting is slow;

- teachers and parents may believe that students can do better if they would only try;

- there are limited testing instruments to measure handwriting skills;

- teachers receive limited training in handwriting instruction (Bain, 1991).

Regardless of the specific reasons why handwriting is not a priority, the fact remains that it is an important skill that deserves more attention from teachers.

Sequence of Handwriting Skills

When teaching students appropriate handwriting, teachers need to follow a sequence of skills. For example, students who have not established a proper pencil grip may not be ready for specific instructional activities related to writing letters legibly. Therefore, teachers need to understand the sequence of handwriting skills, determine where along this sequence students are experiencing problems, and develop intervention plans accordingly.

Polloway and Smith (1992) list ten different skills that comprise a sequence necessary for competence in handwriting. These are:

1. appropriately grasping crayons and paint brushes;

2. appropriately grasping pencils;

3. moving writing instrument in logical patterns;

4. reproducing written patterns;

5. copying letters and words;

6. writing letters and words;

7. developing fluidity of movements required for cursive writing;

8. copying letters and words using cursive;

9. using cursive to write letters and words; and

10. using cursive to write sentences and paragraphs.

Regardless of the list of skills used in teaching handwriting, teachers must be aware of the many different steps and skills required to produce legible, timely written information.

Handedness   One of the first skills that most children develop related to handwriting is the development of handedness. As we are all aware, the majority of people in our society are right-handed. Development of handedness generally occurs before a child starts to school. Most children naturally develop a preference for one hand over the other. Students who have not developed this preference may need to be encouraged to use one hand over the other to facilitate the handwriting process. Continuing not to have a preferred hand only makes the development of handwriting skills more difficult.

Pencil Grip   How students grip their writing utensil is an important skill that should be developed prior to writing activities. Many children will naturally grip a pencil in the proper manner, between the thumb and middle finger, balanced with the index finger. However, some students need assistance in learning proper pencil grip. Ways to assist students develop proper pencil grip include 1. placing a piece of tape or rubber band where the pencil should be gripped, 2. putting a pencil through a practice golf ball with holes to assist in the grip, 3. using a piece of clay around the pencil to assist the grip, and 4. using larger crayons and pencils (Lerner, 1988).

Prewriting Skills   There are numerous prewriting skills that students need to be able to perform before they begin writing in addition to establishing handedness and developing proper pencil grip. These include the ability to:

1. Perform hand movements such as up-down, left-right, and forward-back.

2. Trace geometric shapes and dotted lines.

3. Connect dots on paper.

4. Draw a horizontal line from left to right.

5. Draw a vertical line from top to bottom and bottom to top.

6. Draw a backward circle, a curved line, and a forward circle.

7. Draw slanted lines vertically.

8. Copy simple designs and shapes.

9. Name letters and discern likenesses and differences in letter forms (Mercer, 1987, p. 341).

Printing   The majority of students learn how to print or write using manuscript letters before they use cursive letters. Hagin (1983) noted that the practice of teaching students to use manuscript letters prior to cursive began in the early part of the twentieth century when a manuscript alphabet was developed by Edward Johnson. Think about how you were taught to write. Most likely, the majority of you learned to print with manuscript letters before learning how to write with cursive letters. Most commercial handwriting programs focus initial handwriting instruction on manuscript letters.

Although this practice continues, there has not been conclusive data to show that students should learn printing before cursive. Proponents of teaching manuscript before cursive believe that 1. manuscript letters are easier to learn than cursive letters; 2. printed letters are like the "type" used in books, especially reading books; 3. printed letters are easier to write legibly than cursive; and 4. separate letters help students with spelling more than letters tied together, as in cursive.

Cursive   Teaching students to write using cursive letters normally begins in the latter second or early third grade. However, some professionals advocate teaching students cursive writing before manuscript. Reasons for this viewpoint include:

■ cursive letters are difficult to reverse, unlike manuscript letters that are frequently reversed in the writing of young children;

■ cursive letters enable students to "connect" letters, therefore helping students see the whole word rather than just a group of letters;

■ cursive letters are faster to write than manuscript letters; writing words with cursive is much faster than writing words with manuscript letters;

■ students who learn cursive before manuscript do not have to make the transition from one to the other; this transition causes problems for many students (Graham & Miller, 1980; Hagin, 1983).

Regardless of which is taught first, teachers need to be aware of the strengths and weaknesses of the approaches and realize that some students may actually learn one method more easily than the other. This calls for flexibility on the part of teachers to use which method works best for individual children.

Assessment of Handwriting Skills   Assessment of handwriting skills can be done formally or informally. Formal assessment enables teachers to use commercially prepared tests and compare the child's performance with the "norm" group on which the test was standardized. Unlike the areas of reading and math, there are limited formal tests available for assessing handwriting skills (Luftig, 1989). This may be due to the unpopularity of teaching handwriting, the complexity of handwriting, or the overemphasis of reading and math. In most instances, handwriting is assessed with teachers' observations and informal methods (Graham, Boyer-Shick, & Tippets, 1989).

Regardless of the limited attention paid to assessing handwriting skills, these skills must be evaluated in order to develop appropriate intervention programs. Without adequate assessment data, teachers are unable to determine what to emphasize in an intervention program. Intervention programs in all areas, including handwriting, must be tied to assessment data (Smith, Price, & Marsh, 1986). There are numerous skills that can be assessed when evaluating a student's handwriting ability. These include sensori-motor skills and other prewriting skills, as well as specific, mechanical skills directly related to handwriting. Most formal and informal assessment measures focus on a few specific areas, including:

- letter formation,

- spacing,

- slant,

- line quality,

- letter size and alignment, and

- writing rate (Luftig, 1989).

Formal Assessment of Handwriting   There are a few formal handwriting tests and scales available. These include the Zaner-Bloser Evaluation Scales (1984); Test of Written Language-2 (TOWL-2) (1988); Test of Legible Handwriting (Larsen & Hammill, 1989); Bezzi Scale (1962); and Freeman Scales (1959). Table 6–1 (on page 198) provides a brief description of a few formalized handwriting tests.

One of the major weaknesses of formal handwriting scales is the limited writing sample used in the evaluation; the scales simply do not allow for the evaluation of a broad range of skills (Graham, 1986). Having students write a few sentences for evaluation purposes may not accurately reflect the student's actual handwriting skills. Other weaknesses of handwriting scales include their lack of differentiating performances for girls and boys (Wood, Webster, Gullickson, & Walker, 1987), limited reporting of reliability, and limited proficiency ratings (Graham, 1986).

One of the major limitations of formal handwriting evaluation instruments is the same as for other formal tests, they frequently do not help teachers teach students. While they may result in standard scores, just knowing how a student compares to other students in handwriting skills does not automatically help teachers develop intervention programs for remedial purposes. For example, knowing how a particular student compares with other students does not tell teachers how to remediate the handwriting deficiencies.

Informal Assessment of Handwriting   Informally assessing handwriting can lead to direct interventions by teachers to overcome specific handwriting deficiencies. One of the best ways for teachers to informally evaluate handwriting skills is to use a checklist or observational scale. There are many different varieties of informal handwriting evaluation scales. Table 6–2 (on page 199) presents one example. By using observations and checklists, teachers are capable of determining specific handwriting skills that students exhibit, as

TABLE 6-1 Characteristics of Handwriting Scales

CHARACTERISTICS	FREEMAN (1959)	BEZZI (1962)	ZANER-BLOSER (1979)	TOWL[A] (1983)
1. Grade Levels	1–8	1–3	1–8	Approximately 3–12[b]
2. Style	Manuscript (1–2) Cursive (3–8)	Manuscript	Manuscript (1–2) Cursive (3–8)	Cursive
3. Handedness	Right and left	Right and left	Right and left	Right and left
4. Sex	Male and female	Male and female	Male and female	Male and female
5. General Description	A series of eight 5-step scales	A series of three 5-step scales	A series of eight 5-step scales	A 10-step scale
6. Nature of Scale	Ordinal	Ordinal	Ordinal	Not known[c]
7. Number of Samples Used in Scale Construction	135,491 samples from 162 cities	7,212 samples from all parts of the U.S.	Approximately 500 samples per grade level	Not reported
8. Criterion for Scaling	General excellence	Quality and speed	General excellence	Legibility
9. Procedures for Scaling	Median placement by judges	Quality and speed	Rank-ordered specimens and selected samples on the basis of letter form slant, alignment, spacing, and line quality	Not reported
10. Nature of Specimen Obtained from the Student	Different specimens for each grade level	Different specimens for each grade level	Different specimens for each grade level	A single specimen
11. Directions for Obtaining Student Specimen	Write from copy at usual speed	Copy at usual speed	Write from copy using their best handwriting	Write a story in response to three pictures
12. Method of Scoring Student Specimen	Match student specimen to appropriate scale	Match student specimen to appropriate scale and determine speed of writing	Match student specimen to appropriate scale	Match student specimen to scale

[a]Handwriting subtest of the Test of Written Language.

[b]Normative scores are available for children ages 8-0 to 18-11.

[c]It was not possible to determine the nature of the scale based on the information provided by the authors.

Source: Graham (1986, p. 67). Used with permission.

TABLE 6-2 Informal Handwriting Scale

SKILL	RATING	
	Ok	Needs Work

Prewriting Skills
   handedness
   pencil grip
   paper position
   writing posture

Manuscript Skills
   forms letters properly and legibly
   lowercase and uppercase
   proper spacing between letters
   proper slant
   proper spacing between words
   proper letter size
   copy letters and words
   writes letters and words from memory
   writing speed and fluency

Cursive Skills
   forms letters properly and legibly
   lowercase and uppercase letters
   proper spacing between letters and words
   proper slant and size
   copy letters and words
   writes letters and words from memory
   writing speed and fluency

well as weaknesses that need to be improved. Information gleaned from checklists can lead directly to remediation efforts by teachers.

Informal assessment of handwriting may also reveal more accurately a student's handwriting abilities. As previously noted, requiring students to write passages for the simple purpose of assessment may result in a sample of writing that does not reflect the student's daily writing abilities. On the other hand, informal assessment takes a student's actual handwriting sample and analyzes it according to pre-established criteria. The handwriting is not obtained through an artificial pretext, but is an example of actual, daily ability.

Teaching Handwriting Skills As previously discussed, students need to have competence in handwriting skills to enhance their success in school. Unfortunately, many teachers do not spend a great deal of time in handwriting instruction or remediation (Bridge & Hiebert, 1985; Luftig, 1988). Regardless of the reason, special education teachers need to understand the importance of handwriting instruction and ways to provide intervention for students who have deficits. One reason this is so important for special education teachers is that students with disabilities have more problems with handwriting than their nondisabled peers (Smith *et al.*, 1986; Wallace *et al.*, 1987; Wallace & McLoughlin, 1988).

There are two general approaches to teaching and remediating handwriting skills: individual skills approach and whole language method. Using the individual skills approach, teachers work on specific skills related to handwriting proficiency. These skills, such as proper pencil grip, proper slant, and proper spacing, are taught somewhat in isolation, then combined with other writing skills. The skills approach differs significantly from the whole language approach, which does not focus on individual skills; proponents of this model advocate teaching handwriting skills as part of the overall writing process.

Teachers who use the specific skills approach can rely on commercial and teacher-made programs. The majority of teachers, up to ninety-five percent by some reports, use commercial programs (Wood *et al.*, 1987). There are three handwriting instruction programs that are used extensively in schools. These include the Palmer method, Zaner-Bloser program, and the D'Nealian program (Wood *et al.*, 1987).

The Palmer and Zaner-Bloser handwriting programs are similar in many ways. Printing is taught before cursive; both programs emphasize a few specific curved and straight line strokes; and specific lessons and pages are provided for instructional activities and practice. These programs provide a fairly traditional approach to teaching handwriting skills. A different approach to teaching handwriting is found in the D'Nealian program. This approach, developed in the late 1960s, combines the use of manuscript and cursive letters. Students learn to write using a modified cursive model, thus removing the major hurdle of the transition between manuscript, or printing, and cursive (Wood *et al.*, 1987).

There is no one handwriting program that is best for all children and teachers. Wood and colleagues (1987) investigated the effectiveness of the Palmer, Zaner-Bloser, and D'Nealian programs and found no significant differences in the handwriting skills of students who were taught using one of the three methods. Teachers need to become familiar with the available commercial programs and use whichever results in handwriting improvements by their students. Another reason special education teachers need to be familiar with commercial programs is to support handwriting instruction that occurs in the regular classroom. If the special education teacher is not familiar with the program being used in the regular classroom, contradictory approaches may be used. This could result in confusion and cause more problems for students already experiencing problems with handwriting.

As previously mentioned, some teachers use a whole language model to teach handwriting skills. Teachers using this model do not instruct students in the mechanics of handwriting; they do not teach specific skills involved in handwriting. For example, teachers using the whole language model do not have students practice on letter formation in isolation. Rather than teaching specific, mechanical skills, teachers encourage and reinforce students for their written compositions. The premise is that handwriting skills should be taught as part of the writing process, not as a separate set of skills. The whole language approach will be discussed in greater detail later in this chapter.

Although the whole language approach is gaining popularity in some schools, many teachers continue to rely on teaching handwriting as a separate set of skills, at least part of the time. Regardless of which commercial program is used to teach specific handwriting skills, teachers may teach specific skills with separate instructional activities. Prior to teaching manuscript or cursive skills, teachers need to ensure that students have the necessary prewriting skills to enable them to be successful writers. Some of these skills include proper pencil grip; understanding concepts of left and right, start and stop, etc.; and being able to make movements with a writing utensil. Table 6–3 describes some of the instructional activities that can be used to help students develop prewriting skills.

When teaching basic manuscript and cursive skills, teachers also may want to rely on specific teaching activities. Some of the things teachers can do to enhance development of these skills include:

- modeling appropriate handwriting skills;
- noting critical attributes of handwriting;
- using physical prompts and cues with students;
- tracing appropriately written letters and words;
- copying appropriately written letters and words;
- using self-verbalizations during writing activities;
- writing letters and words from memory;
- using repetition in letter and word formation;

TABLE 6-3 Instructional Activities for Prewriting Skills

Develop Handedness	tape on preferred hand erasable dot on preferred hand connect writing instrument to one side of desk
Proper Pencil Grip	place tape around end of pencil at grip point use pencil "grippers" model appropriate grip use large pencils/crayons use magic markers use a plastic golf ball with holes; place pencil through holes; student grips ball
Visual Motor Skills	tracing activities cutting activities coloring activities manipulative activities for fine motor skill development encourage scribbling

Movement Activities	activities that require left-right and up-down
	    movements
	develop basic strokes by having students copy
	    circles, straight lines, and curved lines
	use templates for practicing strokes
	use cut outs for practicing strokes

- using self-correction and feedback techniques; and

- appropriate use of reinforcement for students (Graham & Miller, 1980).

Modeling appropriate handwriting skills is an excellent teaching method. Students who observe their teachers and peers use proper pencil grip, hand position, and letter formation may model appropriate actions. On the other hand, students are likely to model poor handwriting practices if given the opportunity. Therefore, teachers need to consider which handwriting opportunities are provided for modeling purposes.

There are several remedial handwriting programs available that can be used by teachers. These range from those that have been available for many years, such as the Gillingham and Stillman model (1960) and Fernald method (1943), to programs that are based on the whole language approach where handwriting skills are taught as part of the total writing process. Hagin (1983) described a program called *Write Right—or Left* for handwriting instruction. This program focuses on specific skills, including "posture, position of the paper, the way the pencil is grasped, arm movements across the paper, visual matching of the letter patterns with graphic model, and timing of feedback." (p. 268) The model uses manuscript letters that are designed to facilitate transition to cursive writing. Figure 6–1 depicts the alphabet used by Hagin (1983). It is similar to the D'Nealian alphabet in that letters are a combination of cursive and manuscript forms.

SPELLING

Another important skill that is a component of written language is spelling. Spelling enables the writer to compose words accurately in order to faciliate decoding. If words are spelled so incorrectly that the reader cannot accurately decode the message, then the entire writing process is of limited value. Therefore, spelling is critical to effective written communication (Wallace, Cohen, & Polloway, 1987).

Spelling is a complex task that "depends upon the adequate functioning and integration of multiple phonological, orthographic, and motor processes." (Bailet, 1991, p. 2) Phonemes are the most basic unit in the English language; they are speech sounds that are related to certain letters, or graphemes. Orthography is the spelling system of a particular language. A perfect alphabetical orthography would have only one grapheme, or letter, for each phoneme. In the English alphabet there may be several different graphemes for each phoneme (Bailet, 1991). Spelling is the ability to properly sequence phonemes to represent graphemes necessary for words.

Accurate spelling is important for students for several reasons. First, spelling is a basic skill that is included in most elementary curricula. As a result, students are graded on their spelling abilities. Spelling is also important because it facilitates written expression. As noted, if spelling is so poor that the reader cannot accurately understand what is written, then the entire writing process may be futile. For adults, being able to spell correctly facilitates securing a job, or keeping a job. Although it is a skill that may be totally unrelated to a particular job, an inability to complete a job application without several misspelled words may result in not getting the job. The combination of the complexity of spelling and the language-based problems experienced by many students with mild disabilities makes this group of students prime candidates for spelling disorders (Vallecorsa, Zigmond, & Henderson, 1985; Wallace *et al.*, 1987).

FIGURE 6-1 Alphabet Used in Right Left-Right.

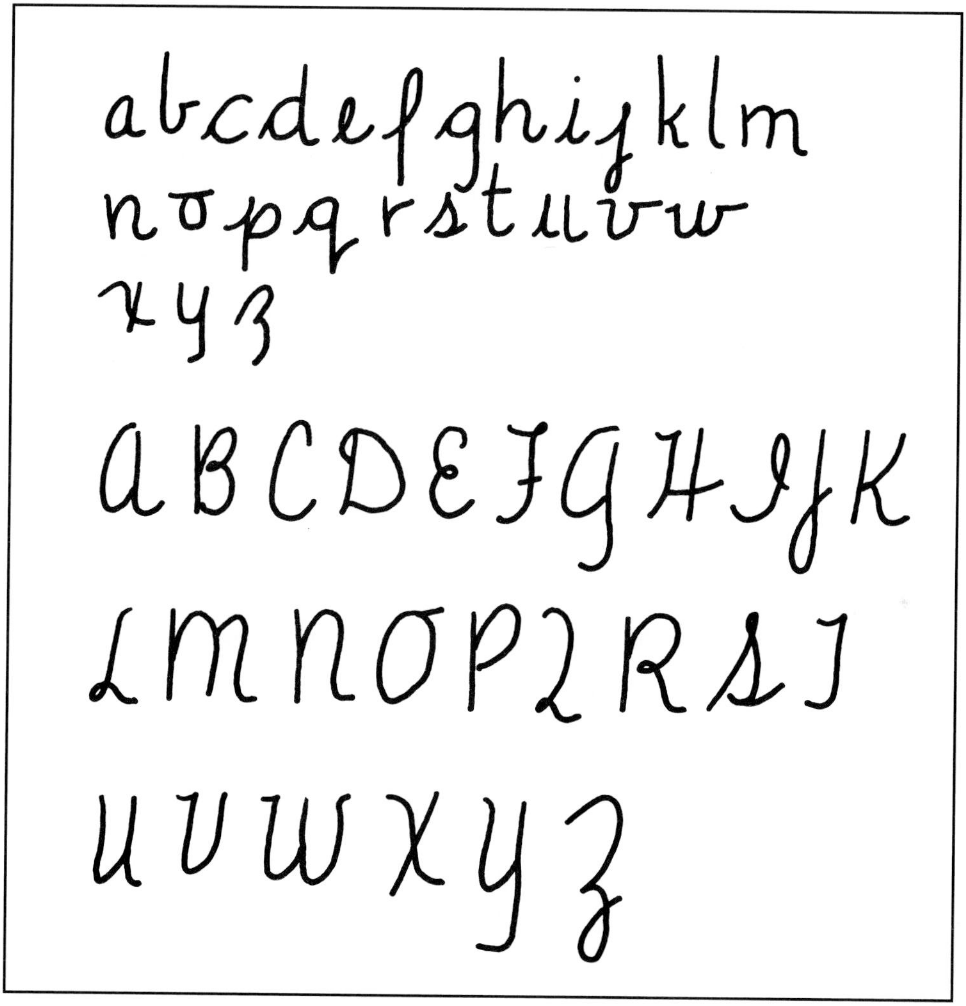

Source: Hagin, 1983, p. 269. Reprinted with permission.

Types of Spelling Errors   Although many students are "good" spellers and know how to spell most words correctly, some students, especially those with mild disabilities, experience significant problems in spelling. For these students, trying to learn how to spell is a "tedious chore" (Gerber & Hall, 1987). It is frustrating and can lead to a negative attitude about other subject areas, especially those that require accurate spelling skills.

There are many different types of spelling errors that students exhibit. These include inserting unneeded letters, omitting needed letters, reversing letters and words, substituting incorrect letters, making phonetic errors, and transposing letters (Polloway & Smith,

1982; Leuenberger & Morris, 1990). For teachers to be in the best position to help students overcome these types of spelling errors, they need to know the type of errors made by students, as well as the spelling skills that are intact. Assessing spelling skills provides this kind of information.

Assessment of Spelling

Spelling can be assessed using formal and informal means. Most standardized, norm-referenced achievement tests include a spelling subtest. For example, the Peabody Individual Achievement Test-Revised (PIAT-R), Wide Range Achievement Test-Revised (WRAT-R), and the Kaufman Test of Educational Achievement (K-TEA) all include components to assess spelling skills. Other formal tests that enable assessment of spelling include tests for evaluating language skills. An excellent example of this type of test is the Test of Written Language-2 (TOWL-2) (Hammill & Larsen, 1988). In addition to tests that have a spelling subtest, some tests specifically focus on the assessment of spelling. The Test of Written Spelling (TWS-2) (Larsen & Hammill, 1986) is an example. The TWS-2 is based on the premises that 1. students must learn certain rules of spelling, and 2. words that violate the general rules of spelling must be learned through rote memorization (Wallace *et al.*, 1987).

In addition to formal assessment instruments, many teachers rely on informal assessment procedures to evaluate spelling skills. Luftig (1989) describes several different ways to informally assess spelling. These include:

- *Observation*   Observe students in a variety of settings and situations. Using a set of guidelines enables the observation to be systematic and reliable and valid.

- *Informal Spelling Inventories*   Relies on a sampling of words the student needs to be able to spell; words are frequently taken from basal reading series. Inventory can also focus on spelling skills rather than specific words.

- *Cloze Technique*   This method uses a fill-in-the-blank format where the student has choices which result in a properly spelled word.

- *Spelling Interview*   Asks students questions regarding their spelling strengths and weaknesses. For example, How do you know if you spell a word correctly?

- *Teacher-Made Spelling Tests*   Similar to informal spelling inventories. Enables teachers to choose any words for sampling purposes.

Instructional Approaches

There are several different ways teachers can teach spelling skills. Research on these various techniques have verified which ones are generally effective and ineffective. Examples of methods that have been determined to be effective include: 1. using high-interest activities, 2. testing students daily, 3. using a test-study-test sequence, 4. emphasizing high frequency words, 5. emphasizing familiar vocabulary, and 6. using a whole-word study approach (Vallecorsa *et al.*, 1985). In addition to these methods, Lerner (1988) describes approaches that focus on auditory perception and memory, visual perception and memory, and multisensory methods. While there is no one best method to teach spelling to students, teachers should understand the various methods and choose which method works best with individual students.

Frank (1987) described a directed spelling instructional model to teach spelling skills. Using this approach, students work directly with the teacher to learn specific spelling words that have been preselected from the school's spelling list, from frequently used words, or from other words deemed important for the student to know how to spell. The approach uses four steps. In step one, students are given an envelope that contains ten word cards, a practice sheet, and a test sheet. In step two, the student looks at the word cards and asks the teacher for assistance with unknown words. The unknown words are then traced with a pencil until the student is ready to spell the word. The word is then written from memory on the practice sheet.

In the third step, students compare their practice sheets with the word cards. Students practice writing the misspelled words several times, then indicate they are ready to be tested. If students spell the words correctly in step four, they are rewarded by having the date of the correct spelling noted on the word card. Another method of using direct instruction to teach specific spelling words was described by Dangel (1987). This particular approach, called the coach's spelling approach, includes several structured steps that focus on students understanding spelling rules about certain words, practicing those words, and keeping detailed records about the ability of the student to spell the words.

There is no one instructional method that works effectively with all students. Some students might even respond better to a combination of approaches rather than a single instructional method. Zylstra (1989) describes a program for students with learning disabilities that was derived from several different methodologies, including Signs for Sounds (Bechthold & Del, 1978); Cloze (Ketchum, 1982); and Auditory Discrimination in Depth (Lindamood & Lindamood, 1975). The combination of these different ways to teach spelling worked very well with the students with learning disabilities described by Zylstra (1989).

In addition to traditional spelling instructional programs, games and other activities can be used to help students develop spelling skills. Wallace *et al.* (1987) described several games that can be used to enhance spelling skills. These include spelling cards, a game where students compete in spelling words on cards; spelling bingo, which uses the bingo format with phonemes heading the columns instead of specific letters; and kinesthetic spelling, where words are written in sand or salt to give a kinesthetic and tactile sense of the correct spelling. The different games and activities that teachers can use to teach spelling are only limited by the teacher's creativity.

WRITTEN EXPRESSION

Written expression has been described as the "culmination of language learning". (Wallace *et al.*, 1987, p. 305) It encompasses all other areas of language, including reading, speaking, and listening. There are three primary components of written expression: prewriting, writing, and postwriting. Prewriting includes skills such as oral receptive and expressive language, legible handwriting, and motivation to write. The writing stage is composed of skills that range from being able to write simple sentences to responding accurately to essay test questions. The final stage, postwriting, includes editing and revising for grammar skills, organization, and content (Wallace *et al.*, 1987).

Importance of Written Expression

Being able to express yourself in writing is critical in our society. For school children, a deficiency in written expression can result in failures in many different subject areas. Not only do deficits in written expression result in poor grades in writing, but they can also lead to poor grades in other subject areas that require competency in written expression. Students may receive poor grades in subjects, not because they do not know the content, but because they are unable to express themselves in writing. Teachers also may develop bias toward students who have poor writing skills. This bias may result in lowered expectations of students, and therefore have a negative effect on the student's total academic performance.

Another major reason why students need to develop skills in written expression is because failure in this area often leads to a withdrawal of effort to learn to write well. Withdrawing from writing activities can "seriously threaten children's potential for learning to write effectively, for in order to become competent writers, they must make and tolerate errors, keep working in the face of frustration, appreciate their own efforts, and see themselves as effective." (Meyer, Pisha, & Rose, 1991, p. 105). For students with disabilities, skills in written expression are critical for success in regular classrooms (Minner, Prater, Sullavan, & Gwaltney, 1989). Too often, however, these students experience significant problems in their writing skills that often have a negative impact on their mainstreamed status (Algozzine, O'Shea, Stoddard, & Crews, 1988).

Assessment of Written Expression

Before developing instructional programs for students in written expression, assessment data need to be collected to determine a student's strengths and weaknesses. Teachers can assess written expression skills using formal and informal methods. Formal methods are generally required to determine the eligibility status of students, while informal assessment results facilitate the development of intervention programs.

Formal Assessment Instruments As in all areas of special education, the number of formal assessment instruments for written expression has increased significantly over the past few years. Many of the tests used to measure written expression are components of more generalized achievement tests; too often these instruments do not provide sufficient information regarding written expression (Polloway, Patton, Payne, & Payne, 1989). Bailet (1991) reviewed several formal instruments currently being used to assess written expression and concluded that, while formal tests can accurately evaluate the many subskills associated with written expression, they may not actually reflect a student's ability in a classroom writing assignment. Table 6–4 summarizes some of the formal tests used to assess written expression. Users of these instruments must keep in mind that some are inappropriate for certain populations and often the technical adequacy of tests are minimal. When using standardized, norm-referenced tests for any assessment, take into consideration the technical adequacy of the test before making critical decisions about results obtained.

Informal Assessment Teachers are able to informally evaluate written expression through observations, checklists, and analysis of spontaneously written materials. When informally assessing written expression skills, teachers should evaluate several components (Minner *et al.*, 1989):

Fluency This is a measure of writing quantity and can be assessed by determining the average sentence length (ASL). This is done by counting the number of words and sentences in a writing sample.

Sentence Types   Determine the types of sentences the student uses. Types include sentence fragments, simple sentences, compound sentences, and complex sentences.

Vocabulary   Written vocabulary is frequently assessed using a type-token ratio (ITR) in which the variety of words used is compared to the number of words used.

TABLE 6–4   Summary of Formal Tests of Written Expression

TEST	PUBLISHER	APPROPRIATE AGES/GRADES*	ADMINIS-TRATION	RELEVANT SUBTESTS OR FOCUS OF ASSESSMENT
SRA Achievement Series (Thorpe, Lefever, & Hasland, 1974)	Science Research Associates	grades 2 to 9	group	usage including capitalization
Stanford Achievement Test (SAT) (Madden, Gardner, Rudman, Karlsen, & Merwin, 1973)	Psychological Corporation	grades 1-5 to 9-5 language subtests, grades 3-0 to 9-5	group	capitalization punctuation usage
Metropolitan Achievement Tests (Durost, Bixler, Wrightstone, Prescott, & Balow, 1971)	Harcourt Brace Jovanovich	grades K to 9-5 language components, grades 3-5 to 9-5		punctuation capitalization usage
Test of Adolescent Language-2 (TOAL-2) (Hammill, Brown, Larsen, Wiederholt, 1987)	PRO-ED	ages 11-0 to 18-5	individual	writing/ vocabulary writing/ grammar
Picture Story Language Test (Myklebust, 1965)	Western Psychological Services	ages 7-0 to 17-0	individual and/or group	scoring areas include the following scales: productivity, syntax, abstract-concrete
Test of Written Language (TOWL) (Hammill & Larsen, 1983)	PRO-ED	ages 8-6 to 14-5	individual word usage style spelling handwriting	vocabulary thematic maturity

*–5 means half; for example, 9–5 means halfway through ninth grade and age 18–5 means eighteen and a half grade

Source: Wallace, G., Cohen, S.B., & Polloway, E.A. (1987). *Language arts.* Austin, TX: Pro-Ed. p. 311. Used with permission.

Structure   This includes the evaluation of mechanical aspects of writing, such as punctuation, grammar, and verb-tense.

Ideation   A subjective assessment of the content of the written work.

One way to evaluate written expression is through written language samples. Similar to spontaneous, spoken language samples described later in the chapter, samples of written work can be analyzed to determine specific strengths and weaknesses of children's writing abilities. Skills that can be assessed in a written language sample include content, vocabulary, punctuation, grammar, and form.

TABLE 6-5   Informal Checklist for Written Expression

Sample Elicitation Procedure: Date: Students' Names	Verbs		Pro-nouns		Words					Sen-tences		Capitals			Puctuation							
	Agreement	Tense	Personal	Possessive	Additions	Substitutions	Modifiers	Negatives	Plurals	Incomplete	Run-on	Beginning sentences	Proper nouns	Inappropriate use	Period	Comma	Question mark	Apostrophe	Colon	Other		Total

Source: Mercer, C.D., & Mercer, A.R. (1985). *Teaching students with learning problems.* Columbus, OH: Merrill. p. 438. Used with permission.

Wallace and Larsen (1978) suggest that teachers should assess the following areas when evaluating students' written samples.

1.   Purpose of the writing—was the main idea clear?

2.   Content—were the ideas consistent with the topic?

3.   Organization—was there an introduction, body of content, and summary?

4.   Paragraphs—were paragraphs properly developed around topics and subtopics?

5.   Sentences—were sentences properly developed, with subject-verb agreement, consistent tense, and logical sequencing?

6. Word choice and usage—were the words appropriate in meaning and complexity?

7. Capitalization—were words capitalized properly?

8. Punctuation—was punctuation used according to rules?

9. Handwriting—was the writing sample legible?

Informal assessment of written expression generally can be enhanced by using checklists. These provide some structure and consistency in the data collection process and assist teachers in collecting germane information. Table 6–5 presents an example of a checklist to evaluate written expression.

Techniques to Improve Written Expression

Similar to handwriting instruction, teaching strategies in the area of written expression can focus on individual skill approaches and holistic approaches. Advocates of the skills approach contend that specific writing skills are more easily learned in isolation (Gould, 1991). Skills taught using this model include 1. punctuation and capitalization, 2. vocabulary and grammar, and 3. sentence and paragraph writing. In contrast, advocates for the holistic or whole language model, believe that the best way to teach written expression is to use the process approach to writing where students learn to write by writing and not by learning specific, isolated skills (Zemelman & Daniels, 1988).

Regardless of the specific approach used, teachers of students with disabilities need to take special care in developing writing skills in their students. Graham and Harris (1988) made ten general recommendations regarding instruction in written expression for students with disabilities. The following describes these recommendations.

■ Time should be allocated for writing. Students with disabilities are capable of learning to write, but only if given an opportunity to write. Therefore, teachers need to allocate specific writing times for students.

■ Students should be exposed to a broad range of writing tasks. This includes helping students acquire basic skills, such as grammar and punctuation; providing opportunities for expressive writing, such as journal writing; and requiring structured writing activities, such as descriptions of things in the environment.

■ Create an appropriate climate for writing. Teachers must create an environment where students feel comfortable writing without the pressure of having red marks all over their papers.

■ Integrate writing and other activities. Writing should be integrated with other academic activities to increase writing opportunities and to tie writing to functional activities.

■ Help students develop basic processes inherent in writing. These include planning what to write, sentence generation, and revising.

■ Help students become automatic in transferring language to written product. Students must develop basic writing skills to such a level that the writing process is not slow and cumbersome.

- Teach students how to know and understand "good writing." Students need to understand the different types of writing and the characteristics of good writing in each.

- Prepare students to carry out more sophisticated writing activities. In order for students to progress in their writing skills, teachers can use conferencing to point out strengths and weaknesses of writing; provide supports to make the writing process easier; and teach students how to use strategies, such as memory skills, to facilitate writing.

- Help students develop goals for the improvement of their writing. Teachers should facilitate students' goal setting in the area of writing.

- Do not focus on instructional activities that do not improve writing. Some practices, such as a heavy emphasis on grammar, are not a prerequisite to good writing. Therefore, teachers should not dwell on teaching grammar skills simply to improve written expression.

In addition to these principles, Polloway *et al.*, (1989) suggest additional general considerations when teaching written expression.

1. Focus on functional writing. Students are able to understand the importance of written expression when they use writing for notes, letters, and functional activities.

2. Teachers should work on increasing the number of words students know by focusing on words outside the students' routine experiences.

3. The basic rules of grammar should be taught to students, as well as how to apply the rules in writing activities.

4. Students should be encouraged to practice their writing skills.

5. Teachers, as well as students who have developed certain writing competence, should serve as role models for other students.

6. Students need to be taught that writing is an enjoyable process, not simply a product.

7. Teachers need to stimulate students to try creative writing.

Teaching Strategies Using a Skills Approach As previously mentioned, there are three general stages to teaching written expression using a skills approach. These are the prewriting, writing, and postwriting stages. During the prewriting period, teachers focus on motivating students for writing and helping them focus on specific purposes for writing (Wallace & McLoughlin, 1988). Probably the most important part of any written expression program is getting students to write (Barenbaum, 1983). Activities that help motivate students should result in their wanting to write.

In addition to getting students motivated to write, teachers need to establish an environment that encourages and reinforces writing efforts. Too often, students are unintentionally intimidated by teachers. They are fearful that if they write something it will be severely scrutinized for spelling, grammar, content, and every other conceivable area that can be judged. Students must feel comfortable and "safe"; they must believe that they can risk making errors without undue negative results should they not perform well. This means that teachers should not overly emphasize mechanical components of writing, such as punctuation, until students feel secure in their writing efforts. Part of the "safe" environment that teachers establish should have a system for providing students with regular, positive reinforcement (Barenbaum, 1983).

During the writing stage, teachers emphasize specific skills, including enhancing expressive vocabulary, proper sentence structure, and developing complete paragraphs (Wallace & McLoughlin, 1988). Again, while these skills are stressed during this component of the writing process, teachers should not place an unreasonable demand on this area; getting students to write and to enjoy the writing process is still a major consideration during the writing stage.

Table 6–6 (on page 212) summarizes the commercial programs available for teaching written language skills. Although commercial programs are used by some teachers, the majority rely on teacher-made activities that focus on specific skill building.

There are several activities teachers can use in their classrooms to improve overall writing skills of students. Davis and Winek (1989) described a program to improve the writing skills of students by increasing their knowledge about a writing topic. Think about your own writing ability. You are more likely to write well if you are familiar with your subject. Trying to write about a topic that you know little about will likely result in writing that is stilted and awkward. In the program described by Davis and Winek (1989), students took several weeks to develop extensive background information about a topic before attempting to write about that topic. As a result of improving their knowledge base of a topic, students were better prepared to write papers about that topic.

In another program, Fortner (1986) increased the ability of students to write about various topics as a result of their participating in creative productive-thinking training. Students with learning disabilities were involved in creativity development activities for thirty minutes per day, three days a week, for nine weeks. The results indicated that training in creativity directly correlated with increased skills in written expression.

Holistic Instruction in Written Expression   Using the holistic approach, students are taught written expression skills through their own writing efforts. This instructional model is called the process approach to writing; it has been shown to be effective with students with disabilities (Gaustad & Messenheimer-Young, 1991; Vallecorsa, Ledford, & Parnell, 1991). Gould (1991) identified five distinct steps in the writing process.

1. *Rehearsal (Prewriting) Stage*   This is the stage when students think about what they are going to write. They rely on their own experiences and interests to develop a topic and generally outline their writing product.

2. *Drafting (Writing) Stage*   During this stage students put their ideas on paper. Teachers can facilitate this difficult transition by having students rehearse the materials orally. Having students write daily journals and modeling the teacher's writing activity can also help students during this stage.

3. *Revision (Rewriting) Stage*   This stage is where the student refines what has been written to make it sound better and to enhance the content. Correcting for poor mechanics also occurs during this stage.

4. *Editing (Proofreading) Stage*   During this stage, final corrections are made, including spelling, grammatical, and punctuation corrections. A final check of the content is also made. Teachers, students, or peers may be involved in this stage.

5. *Publishing (Recopying) Stage*   The final stage of the writing process is when students recopy their work in final form. Writing is neat and mechanics of the writing process are checked for final format. Students may be allowed to "publish" this final copy.

Editing and rewriting materials are tedious and time consuming tasks that students may not enjoy. Still, if written materials are to communicate maximally with the reader, the writing must be as polished as possible. Tompkins and Friend (1988) describe several activities that teachers can use to improve the editing and rewriting skills of students. These include encouraging proofreading and the use of proofreader's marks, working with students during the correcting stage, and evaluating the final product of the student. Students seem

TABLE 6-6   Commercial Programs for Teaching Written Expression

PROGRAM	PUBLISHER	DESCRIPTION
Lessons for Better Writing	Curriculum Associates	writing improvement program writing and editing exercises grades 6–12
Moving up in Grammar	DLM	focuses on grammar skills elementary and intermediate grades contains 6 kits of 16 units 6 kits include: sentences, pronouns, nouns and verbs, capitalization and punctuation, adjectives and adverbs, and word usage
Phelps Sentence Guide Program	Teraski & Phelps, 1980	language remediation in written expression elementary ages students develop sentences from picture stimulus sentences structured using who, what, when, where, how guide extensive teacher-student dialogue

Source: Mercer, 1987.

to enjoy proofreading more if they are allowed to use the "professional" proofreader's marks in editing their own papers. This can lead to corrections, which when supervised by the teacher, provide additional positive feedback to the student.

Sometimes a major problem for students is selecting a topic. Often students simply go blank when trying to decide what to write about. One way of introducing students to ideas for writing is through storytelling (Houston, Goolrick, & Tate, 1991). This technique provides ideas for content for students and motivates them to write about the story or something similar. Teachers can use storytelling by having students sit in a circle and tell stories to each other. Following this activity, students should generate a writing topic related to someone's story. Storytelling by the teacher can also be used to generate writing topics. Other ways to help students select topics include 1. having students focus on their past experiences, such as "last summer" or "vacation" or "their family"; 2. having students focus on a theme, such as science fiction; and 3. having students describe the world in ten years.

Although there are some advocates of the skills approach and the whole language approach who advocate their model at the exclusion of the other, many professionals consider both approaches as sound ways to teach written expression. The models do not have to be self-exclusionary. Teachers can select parts of the skills approach and parts of the whole language approach to meet the needs of individual students. Some of the activities of the two approaches, such as practice writing, are not that different from each other.

Regardless of which method is used, and how "purely" it is used, the hope during the writing process is that students' skills will increase with their practice. Since written expression is a complex task that is learned, it is assumed that practicing good writing skills will result in students becoming better writers than those that simply learn the mechanics of writing in isolation. Therefore, even if a skills approach is used, students need to practice their writing ability. Figures 6–2, 6–3, and 6–4 (on pages 214, 215, and 216) provide examples of student's work at various stages of the writing process.

Oral Language

Expression of language through oral means is just as critical to individuals as written language. Oral language enables persons to communicate without any devices that may be required with written language. Students routinely use oral expression in academic settings. They respond orally to questions, ask questions for clarification, enter into discussions to further understand concepts, and make oral reports for specific assignments. In addition to these academic-related purposes, oral language serves important social purposes. Oral expression enables individuals to communicate in social settings and facilitates getting to know others and engage in "friendly" conversations.

Oral language is important for adults also. Adults use oral language extensively for vocational and social purposes. Without adequate oral language skills, individuals would have problems in many jobs. Likewise, impaired ability in oral language would impede social relationships by simply making communication among individuals difficult.

FIGURE 6-2 The Enemy Dragon, Written by a Boy Aged Nine

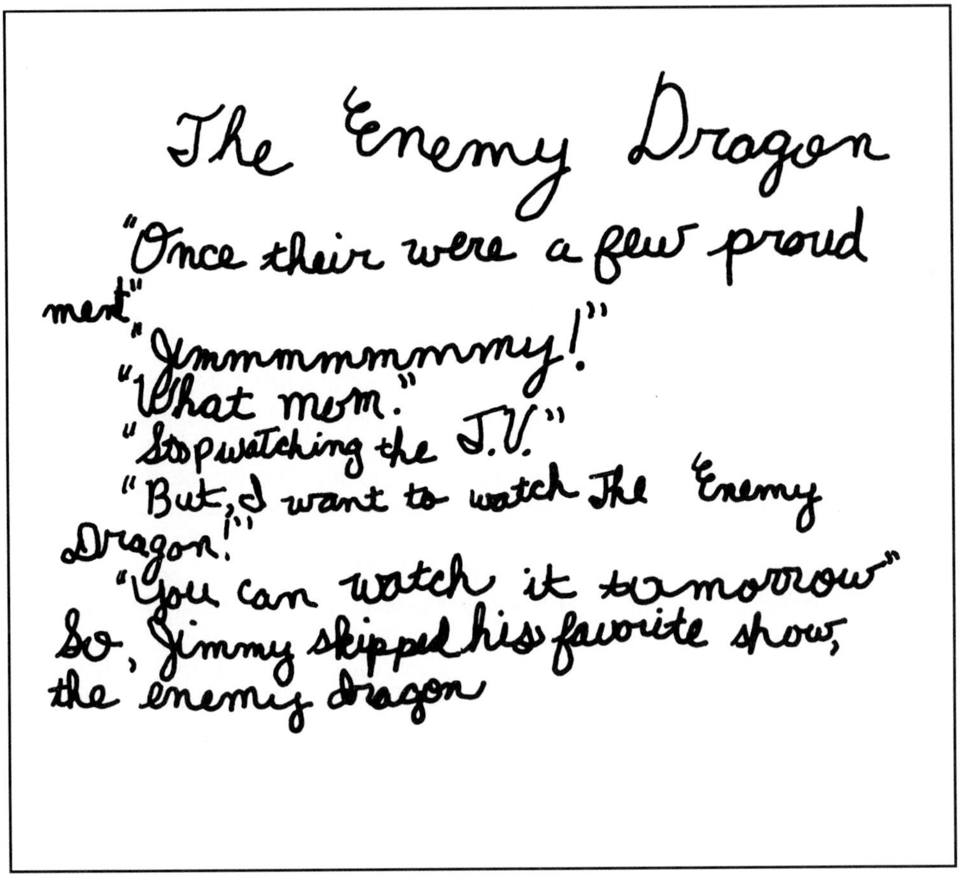

> The Enemy Dragon
> "Once their were a few proud
> men"
> "Jimmmmmmmy!"
> "What mom."
> "Stop watching the T.V."
> "But, I want to watch The Enemy
> Dragon!"
> "You can watch it tomorrow"
> So, Jimmy skipped his favorite show,
> the enemy dragon

Although difficulties in oral language can result in academic and social problems for students, there has not been a great deal of emphasis in schools placed on enhancing skills in oral language. Reasons for this limited attention include:

- difficulty in breaking down the skills necessary for oral expression for instructional purposes (Morley, 1972);

- emphasis placed on academic skill instruction (Smith, 1990);

- lack of training in oral expression intervention techniques for regular and special education teachers (Polloway & Smith, 1992);

- most children develop oral language skills without any major problems; those that do not may be thought of as shy (Polloway & Smith, 1992).

FIGURE 6-3 If I Were a Bug, Written by a Boy Aged Eight

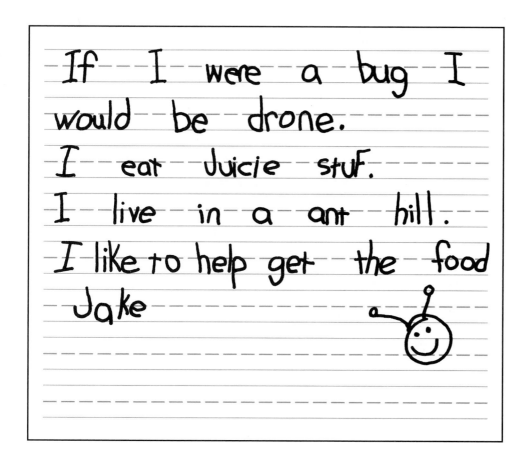

> If I were a bug I
> would be drone.
> I eat Juicie stuf.
> I live in a ant hill.
> I like to help get the food
> Jake

There appears to be a trend for schools to pay more attention to teaching oral skills than in the past. This trend is the result of recent research revealing the significant relationship between oral language skills and academic success. For example, recent studies have determined that positive relationships exist between reading skills and oral language abilities (Wesson, Otis-Wilborn, Hasbrouck, & Tindal, 1989; Mann, Cowin, & Schoenheimer, 1989; Eisenson, 1990; Scarborough & Dobrich, 1990).

THE NATURE OF ORAL LANGUAGE

Speaking is the obvious means of oral language. Although it may seem like a simple skill, speaking "involves a complex process of identifying ideas or feelings, formulating these into an appropriate and grammatical sequence of words and sentences, and finally coordinating the speech-producing mechanisms of human anatomy to produce speech sounds,

FIGURE 6-4 Indian Blood, Written by a Girl Aged Eight

I have some
indein blad
my ansesters
wer from
indana and
ierled my indein
anseter was
a girl she
was on my
mom's side of
the famely
and she was
a chericy indein

intonation, pitch, stress, and juncture." (Hammill & Bartel, 1990, p. 33) Speaking is a complicated process. Just think about all the things you have to do in order to speak. Most of the time we actually speak without even consciously thinking about what we want to say. The process is so automatic that it seems to "just happen." As noted by Hammill and Bartel (1990), however, the process is quite complex and requires a high level of integration of cognitive and motor activities.

PROBLEMS IN ORAL EXPRESSION

Many students experience problems with oral expression. While these kinds of problems do not restrict themselves to particular types of children, those with disabilities have a higher prevalence of problems in oral language than other students. Gibbs and Cooper (1989) noted that more than ninety percent of students classified as learning disabled experience problems with oral language. These kinds of problems are also more likely in students with sensory deficits and mental retardation than in the nondisabled populations (Patton, Payne, & Beirne-Smith, 1986; Smith, Price, & Marsh, 1986).

There are four basic components of oral language. These include phonology, morphology, syntax, and semantics. Phonology is the study of speech sounds; phonemes are basic speech sounds which make up expressive oral language. Expressive phonology is articulation. Morphology combines sounds into meaningful units, such as words, suffixes, and prefixes. The combination of words into meaningful word order, such as sentences and phrases, is syntax. The fourth component, semantics, is how language is used to communicate a message (Luftig, 1989).

A fifth component, pragmatics, has recently received a great deal of attention. Pragmatics is the appropriate use of language in context. Knowing when to speak, how to speak, and what type of slang is appropriate are included in the pragmatics component (Polloway & Smith, 1992). The selection of the form and content of the spoken message is made by the speaker to best meet the intent of the effort (Shames & Wiig, 1990). For example, a college graduate who returns home to a family of lesser educated individuals might make an effort to speak in the local slang rather than sounding like an erudite. Also, the language used in a football locker room would likely differ significantly from language used in a formal speech.

Pragmatics include a wide variety of language patterns. "Specific acts stemming from those functions, such as thanking, promising, answering questions, greeting another person, asking for assistance or clarification, and ingratiating oneself for some purpose, all fall within the generic concept of pragmatics." (Polloway & Smith, 1992, p. 14) Helping students with pragmatics is therefore a daily activity.

Assessment of Oral Expression Problems

By its very complexity, oral expression is difficult to evaluate (Wesson *et al.*, 1989). However, if appropriate intervention strategies are to be developed, adequate oral language assessments must be completed. The relationship between assessment and intervention has been established for all areas, including math, reading, written expression, and oral expression (Patton *et al.*, 1986; Smith, Price, & Marsh, 1986; Wallace *et al.*, 1987; Lerner, 1988; Luftig, 1989).

There are three goals for oral language assessment. These include:

1. To determine if the child has functional language in several different environments;

2. To determine if the child has functional language with several different groups of people, for instance, age peers, parents, teachers;

3. To determine if the student understands reasons for communicating (Hammill & Bartel, 1990).

When assessing language, it is important to remember that when at all possible, the assessment should occur in natural settings (Taenzer, Cermak, & Hanlon, 1981). Determining a child's language skills in a clinical, isolated environment may not reflect the true language functioning of the child (Blau, Lahey, & Oleksiuk-Velez, 1984). In such an unnatural environment, students will likely feel intimidated. This may result in their verbal withdrawal, or efforts on their part to impress the evaluator. In either case, the child's normal language functioning will not be evaluated. When possible, spontaneous language during play should be part of the assessment process (Allen, 1989). This is an excellent way to determine the actual language abilities of the child. Children in natural play settings are more likely to display their actual language abilities than when they are in other environments.

Formal Assessment Methods   There are not nearly as many assessment instruments available for oral expression as for other skills, such as reading and math. This is due to the complexity of oral expression and the traditional place of oral language instruction in the curriculum, as previously noted. Still, there are some formal assessment instruments to evaluate oral expression. Table 6–7 describes some of the formal assessment instruments available to evaluate oral expression.

Informal Assessment Methods   Collecting information about students' oral language skills that will facilitate intervention programs may best be accomplished using informal assessment procedures. As opposed to formal assessment practices, informal methods generally occur in a natural setting rather than structured, include flexible activities rather than ordered, and result in descriptive rather than numerical data (Guerin & Maier, 1983).

Informal oral language assessment should be an ongoing process. Teachers need to be attuned to the oral expressions of the child and note specific strengths and weaknesses related to phonology, morphology, syntax, semantics, and pragmatics. One way to facilitate this is to use a structured format when informally assessing oral language. Table 6–8 (on page 220) provides an example of an oral language profile. All of the ratings can be completed as a result of observing children's spontaneous oral expression in natural environments.

Language samples provide an excellent way teachers can evaluate oral language skills. Language samples are an actual record of a child's oral language that has been collected during spontaneous speech. While they are relatively simple to use, research has shown that results obtained from language samples are frequently correlated with the results from formal, norm-referenced evaluations (Blau *et al.*, 1984). When using language samples, teachers record the spontaneous speech of students, transcribe the spoken language to a written record, then analyze the content of the sample. There are many ways

TABLE 6-7 Formal Tests for Oral Expression

TEST	AGE/GRADE	GROUP/INDIVIDUAL
Brigance (1978)	0–7 years	individual
Clinical Evaluation of Language Fundamentals-Revised	5–16-11	individual
Test of Adolescent Language-2 (1987)	12–18-5	varies by subtest
Test of Early Language Development (1981)	3–7-11	individual
Test of Language Development-2 Intermediate (1988)	8-6–12-11	individual
Test of Language Development-2 Primary (1988)	4–8-11	individual
Woodcock Language Proficiency Battery (1980)	3–80+	individual
Arizona Articulation Proficiency Scale (1986)	1-6–13-11	individual
Goldman-Fristoe Test of Articulation (1986)	2–16+	individual
Photo Articulation Test (1984)	3–12	individual
Test of Articulation Performance (1983)	3–8-11	individual
Carrow Elicited Language Inventory (1974)	3–7-11	individual
Let's Talk Inventory for Adolescents (1982)	9–adult	individual
Let's Talk Inventory for Children (1988)	4–8	individual
Test of Pragmatic Skills (1986)	3–8-11	individual

Source: McLoughloin & Lewis, 1990

TABLE 6-8 Oral Language Checklist

Voice Quality

_____ pleasant

_____ unpleasant

_____ hoarse

_____ quiet

_____ loud

_____ high pitched

_____ low pitched

_____ nasal

Speech Fluency

_____ very fluent

_____ generally fluent

_____ nonfluent

Sound Production (circle letters of sounds usually produced)

p, m, f, w, g, d, h, n, b, k, t, ng, y

r, l, s, z, v, th, ch, sh, j, th, zh

Source: Lewis & Doorlag (1992).

spontaneous language samples can be generated. Wiig & Semel (1984) describe a variety of questions and requests that can be used.

- ■ Tell me about "The Three Bears" (or some other familiar story).
- ■ Tell me about a television program you recently watched.
- ■ Tell me about something that is funny.
- ■ Tell me about your pet (or hobby or favorite sport).
- ■ Tell me about your last birthday party (or some other special event).
- ■ Complete the end of the story I am about to start telling.

Oral language samples can be analyzed several different ways. These include 1. mean length of utterances (MLU), which assesses language development; 2. developmental sentence analysis, which provides a quantitative evaluation of syntactic structures; 3. the fourteen morpheme analysis, which analyzes the use of fourteen specific morphemes;

4. syntactic analysis by distribution to determine distribution of simple and complex sentences; 5. case grammar analysis, which uses a grammar system; and 6. structural analysis of illustrative language samples, which is a complex analysis of language samples (Wiig & Semel, 1984).

The different analyses of language samples range from simple to complex. A simple, cursory analysis of the sample can be made by determining if the vocabulary used matches the intent of the speaker and the meaning that can be determined by the sentences (Wesson, Otis-Wilborn, Hasbrouck, & Tindal, 1989). A more complex analysis could use the dysfluency and word-finding analysis model that reviews samples for several different types of problems. For further detail about how to conduct a language analysis, see Wiig and Semel (1984).

Types of Oral Expression Problems

There are numerous problems in oral expression that some children display. These include problems in all five basic components previously noted: phonology, morphology, syntax, semantics, and pragmatics. Wallace and McLoughlin (1988) organize oral expression problems into four major groups: 1. expressing speech sounds, 2. formulating words and sentences, 3. word finding, and 4. pragmatic deficits.

Problems expressing speech sounds result when there is an inability to make certain sounds. These problems with phonology may be manifested through the omission of certain sounds, substitutions of one sound for another, or simple distortions of sounds (Mandell & Gold, 1984). Some students experience difficulties with formulating words and sentences. They may be able to say words in isolation, but have problems when words have to be sequenced together to form sentences. Students who display these kinds of problems are likely to:

use simple sentences;

sequence isolated words and phrases;

exhibit grammatical errors, such as improper use of plurals, unmatched verb tense, and prepositions that do not agree with antecedents (Wallace & McLoughlin, 1988).

Other characteristics associated with students who have problems formulating words and sentences include the overuse of indefinite words, such as "this" and "that"; overuse of functional definitions; and frequently changing the topic of conversation (Wiig & Semel, 1984).

Word finding is another area that creates problems for students. Students who experience this type of problem are not able to "find" the right word when speaking or answering questions. The frequent result is verbal expression with poor grammar and inadequate words (Wiig & Semel, 1984). Table 6–9 (on page 222) provides an example of a word-finding problem in a ten-year-old student.

Pragmatic deficits present problems for many students with mild disabilities. Pragmatics, or the proper use of language, is critical for the success of students in school and in social settings. Knowing what to say and when to say it is an important, functional social skill. Examples of problems in pragmatics include 1. not taking your turn in a conversation, 2. difficulty opening, maintaining, and ending a conversation, 3. problems continuing

TABLE 6-9 Example of Word-Finding Problem

1. First they had, they sang a song.
2. Then they had a commercial.
3. Then Cher was on top of the piano.
4. She was singing and went to all these things.
5. And once Chastity had a turn.
6. She's the little daughter.
7. And then Cher came back and she turn.
8. And then Dennis Weaver sang a song.
9. And then they had "Mr. and Mrs."
10. Cher was the wife and Sonny was the husband.
11. And then some guy, I forget what his name was, he comes in and he says "Barney Sue is drunk."
12. She says "I had a wonderful macaroni and cheese" something like that.
13. And all she does is she drank the wine sauce and she hit me in the face for no reason.
14. And then he comes in there.
15. And then she comes in and she says: "Oh there you are."
16. And then they say: "Will you do something about her?"
17. And then she starts kung fuin' everything.
18. And then sheriff tries to calm her down.
19. And then when she goes like that, she just touches like that, she falls down.
20. And then the guy says: "Look what you did."
21. And that was the end.
22. And they walked off.
23. And then they had "at the laundromat."
24. What they had was, they tell jokes like they were talking about what their husbands do.
25. And then after that they go into this thing like the wonder driers.
26. And then there's Cher and she's singing a song.

Used with permission. Wiig & Semel, 1984, pp. 108–109.

with the same topic, 4. difficulty contributing to the conversation (Shames & Wiig, 1990), using appropriate language codes or styles with different groups of people, and understanding your role in a conversation.

With the current emphasis in special education on the transition of students with disabilities into young adults who are capable of living as nearly normal lives as possible, the emphasis on pragmatics becomes obvious. Students and young adults with disabilities must be able to use language appropriately in different settings in order to achieve their maximum levels of assimilation into society.

INTERVENTION PROGRAMS FOR STUDENTS WITH PROBLEMS IN ORAL EXPRESSION

There are several intervention approaches and training procedures that are effective with students exhibiting oral language problems. These include direct instruction, milieu training, interactive approaches, imitation, and modeling. These models vary significantly. For example, the direct instruction model focuses on specific oral language skills with which students need assistance. The help comes in the form of practice and drill. The milieu training, on the other hand, focuses on altering the environment to enhance oral language skills. Studies comparing the effectiveness of these various methods have not revealed any one particular method as most effective. In fact, "the few studies that have directly compared intervention methods have not been particularly illuminating" (Weismer, 1991, p. 235). Rather than focusing on one particular approach, Weismer (1991) suggests that teachers use whatever works for them with particular students. There are a few commercial programs available to use in oral language development. However, most teachers use teacher-designed activities and natural practices to improve students' oral expression skills.

General Instructional Considerations

When working with students to improve their oral expressive abilities, teachers should consider the following.

1. All persons who interact with the child should help teach oral language skills, including parents, grandparents, and teachers (McCormick & Goldman, 1984).

2. Modeling appropriate oral language expression is an excellent instructional approach.

3. Instruction in oral language skills should occur wherever the student will use language (Spinelli & Terrell, 1984; Allen, 1989). Generalizations from a structured, clinical setting, may not transfer to a more natural environment (Fey, 1988).

4. Oral language intervention should be initiated as soon as possible and should be provided continuously in all settings (Pigford, 1988).

5. Materials used in oral language intervention programs should be those natural materials found in the child's routine environment.

6. Functional language should be a focus on language intervention; function should be stressed over form (McCormick, 1986).

7. Train students in oral language skills across activities; do not just teach language during a language period (McCormick, 1986).

8. Be sensitive to students' oral language patterns (Pigford, 1988).

Teachers must create an environment that is conducive to oral language development. This includes arranging the physical setting to facilitate students talking among each other. While getting students to talk is not generally a problem, teachers need to promote talking through physical room arrangements and giving students specific topics to talk about. For example, having students sit in neat, straight rows, and forbidding them to turn and face each other during conversations and discussions does not promote talking. On the other hand, arranging the seating so students can see each other and are in smaller, more "secure" groups does promote talking.

A second thing teachers can do to facilitate oral language is to provide opportunities for students to interact verbally during their learning activities. Classroom discussions about specific topics help achieve this goal. Teachers can encourage discussions through questioning procedures that are designed to elicit oral responses from students. One method of encouraging interactions among students with oral language problems and other students is through storytelling. As noted in Chapter 5, storytelling is an old method of getting students involved in language experiences. By providing opportunities for students to engage in storytelling, teachers facilitate oral language interactions among all students. During these storytelling activities, students with oral language deficits have a chance to observe and model appropriate oral language expression. They may also feel more comfortable with oral language in an informal storytelling situation.

Teachers can also facilitate oral language in the classroom by providing a variety of audiences for students. Peers, other teachers, younger students, and parents make a good variety of audiences. Without this variety, students may get very comfortable speaking in front of some audiences, but have significant problems with other groups and other settings. Finally, teachers need to reinforce verbal communication among students and encourage them to continue to talk and discuss various topics (Dudley-Marling & Searle, 1988).

Commercial Oral Language Programs

Several commercial language programs are available for teachers wishing to use a formalized approach to language instruction. These include:

Clinical Language Intervention Program (1982).   This program focuses on instructional activities related to semantics, syntax, memory, and pragmatics. The program is for students in kindergarten through eighth grade. Over two thousand stimulus pictures, as well as a teacher's guide suggesting specific activities, make up the program.

DISTAR Language Program (1976).   The DISTAR language program was originally designed for children from culturally disadvantaged environments. Additionally, it has been used for students with various language problems. The program is very structured, targets students from preschool through third grade, and focuses on receptive and expressive language and cognitive development. Group drills in a highly structured atmosphere is the primary approach.

Fokes Sentence Builder Kit (1975).   This program focuses on the development of verbal expression, comprehension, and sentence construction. Different kinds of sentences in different time frames (past, present, future) are taught. Although this program was designed for students with severe disabilities, it can be modified and used effectively with students who are experiencing milder disabilities.

Let's Talk: Developing Pro-Social Communication (1982).   This program was developed by Wiig for students ages nine through adulthood. It teaches prosocial communication skills through practicing functional communication (Mercer, 1987).

Instructional Activities for Oral Language Intervention

Although some commercially developed programs, like those described above, are used by some teachers to facilitate oral language development, many teachers use a variety of different techniques to improve oral language skills. Manning and Wray (1990) describe several ways to use figurative language to enhance oral language skills. Figurative language can be described as the use of words for multiple purposes. Examples include metaphors, similes, proverbs, idioms, and verbal humor.

Three guidelines are suggested for using figurative language. These are:

1. *Isolate terms*   Teachers should focus on specific, key words in a phrase.

2. *Analyze Semantic-Syntactic Contexts*   For example, if the topic were "rat," the student would analyze conceptions of a "rat."

3. *Compare Shared Features*   Teach students to use both figurative and literal interpretations and compare the two.

Lerner (1988) describes numerous activities that are useful in teaching oral language skills. The following provides a brief description of some of these activities.

- Activities to Build Oral Vocabulary
  a. Have students name common objects.
  b. Play "department store" where students use simulated "shopping" to use oral language.
  c. Give students a limited time frame to name all the objects in the room.
  d. Use the cloze method, having students complete sentences or phrases.
  e. Focus specific lessons on words that are difficult.

- Activities to Produce Speech Sounds
  a. Have students "exercise" mouth and facial muscles involved in speech.
  b. Use mirrors and vibrations to help students relate sounds with vibrations and lip movements.

- Activities to Teach Linguistic Patterns
  a. Teach students general morphological rules, such as adding *s*, *es*, and other endings to make plurals.
  b. Use pictures to teach morphological generalizations, such as a picture showing a boy painting a picture and a picture showing a completed picture.

- Activities to Teach Formulating Sentences
  a. Show students how to use different forms of sentences, such as simple, comlex, compound.
  b. Substitute a single word in a sentence to change the sentence content.

- Activities to Facilitate Practice in Oral Language
  a. Have students tell about various objects.
  b. Have students tell how to do something, such as "brush your teeth."
  c. Begin a story and have students complete the story.

Boucher (1986) described a way to enhance oral language skills using a pragmatics approach. Using this model, teachers do more than simply model appropriate oral language skills; they involve the students directly in the process. One way teachers can involve students pragmatically is through coaching. This approach requires the teacher to actively work with a student's oral language skills. Role play situations, rehearsals, and self-evaluations through videotapes are also intervention methods.

SUMMARY

This chapter has focused on expressive language skills. Content in the chapter was developed around two primary components of expressive language—written expression and oral expression. It was noted that the ability of humans to express themselves with language is one of the most important skills that separates humans from other animal species.

Written expression is critically important for students as well as adults. In school, students must be able to respond in writing to tests and perform other written assignments. Adults must possess certain competencies in written expression to function in certain jobs as well as get along socially. Unfortunately, although written expression is very important, teaching students writing skills is not a high priority in most schools.

There are several subcomponents of written expression. These include handwriting, spelling, and writing compositions (also called written expression). Each of these areas was discussed in regards to assessing strengths and weakness and specific intervention techniques. It was noted that there are commercially prepared assessment devices and intervention programs for all written expression skills. However, many teachers use their own informal, teacher-made tests and activities to evaluate and remediate written expression skills.

There are two main orientations to intervention in written expression. Teachers who use the skills approach teach specific skills related to written expression, such as spelling and handwriting. Advocates of the holistic or whole language model emphasize teaching writing skills through the "process of writing." This model supports students learning to write through their writing efforts rather than having teachers focus on isolated skills.

The second major section of the chapter dealt with oral expression. This skill, similar to written expression, is extremely important for students in school and adults in the work force. In school, students must use oral expression to make their feelings known, enter into discussions in class, ask questions, respond to questions, and interact socially. For adults, the ability to express yourself orally is vitally important for vocational and social success.

Improving students' skills in oral expression is often overlooked as an integral part of the curriculum. For teachers and schools that choose to include this area in the curriculum, there are numerous commercial tests and programs available. However, as in the area of written expression, teachers frequently use teacher-made assessment devices and teaching activities to enhance oral expression.

REFERENCES

Alexander, N. (1983). A primer for developing a writing curriculum. *Topics in Learning & Learning Disabilities, 3,* 55–62.

Algozzine, B., O'Shea, D.J., Stoddard, K., & Crews, W.B. (1988). Reading and writing competencies of adolescents with learning disabilities, *Journal of Learning Disabilities, 21,* 154–160.

Allen, D.A. (1989). Developmental language disorders in preschool children: Clinical subtypes and syndromes. *School Psychology Review, 18,* 442–451.

Bailet, L.L. (1991). Development and disorders of spelling in the beginning school years. In A.M. Bain, L.L. Bailet, & L.C. Moats (Eds.), *Written language disorders.* Austin, TX: Pro-Ed.

Bain, A.M. (1991). Handwriting disorders. In A.M. Bain, L.L. Bailet, and L.C. Moats (Eds.), *Written language disorders.* Austin, TX: Pro-Ed.

Barenbaum, E.M. (1983). Writing in the special class. *Topics in Learning & Learning Disabilities, 3,* 12–20.

Bechthold, C., & Del, L. (1978). *Signs for sounds.* Hillsborough, CA: Educational Support Systems.

Blau, A.F., Lahey, M., & Oleksiuk-Velez, A. (1984). Planning goals for intervention: Language testing or language sampling? *Exceptional Children, 51,* 78–79.

Bos, C.S. (1988). Process-oriented writing: Instructional implications for mildly handicapped students. *Exceptional Children, 54,* 521–527.

Boucher, R. (1986). Pragmatics: The meaning of verbal language in learning disabled and nondisabled boys. *Learning Disability Quarterly, 9,* 285–294.

Bridge, C.A., & Hiebert, E.H. (1985). A comparison of classroom writing practices, teachers' perceptions of their writing instruction, and textbook recommendations on writing practices. *Elementary School Journal, 86,* 155–172.

Dangel, H.L. (1987). The coach's spelling approach. *Teaching Exceptional Children, 19,* 20–22.

Davis, S.J., & Winek, J. (1989). Improving expository writing by increasing background knowledge. *Journal of Reading, 33,* 178–181.

Dudley-Marling, C. & Searle, D. (1988). Enriching language learning environments for students with learning disabilities. *Journal of Learning Disabilities, 21,* 140–143.

Eisenson, J. (1990). Impairments and delays for spoken and written language children. *Education, 109,* 419–423.

Fernald, G.M. (1943). *Remedial techniques in basic school subjects.* New York: McGraw-Hill.

Fey, M.E. (1988). Generalization issues facing language interventionists: An introduction. *Language, Speech, and Hearing Services in Schools, 19,* 272–281.

Fortner, V.L. (1986). Generalization of creative productive-thinking training to LD students' written expression. *Learning Disability Quarterly, 9,* 274–284.

Frank, A.R. (1987). Directed spelling instruction. *Teaching Exceptional Children, 20,* 10–13.

Gaustad, M.G., & Messenheimer-Young, T. (1991). Dialogue journals for students with learning disabilities. *Teaching Exceptional Children, 23,* 28–32.

Gerber, M.M, & Hall, R.J. (1987). Information processing approaches to studying spelling deficiencies. *Journal of Learning Disabilities, 20,* 34–42.

Gibbs, D.P., & Cooper, E.B. (1989). Prevalence of communication disorders in students with learning disabilities, *Journal of Learning Disabilities, 22,* 60–63.

Gillingham, A., & Stillman, B. (1970). *Remedial training for children with specific difficulty in reading, spelling, and penmanship* (7th ed.). Cambridge, MA: Educators Publishing Service.

Gould, B.W. (1991). Curricular strategies for written expression. In A.M. Bain, L.L. Bailet, & L.C. Moats (Eds.), *Written language disorders.* Austin, TX: Pro-Ed.

Graham, S. (1986). A review of handwriting scales. *Journal of School Psychology, 24,* 63–71.

Graham, S. & Miller, L. (1980). Handwriting research and practice. *Focus on Exceptional Children, 13,* 1–16.

Graham, S., & Harris, K.R. (1988). Instructional recommendations for teaching writing to exceptional students. *Exceptional Children, 54,* 506–512.

Graham, S., & Harris, K.R. (1989). Improving learning disabled students' skills at composing essays: Self-instructional strategy training. *Exceptional Children, 56,* 201–214.

Graham, S., Boyer-Schick, K., & Tippets, E. (1989). The validity of the handwriting scale from the test of written language. *Journal of Educational Research, 82,* 166–170.

Gregg, N. (1991). Disorders of written expression. In A.M. Bain, L.L. Bailet, & L.C. Moats (Eds.), *Written language disorders.* Austin, TX: Pro-Ed.

Guerin, G.R., & Maier, A.S. (1983). *Informal assessment in education.* Palo Alto, CA: Mayfield Publishing.

Hagin, R.A. (1983). Write right—or left: A practical approach to handwriting. *Journal of Learning Disabilities, 16,* 266–271.

Hammill, D.D. & Bartel, N.R. (1990). *Teaching students with learning and behavior problems*, 5th Ed. Boston: Allyn & Bacon.

Houston, G., Goolrick, F., & Tate, R. (1991). Storytelling as a stage in process writing: A whole language model. *Teaching Exceptional Children, 23*, 40–43.

Ketchum, P.J. (1982). *Cloze stories for drill*. Wilkinsburg, PA: Hayes School Publishing Co.

Larsen, S., & Hammill, D.D. (1989). *Test of legible handwriting*. Austin, TX: Pro-Ed.

Larsen, S., & Hammill, D. (1986). *Test of Written Spelling*. Austin, TX: Pro-Ed.

Lerner, J. (1988). *Learning Disabilities*, 5th Ed. Boston: Houghton-Mifflin.

Lewis, Doorlag, *Teaching special students in the mainstream*, (Ed.). Columbus, OH: Merrill.

Lindamood, C.H., & Lindamood, P.C. (1975). *The A.D.D. program, auditory discrimination in-depth*. Hingham, MA: Teaching Resources.

Luftig, R.L. (1989). *Assessment of learners with special needs*. Boston: Allyn & Bacon.

McCormick, L.P. (1986). Keeping up with language intervention trends. *Teaching Exceptional Children, 18*, 123–129.

McCormick, L. & Goldman, R. (1984). Designing an optimal learning program. In L. McCormick & R.L. Schiefelbusch, (Eds.). *Early language intervention*. Columbus, OH: Merrill.

Mandell, C.J., & Gold, V. (1984). *Teaching handicapped students*. St. Paul, MN: West.

Mann, V.A., Cowin, E., & Schoenheimer, J. (1989). Phonological processing, language comprehension, and reading ability. *Journal of Learning Disabilities, 22*, 76–89.

Manning, A.L., & Wray, D. (1990). Using figurative language in the classroom. *Teaching Exceptional Children, 22*, 18–21.

Mercer, C.D. (1987). *Students with learning disabilities* (3rd Ed.), Columbus, OH: Charles E. Merrill.

Meyer, A., Pisha, B., & Rose, D. (1991). Process and product in writing: Computer as enabler. In A.M. Bain, L.L. Bailet, & L.C. Moats (Eds.). *Written language disorders*. Austin, TX: Pro-Ed.

Miller, L. (1989). Classroom-based language intervention. *Language speech, and hearing services in schools, 20*, 149–152.

Minner, S., Prater, G., Sullavan, C., & Gwaltney, W. (1989). Informal assessment of written expression. *Teaching Exceptional Children, 21*, 76–79.

Morley, J. (1972). *Improving aural comprehension*. Ann Arbor, MI: University of Michigan Press.

Patton, J.R., Beirne-Smith, M., & Payne, J.S. (1989). *Mental Retardation* (3rd Ed.). Columbus, OH: Charles E. Merrill Publishing.

Phelps, J., Stempel, L., & Speck, G. (1985.). The children's handwriting scale: A new diagnostic tool. *Journal of Educational Research, 79*, 46–50.

Pigford, A.B. (1988). Teachers, let students talk. *Academic Therapy, 24*, 193–198.

Polloway, E.A., Patton, J.R., Payne, J.S., & Payne, R.A. (1989). *Strategies for teaching learners with special needs*, 4th Ed. Columbus, OH: Merrill.

Polloway, E.A., & Smith, T.E.C. (1992). *Language disorders in students with mild disabilities*, 2nd Ed. Denver: Love Publishing.

Scarborough, H.W., & Dobrich, W. (1990). Development of children with early language delay. *Journal of Speech and Hearing Research, 33*, 70–83.

Shames, G.H., Wiig, E.H. (1990). *Human communication disorders*. Columbus, OH: Merrill.

Smith, T.E.C. (1990). *Introduction to education*, 2nd Ed. St Paul: West Publishing.

Smith, T.E.C., Price, B.J., & Marsh, G.E. (1986). *Mildly handicapped children and adults*. St. Paul: West Publishing.

Spinelli, F.M., & Terrell, B.Y. (1984). Remediation in context. *Topics in Language Disorders, 5*, 29–40.

Taenzer, S.F., Cermak, C., & Hanlon, R.C. (1981). Outside the therapy room: A naturalistic approach to language intervention. *Topics in Learning and Learning Disabilities, 1*, 41–46.

Tompkins, G.E., & Friend, M. (1988). After your students write: What's next? *Teaching Exceptional Children, 20,* 4–9.

Vallecorsa, A.L., Ledford, R.R., & Parnell, G.G. (1991). Strategies for teaching composition skills to students with learning disabilities. *Teaching Exceptional Children, 23,* 52–55.

Vallecorsa, A.L., Zigmond, N., & Henderson, L.M. (1985). Spelling instruction in special education classrooms: A survey of practices. *Exceptional Children, 52,* 19–24.

Wallace, G., Cohen, S.B., & Polloway, E.A. (1987). *Language arts.* Austin, TX: Pro-Ed.

Wallace, G., & Larsen, S.L. (1978). *The educational assessment of learning problems: Testing for teaching.* Boston: Allyn & Bacon.

Wallace, G., & McLoughlin, J.A. (1988). *Learning disabilities: Concepts and Characteristics,* 3rd Ed. Columbus, OH: Merrill.

Weismer, S.E. (1991). Child language intervention: Research issues on the horizon. In J. Miller Ed.), *Research on Child Language Disorders,* Austin, TX: Pro-Ed.

Wesson, C., Otis-Wilborn, A., Hasbrouck, J., & Tindal, G. (1989). Linking assessment, curriculum, and instruction of oral and written language. *Focus on Exceptional Children, 22,* 1–12.

Wiig, E.H., & Semel, E. (1984). *Language assessment and intervention for the learning disabled.* Columbus, OH: Merrill.

Wood, R.W., Webster, L., Gullickson, A., & Walker, J. (1987). Comparing handwriting legibility with three teaching methods for sex and grade differences. *Reading Improvement, 24,* 24–30.

Zemelman, S., & Daniels, H. (1988). *A community of writers.* Portsmouth, NH: Heinemann.

Zylstra, B.J. (1989). Combined spelling—It works. *Academic Therapy, 24,* 315–320.

Teaching Mathematics to Students with Mild Disabilities

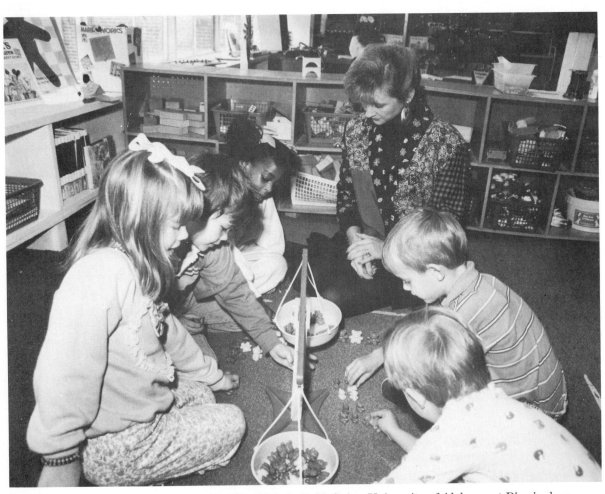

Chapter 7 was written by: Michele D. McGuire, University of Alabama at Birmingham

Outline

Introduction

Sources of Math Difficulty
  Mathematics Anxiety
  Math Myths and Teacher Bias
  Instructional Issues
  Instructional Logistics and
    Curriculum Issues
  Learner Characteristics (or, Issues
    We Tend to Overlook)
  Erroneous or Faulty Learning

Mathematics Curricula
  Mathematics as a Knowledge Base
  Curriculum Development

Readiness for Mathematics Instruction
  Math Skills, Learning, and Child
    Development
  Maturation and Readiness

Assessment
  Sequences of the Assessment Process
  Standardized Assessments
  Assessment for Instructional
    Planning

Instructional Techniques
  Instruction and Sequences
  Teaching Mathematics Skills

Instructional Materials

OBJECTIVES

After reading this chapter, you should be able to:

- identify the potential sources of mathematics difficulty and anxiety experienced by teachers and students;

- identify the mathematical skills and competencies included in an effective mathematics curriculum;

- identify the various levels of learning and skills acquisition associated with mathematics instruction;

- identify and implement the sequence of assessment-evaluation-instructional planning procedures;

- select and implement effective instructional practices.

Introduction

Teachers of mathematics are faced with the challenge of preparing children for an increasingly complex, technological society. Since the Sputnik era of the 1950s and early 1960s, technological advancements have had a significant impact on all aspects of our lives and the multiple contexts in which daily life activities occur. Cooking, handling money, even programming a VCR are examples of commonplace activities that incorporate various levels of mathematics principles and likely involve some level of technological skills.

There is little dispute that a meaningful knowledge of mathematics plus the ability to apply that knowledge in typical life situations are essential skills. For teachers of mathematics, particularly teachers of children with learning challenges or mild disabilities, this presents an enormous instructional responsibility. Not only must these educators provide children with the critical skills needed today; but, the rapid rate of technological growth demands that teachers also predict and provide skills that will enable children to cope with unknown challenges of the future. Instruction, therefore, must be designed to help children develop a functional understanding of mathematics that will enhance learning as a life skill in the context of an ever-changing world.

Teachers who work with pupils with mild learning disabilities understand the difficulties of imparting a largely abstract body of knowledge in a functional context. Bridging the cognitive gap between math abstractions and practical applications poses a challenge for both the students and their teachers. However, it is this critical component of mathematics education that is frequently neglected—perhaps because such instruction is so difficult.

This chapter presents a consolidated view of math instruction that involves the integration of skills and structural knowledge, and, will help teachers meet the instructional challenge posed by mathematics. Learning effectiveness will be discussed as related to sources of difficulty and attitudinal issues, curriculum concerns, developmental factors and readiness, learning levels and levels of teacher presentation, effective assessment and evaluation practices, and instructional methodologies. The approach is holistic and stresses the belief that math is and should be taught as an applied life science; one that is applied across multiple contexts. The information presented not only has been empirically tested, but has been implemented in classroom settings for the true acid test.

Sources of Math Difficulty

Difficulties in mathematics stem from a range of sources including intellectual, sensory, cultural, instructional, and attitudinal factors. A typical math class, in either regular or special education, may include students who are gifted mathematicians and those who are struggling to understand. Teachers can relate to the frustration, if not exhaustion, such a classroom configuration imposes on both students and teachers. Nonetheless, math teachers are expected to accommodate the various individual needs of students while ensuring that yearly "scope and sequence" requirements are met. It is critical, therefore, for teachers to approach mathematics instruction with a positive attitude, make every effort to reduce their own anxieties about math, and create a learning environment in which students find mathematics an exciting challenge.

MATHEMATICS ANXIETY

Some people read for pleasure or write to relax, but very few people compute math problems as a source of entertainment. Math anxiety is a serious problem for many (Tobias, 1981). Few children or adults share fond recollections of math classes. Rather, most people tend to recall math courses with negative and self-derogatory comments (Tobias, 1981; Kennedy & Tipps, 1991). Ironically, some teachers fall into this category, and teachers who hold negative attitudes toward math readily convey negative messages to their students.

Math anxiety can be described as an intense dislike, fear, or emotional reaction to mathematics in any form. Typically, the source of anxiety is not related to an individual's ability to learn, even when considering children with mild learning difficulties. More often the problem is related to the ways in which math is taught and to the nature of the demands placed on the learner. Particular teaching methods can create anxiety and leave many students feeling inadequate and ineffective in using mathematics.

Kennedy and Tipps (1991) identified five faulty teaching practices that are commonly used in mathematics classrooms that contribute to math anxiety: 1. lack of variety in teaching-learning process, 2. emphasis on memorization, 3. emphasis on speed, 4. emphasis on doing one's own work, and 5. authoritarian teaching. They found that more than seventy percent of instructional time is commonly allocated for independent practice, most frequently with workbook-type assignments. Also, children are typically laden with extensive homework assignments that are merely more of the same. This suggests that students are receiving very little direct instruction in the concepts and skills they are to practice. For children who are unable to grasp new material based on minimal instruction, this approach can be boring and frustrating. Further, without guided practice, students often apply erroneous procedures, then drill-and-practice their errors and become quite good at computing problems incorrectly! Clearly, unlearning a faulty method can be more difficult than learning the correct procedure during initial instruction.

An emphasis on memorizing facts leads children to believe math is a series of isolated processes rather than a logical knowledge base. Few children, particularly those with learning problems, are able to independently understand the interconnections among math skills and concepts when memorization is the primary learning mode. In the early elementary grades, rote processes are adequate for completing simple math tasks. As students approach the upper elementary grades, however, memorized facts and rules take on overwhelming proportions and often become confused or forgotten. Students experience increasing difficulty in sorting through facts and rules to select an appropriate strategy for solving more complex problems.

Similarly, an emphasis on speed can have a negative impact on children's learning and enjoyment of math. Timed tasks pose high risks for failure. The child with learning problems may need extended time to complete assignments or may work in a systematic, deliberate fashion. Under such circumstances, a child is likely to become anxious and apprehensive about timed conditions, and a negative effect on performance can be expected. In some instances, children with learning problems choose not to complete or even attempt tasks rather than risk failure.

"Keep your eyes on your own paper" is commonly heard in classrooms. It is customary for teachers to expect children to work independently rather than ask others for assistance. Yet, cooperative learning and peer coaching are sound instructional procedures. Mathematics is a subject that lends itself to such practices—collaboration encourages the development of global mathematical thinking skills in addition to diverse problem solving strategies and abilities.

When teachers encounter children who have difficulty learning mathematics skills and concepts, they too often adopt an authoritarian, inflexible teaching style. Each of the faulty practices described by Kennedy and Tipps are found in such teachers' classrooms. The less typical the child, the more teachers tend to emphasize step-by-step procedures, rules, correctness of responses, and memorization drills rather than using unique instructional methodologies. Oddly, the very techniques that teachers embrace are the methods least likely to have a positive learning impact on students with special needs (Love & McGuire, 1990). When teachers abandon variations in the teaching-learning process and encourage the belief that there is only one way to solve a problem, they are promoting an environment prime for math anxiety. As a result, students progressively become more discouraged and frustrated, develop negative attitudes toward math, and generally become increasingly less receptive to mathematics instruction.

MATH MYTHS AND TEACHER BIAS

Reducing the potential for math anxiety involves more than changing students' attitudes; there must also be a change in the attitudes teachers hold about mathematics teaching and learning. Kogelman and Warren (1978) and later Frank (1990) examined teachers' beliefs about math in an attempt to clarify issues related to revising mathematics curricula and changing customary instructional patterns. In descending order (most believed by teachers to least believed) the following twelve myths were commonly identified.

1. Men are better at math than women.

2. Math requires logic, not intuition.

3. You must always know how you got your answer.

4. Math is not creative.

5. There is a best way to complete a math problem.

6. It is always important to get the answer exactly right.

7. It is bad to count on your fingers.

8. Mathematicians do problems quickly, in their heads.

9. Math requires a good memory.

10. Math is done by working intensely until the problem is solved.

11. Some people have a "math mind" and some don't.

12. There is a magic key to doing math (Frank, 1990, p. 11).

Kogelman and Warren (1978) proposed that teachers are influenced by their beliefs and convey their attitudes to students through the instructional practices employed. Essentially, teachers set up a self-fulfilling prophecy either by subliminal messages or overt reinforcement of behaviors related to the twelve identified myths. Frank contended that disrupting "mathematics myths" believed by teachers is an essential precursor to improving students' acquisition of math knowledge and skills. That is, effectively changing mathematics curriculum and instruction can occur only when teachers recognize their attitudinal barriers that are influencing math education.

INSTRUCTIONAL ISSUES

The recent call for "back to basics" teaching reemphasized the use of basic facts memorization and rote drill and practice procedures that are common to traditional math instruction (Ashlock, 1990; Smith, 1990). While many teachers elect to use this method, a growing number of educators believe that rote procedures are insufficient for children to adequately solve real-life problems. These educators promote instruction that emphasizes mathematics principles and concepts and deemphasizes computational skills. Unfortunately, both teachers and math texts tend to accept the two perspectives as mutually exclusive (Wilson, 1990), despite common sense knowledge plus empirical evidence that effective teaching-learning practices integrate these two essential components of mathematics knowledge (Ashlock, 1990; Kennedy & Tipps, 1991).

Classroom teachers know that a dichotomous approach to mathematics teaching-learning does not work. Mere drill and practice does not ensure functional learning; in other words, the mastery of computational skills does not ensure children will understand and therefore generalize mathematics concepts and principles in more complex thinking and problem solving tasks. Similarly, the acquisition of a structural-conceptual knowledge of math does not assure children will know when and how to appropriately use computational skills as problem solving tools. Thus, the failure to consolidate conceptual learning with computation skills leaves students with incomplete, incorrect, and inefficient mathematics strategies (Ashlock, 1990; Cawley & Parmar, 1990; Kennedy & Tipps, 1988, 1991).

INSTRUCTIONAL LOGISTICS AND CURRICULUM ISSUES

In recent years, public school programs have telescoped mathematics curricula; that is, abstract concepts and advanced content are taught at earlier and earlier grade levels. While the intention is to accelerate the acquisition of mathematics abilities, compressed curricula have posed significant difficulty for teachers and students and can conflict with a child's readiness for learning. Essentially, presenting more information at a more rapid rate cannot also accelerate developmental processes, such as learning readiness.

Ironically, research has demonstrated that telescoping efforts have resulted in an overall, modest decline in mathematics achievement, rather than the anticipated improvement (National Commission on Excellence in Education, 1983; McKnight, Travers, Crosswhite,

& Swafford, 1985; Love, 1987). Further, there has been a substantial increase in the number of students who are referred for special education services specifically on the basis of mathematics difficulties (Fleischner, Nuzum, & Mazzola, 1987; Love, 1987). Such trends have led many educators to examine the relevance of math curricula in general, and to re-examine available, diverse instructional methodologies that may enhance mathematics learning efficiency.

LEARNER CHARACTERISTICS (OR, ISSUES WE TEND TO OVERLOOK)

Children enter school with varied notions about numbers that reflect differing degrees of cognitive maturity. Some children will have had opportunities to explore concrete materials toward constructing an understanding of basic concepts while other children will not (Piaget, 1965; Kamii, 1990). Consequently, a common knowledge or level of competence in understanding and using numerical concepts cannot be assumed. Nevertheless, the content of instructional programs is typically structured on such an assumption. Many children, in fact, are not cognitively ready to learn about numbers at the time numerical tasks are introduced in instructional programs.

Readiness

When any individual is asked to perform a task or skill they do not understand, the experience is highly frustrating. Adults generally have the option to not participate or to find an alternative challenge. Children in classrooms have fewer options. However, Tobias (1981) found that students do elect not to participate in math; they "shut down" learning and substitute math mechanics for understanding. This has a serious, cumulative effect.

As mathematics knowledge becomes more complex, applications of math skills become more implied than implicit, and the pressure to perform increases. At this stage of math education, typically during upper elementary and middle school years, mechanical procedures become increasingly less adequate. Students who have "shut down" often resign themselves to confusion and believe they are unable to learn or understand math (Tobias, 1981). In some instances, frequently during the middle or high school years, these students suddenly appear to have specific math disabilities and are referred for special education services. The resulting frustration, for students and their teachers, is self-perpetuating and can be educationally damaging.

Learning Problems

Certainly, there are students who do have specific learning disabilities or associated learning problems. It is essential for teachers of the earliest grades to be attuned to potentially troublesome characteristics children exhibit in the classroom. Herold (1979) identified several such factors that more commonly affect learning in mathematics and associated evidence to suggest a potential concern:

- Spatial perception: difficulty in perceiving size and quantity relationships.

- Visual perception: difficulty learning and discriminating process signs (e.g., =, +, −), clutter confusion (e.g., too many items on a single page), shape discrimination problems (e.g., squares and rectangles).

- Visual spatial relationships: difficulty discriminating differences in size, quantity, length, figure-ground discrimination, place value.

- Directionality: right-left and/or top-bottom confusion, reversals, place value, location of where to start computation.

- Memory: difficulty memorizing facts, procedures, rules.

- Sequencing: difficulty remembering the order of steps in operations and/or distinguishing patterns.

- Visual-motor coordination: difficulty in writing numbers, drawing shapes; messy work products.

- Auditory reception: difficulty understanding or confusion of aural information; not due to an acuity deficit.

- Perseveration: difficulty shifting from one activity to another.

- Hypoactivity: time consuming work habits, unable to complete tasks in allocated time periods despite intellectual ability, skills, and knowledge to meet task demand (pp. 52–53).

Nearly everyone exhibits one or more of these characteristics at some point in their lives. Therefore, it is important that teachers exercise caution and not assume a learning disability exists merely on the basis of random or isolated student errors. Rather, they should employ multiple instructional techniques and task response designs to 1. better assure that various learning styles are accommodated and 2. determine whether or not a concern is consistent and pervasive.

ERRONEOUS OR FAULTY LEARNING

Not all errors in mathematics are due to carelessness or lack of knowledge about processes and rules. In fact, many children believe math is a system of rules and procedures applied for the purpose of reaching an answer. In their efforts to "come up with the answer," students systematically apply simplistic processes they can remember or procedures they have practiced, even when the application is faulty. Curiously, children have a high degree of confidence in their erroneous procedures. Ashlock (1986) observed: "Because incorrect algorithms do not usually result in correct answers, it would appear that a child [would receive] limited positive reinforcement for the continued use of erroneous patterns. However, children sometimes hold tenaciously to incorrect procedures even during remedial instruction" (pp. 7–8).

Several significant implications can be examined. First, teachers tend to score written work on the basis of correctness of responses—problems are graded as right or wrong. The problem-attack procedures children employ are not examined; consequently, neither the teacher nor the students know when an appropriate or inappropriate problem solving strategy has been learned and used. Even faulty procedures often result in correct responses. Therefore, when grading is focused on responses alone, students can be led to believe their errors were random or careless mistakes rather than the result of erroneous strategies.

This belief is reinforced when teachers fail to provide instruction to remediate or correct procedural errors that have been learned and routinely practiced. Exploring the procedures a child uses, however, actually creates the teachable moment. Knowing which problem-attack and solving skills a child has and has not adequately learned identifies where instruction is needed and should begin.

Learning Patterns of Error

It is commonly assumed that children with mild disabilities characteristically experience difficulties in mathematics. The nature of their learning patterns and the very nature of mathematics as a subject leads educators to expect and even reinforce difficulties when they occur. However, research suggests that effective teaching practices will enable most children to learn and apply math skills.

There are numerous reasons why children learn error patterns. Certainly, learning difficulties influence the efficiency with which a child learns; but, the instructional practices used can either help a child overcome learning hurdles or reinforce inefficient learning.

Constructing a Knowledge Base Children learn erroneous math concepts and procedures in basically the same way they learn ideas and processes that are appropriate. Effective learning builds on prior experiences with interrelated concepts and activities (at concrete, graphic, and symbolic levels), and students seek to find commonalities among the characteristics of new information and information they have stored in memory. However, when the prerequisite knowledge base is inadequate, they are apt to form incomplete or ineffective concept constructions. As a result, subsequent learning is based on fragmented knowledge, erroneous premises, or faulty logic; learning is significantly impaired; and, ultimately, students "shut down" (Tobias, 1981).

This commonly occurs when students attend several different schools, when school attendance is sporadic, or, in some instances, when the learning process has not been adequately monitored by classroom teachers. The addition of simple fractions may present a vivid example. Suppose that a child has learned to combine simple fractions containing common denominators, such as:

$$\frac{1}{5} + \frac{3}{5} = \frac{4}{5}$$

At a later date, combining fractions with unlike denominators is introduced. The child may have been absent or perhaps did not fully understand the lesson. Given a problem set to complete, he or she is likely to search for similarities between the new tasks and prior knowledge—unaware of critical differences and the need to seek teacher assistance. Thus, the student innocently relies on comfortable, previously successful procedures to complete the assignment. Imagine the child's confusion and frustration when a reliable technique suddenly results in a poor performance!

Consider the following computations completed by a ninth-grade student. Eddie explained that he had "... learned that when the numbers are the same in the top or the bottom you keep it. When they are different you add them together. Then you reduce ... if you can."

$$\frac{1}{4} + \frac{3}{5} = \frac{4}{9} \qquad \frac{2}{3} + \frac{2}{5} = \frac{2}{8} = \frac{1}{4}$$

Eddie had pieced together fragments of rules to formulate a strategy; and, albeit faulty, the logic he applied made sense to him. Because he had not received effective direct or corrective instruction, Eddie received considerable practice over the years in using (learning?) an incorrect process. Thus, he came to believe his strategy was correct but that "...I make mistakes somehow. Sometimes I get it right. I'm not sure what I do wrong."

Generalization for Learning   In the absence of extended experiences with diverse representations of concepts, efforts to draw meaningful relationships are frustrated. For example, suppose a child was first taught the concept of "three" using a linear configuration of blocks. The child consistently indicated the correct numerical value when shown the aligned blocks. The teacher then presented a flash card with three black dots in a triangular configuration, but, the child was unable to produce the response three. For the child, this "new" picture was unique; it did not "look like" three.

One classic example is computation via vertical and horizontal processes. A child may be able to solve Problem A with ease; yet when given Problem B, may appear completely baffled.

$$
\textbf{A.} \quad \begin{array}{r} 7 \\ + 8 \\ \hline \end{array} \qquad \textbf{B.} \quad 7 + 8 =
$$

Children typically believe that the answers cannot be the same because the problems "look" different.

When teachers assume generalization, faulty learning can occur. Children will seek any commonalities among new concepts and previous knowledge to construct a personally meaningful knowledge set. In the absence of a range of experiences and appropriate instructional examples, children tend to form concept constructions based on attributes sometimes disassociated with what the teacher has in mind. Consider the blocks example; if the child, after several trials with three blocks had been given five blocks similarly aligned, it is probable that the child would have initially answered three. Such a response would be activated by the objects and the configuration, rather than the attribute of quantity.

In math, helping children draw appropriate generalizations is an essential component of effective instruction. Teachers need to provide multiple examples and opportunities for exploration of the relationships among new concepts and previous knowledge, regardless of the grade placement or level of math instruction. When instruction proceeds without clarification of relationships, children are encouraged to rely on what they remember and often patch together rules and procedures that seem related. Ashlock (1990) suggests this encourages children to invent rules and procedures for problem solving. Because these rules and procedures are derived of a search for meaning, the learning process (though not the content) is logical, and students become rather loyal to their creations.

Teacher Behaviors   Teachers, operating under positive intentions, often initiate erroneous learning patterns through instruction of partial rules or mathematical "white lies." Teachers are aware that children may not be cognitively ready for abstract concepts, and base instructional plans on what they believe is sensible and logical for their students. Thus, the underlying intentions are positive, yet the effects are frequently realized in faulty learning outcomes. One such example is when teachers introduce the concept of zero; a source of many students' misconceptions. When teaching zero as the first counting numbers, teachers tend to emphasize that zero is the smallest number; there is nothing less than zero. Pity the poor teacher who later must explain that this is not true and teach the concept of number values less than zero! A further assault on zero occurs when teachers define zero as nothing. To use the term "nothing" rather than explaining the concept of "none" implies no value whatsoever; it is no wonder that many children become confused with place values, or simply ignore zeroes in multidigit problems.

Teachers tend to introduce rules in increments, gradually leading to more complex rules and procedures. The intention is to ensure children will systematically apply the rule for current instructional purposes. However, many rule increments have significant exceptions, or are only a portion of the more complex concept.

When increments, or partial rules are introduced as absolutes teachers lay the foundation for error patterns. Terms such as *always* and *never* set up learning confusion. During initial instruction in subtraction, for example, teachers routinely state that the larger numeral "always goes on the top...*never, never, never* use the smaller numeral as the minuend (top numeral)." Among the many problems related to this rule, the defective subtraction algorithm pictured is one of the most common.

Student's problem solving process:

573
− 638
145

- 8 take away 3 is 5
- 7 take away 3 is 4
- 6 take away 5 is 1

Essentially, children subtract the smaller number from the larger whether it is the minuend or subtrahend (bottom numeral). In more advanced instruction, the subtraction of numbers resulting in negative (less than zero) values becomes almost too much for students to comprehend—there is a conflict between the new information and the "always" rule they have ingrained.

Many of the defective algorithms used by students in upper elementary, middle, and high schools can be traced to "rule confusion" (Love & McGuire, 1985). When this occurs, students attempt to make sense of new information in the framework of procedures they can remember and resort to using more simplistic procedures they have memorized. Usually, as many teachers and students can attest, the procedures are inadequate for solving tasks at hand. Nonetheless, students will continue to use procedures with which they are comfortable.

To investigate students' math error patterns and learning, Love and McGuire interviewed upper elementary, middle, and high school students from several states. Participants in the study were identified as mildly learning handicapped or learning disabled and were receiving special education services. Interestingly, they found that the students commonly believed teachers had lied or withheld information, as though math were a great mystery to be solved. In fact, most of the students interviewed suggested that teachers, when introducing new rules, should inform students that they are learning but a part of a larger picture, "like a puzzle where all the pieces together make sense."

Finally, teachers often use paper-and-pencil computations as the primary strategy in the teaching-learning process. This not only ignores the need for students to explore concepts, but also encourages students to believe math is a series of memorized, mechanical procedures (Ashlock, 1990). In the attempt to memorize such sequences, students often become confused and discouraged, and rely on simplistic methods they are able to recall. When these invented procedures intermittently produce correct responses, students are reinforced in believing that their problem solving strategies are procedurally correct, and that incorrect responses are due to random, careless computational errors (Love & McGuire, 1985; Ashlock, 1986).

Again, it is important to note that unless the problem-attack procedures children employ are examined, neither the teacher nor the students know when erroneous strategies are consistently used. Grading the correctness of solutions does not provide instructional planning information; rather, a more efficient instructional practice is to invest time analyzing the ways in which children compute.

Mathematics Curricula

Efforts to evaluate and restructure curricula in the context of future based, functional adult needs have influenced a transition in educators' thinking about math instruction. Instead of the rote memorization of facts or an exclusive emphasis on understanding mathematics concepts and principles, educators are pursuing methods to teach mathematics as a way of thinking and problem solving, wherein computational skills are problem solving tools (Cawley, Miller, & Carr, 1988; Kennedy & Tipps, 1988; Ashlock, 1990). Nonetheless, the availability of technology, such as hand-held calculators and home computer systems, has influenced a decrease in the perceived importance of teaching and learning computational skills. It is the very use of computation aids, however, that increases the need for students to learn 1. estimation skills, 2. procedures for determining correct responses, and 3. methods for determining the reasonableness of responses obtained (Kennedy & Tipps, 1988; Ashlock, 1990). Underpinning these computational skills are logical mathematical concepts and principles.

MATHEMATICS AS A KNOWLEDGE BASE

The acquisition of structural knowledge (concepts and principles) forms the basis for integrating and understanding the use of computation skills. This premise is clarified by reports and curriculum recommendations issued by professional organizations such as the National Council for Supervisors of Mathematics (NCSM), and National Council for Teachers of Mathematics (NCTM) (1989). Mathematics competencies identified by these organizations primarily address generalized applications of skills and computational aspects of math knowledge. A compilation of the competencies delineated by NCTM and NCSM includes abilities in the following twelve domains.

1. Problem solving

2. Communicating mathematical ideas and concepts

3. Mathematical reasoning

4. Mathematics applications in everyday situations

5. Alertness to the reasonableness of results

6. Estimation

7. Selecting and applying appropriate computational skills

8. Algebraic thinking

9. Geometric properties and applications

10. Measurement

11. Statistics and probability

12. Computer literacy (Carl, 1989, p. 41)

Based on these domains, students' proficiency in each can be observed and measured as applied skills. Learning outcomes would be demonstrated as abilities to:

- analyze situations and seek alternative solutions;

- demonstrate and discuss mathematical ideas;

- solve ratio and percentage problems;

- compute and estimate measurements (volume, mass, length, and area);

- use mental arithmetic (addition, subtraction, multiplication, and division);

- compute mathematical function using equations, tables, and graphs;

- demonstrate applications of geometric principles;

- use known probabilities to analyze previous research and predict future events;

- use technological devices for calculating and problem solving (Carl, 1989, p. 41).

CURRICULUM DEVELOPMENT

The identified curricular domains and math competencies provide a conceptual framework for developing a functional mathematics curriculum. When and where specific skills should be introduced within this framework are determined by several factors including child learning characteristics, local district learning outcome goals, and the adopted curriculum. Resources including mathematics textbooks, scope and sequence materials, and local and state minimum competency requirements provide empirically sound guidelines for establishing a comprehensive skills hierarchy or sequence. Figure 7–1 provides an example of the curriculum sequence proposed by the NCTM Curriculum Standards. Using such a hierarchical guide, it is possible to formulate a localized, district-wide curriculum plan that integrates global math hierarchies and competencies with local instructional goals and objectives. An internally consistent curriculum offers at least two benefits: 1. mathematics will be taught and learned as a continuous system of interrelated skills and competencies, therefore 2. teaching and learning are more likely to occur in a logical progression across all grade levels.

FIGURE 7-1 NCTM Curriculum Standards/Content by Grade Classification

Grades K-4

Standard	1:	Mathematics as Problem Solving
Standard	2:	Mathematics as Communication
Standard	3:	Mathemetics as Reasoning
Standard	4:	Mathematical Connections
Standard	5:	Estimation
Standard	6:	Number Sense and Numeration
Standard	7:	Concepts of Whole Number Operations
Standard	8:	Whole Number Computation
Standard	9:	Geometry and Spatial Sense
Standard	10:	Measurement
Standard	11:	Statistics amd Probability
Standard	12:	Fractions and Decimals
Standard	13:	Patterns and Relationships

Grades 5-8

Standard	1:	Mathematics as Problem Solving
Standard	2:	Mathematics as Communication
Standard	3:	Mathemetics as Reasoning
Standard	4:	Mathematical Connections
Standard	5:	Number and Number Relationships
Standard	6:	Number Systems and Number Theory
Standard	7:	Computation and Estimation
Standard	8:	Patterns and Functions
Standard	9:	Algebra
Standard	10:	Statistics
Standard	11:	Probability
Standard	12:	Geometry
Standard	13:	Measurement

Grades 9-12

Standard	1:	Mathematics as Problem Solving
Standard	2:	Mathematics as Communication
Standard	3:	Mathemetics as Reasoning
Standard	4:	Mathematical Connections
Standard	5:	Algebra
Standard	6:	Functions
Standard	7:	Geometry from a Synthetic Perspective
Standard	8:	Geometry from an Algebraic Perspective
Standard	9:	Trigonometry
Standard	10:	Statistics
Standard	11:	Probability
Standard	12:	Discrete Mathematics
Standard	13:	Conceptual Underpinnings of Calculus
Standard	14:	Mathematical Structure

A functional curriculum is driven by essential mathematical competencies and life skills; therefore, adherence to sequencing guidelines is critical to ensure curriculum relevance and promote effective teaching practices. Sequencing mathematics concepts and skills for classroom instruction purposes are directly related to the learning and response demands placed on learners. Readiness variables, students' prior knowledge, current levels of skill development, and learning efficiency are among the broad concerns to be considered. Each of these concerns is addressed and instructional implications are clarified in subsequent sections of this chapter.

Readiness for Mathematics Instruction

Focusing on future-based, adult needs highlights the importance of NCTM and NCSM proficiencies and recommendations as well as the need to create and teach a comprehensive, functional mathematics curriculum. To meet such challenges, teachers must reorganize their thinking about and instructional approaches to mathematics. Teachers need to recognize that students learn math more efficiently through active-interactive processes than traditional passive-receptive methods. Further, they must develop an understanding of mathematics as a cumulative, integrated thinking and problem-solving process. Typically, students view math as a set of unrelated skill exercises, rather than a system where each new skill overlaps and builds upon previous information. This outcome is largely due to "train and hope" instruction. That is, teachers teach or train the use of number facts and computation procedures as isolated skills, then hope students will infer interrelationships among skills to derive problem-solving procedures. One would hardly teach an individual the names and uses of various auto parts and tools used for repairs, then assume that individual could independently determine how to repair an engine. Such a method is based on faulty logic and poor pedagogical practice. In math, complex applied abilities cannot be assumed to have been learned merely because students are able to complete drill and practice exercises with relative success.

An understanding of the relationships among skills and applications must be taught, not implied or assumed. Few school-aged children possess the ability to process, analyze, synthesize, and use new information as simultaneous functions; they are often developmentally not yet ready. Nonetheless, many teachers continue to frustrate themselves and their students by routinely using train and hope techniques.

MATH SKILLS, LEARNING, AND CHILD DEVELOPMENT

Research into learning theory provides a valuable foundation for developing a meaningful and effective mathematics program. Cognitive theorists, such as William Brownell, Jean

Piaget, Robert Gagné, and Jerome Bruner, posture learning as a continuous, developmental process. From this perspective, effective learning is dependent upon one's level of readiness for new information. The acquisition of mathematics knowledge and proficiency is such a process. Developing the ability to think mathematically requires a learning environment that is sensitive to and parallels each child's level of conceptual development and learning readiness.

In the 1930s, Brownell introduced the *meaning theory*, which suggested children must understand what they are learning if learning is to be permanent. Brownell (1986, 1987) concluded that children need opportunities to explore and manipulate objects as a basis for assigning meaning to new concepts and skills. Piaget, Gagné, and Bruner also believed children must have meaningful experiences in preparation for learning to occur. These theorists suggested that children use experiences to construct a reference field—a prior knowledge set—needed to analyze and make sense of new information.

The contributions of these theorists have significantly influenced the nature and direction of mathematics education. For example, Gagné (1977) suggested the use of task analysis procedures as a means to teach mathematics tasks as a sequence of clearly identified subtasks. According to Gagné, task analysis provides a teaching-learning sequence of successive approximations or increments of learning toward understanding more complex tasks. Figure 7–2 (on page 246) is a representation of one way to task analyze and sequence the skills subsumed under the addition of whole numbers.

Bruner not only was an advocate of discovery learning as a critical component in math education, but he believed it was important to observe ways children represent their understanding. Bruner (1966) identified three graduated levels of representation: 1. *enactive*, involving the manipulation of concrete materials; 2. *iconic*, utilizing pictures and graphic representations, and 3. *symbolic*, referring to numerals, words, and similar symbols used to represent abstractions. According to Bruner, attending to the representations children use to demonstrate knowledge provides direct clues to his or her way of organizing and understanding information. These clues are strong indicators for selecting an appropriate instructional mode. For example, the child who uses a finger-counting strategy is relying on a concrete format for organizing an addition task. For this child the use of concrete or manipulative objects would be the preferred instructional method.

Among the cognitive theorists, Jean Piaget has likely had the most significant influence on the nature and direction of mathematics education. Piaget (1952, 1965) believed that learners sequentially progress through four stages of development as they achieve intellectual maturity. Figure 7–3 (on page 247) provides a description of these stages and a cursory review of the child characteristics associated with each. Piaget's theory of learning, *constructivism*, is based on the belief that children construct and learn concepts through active experiences with real objects, rather than through passive internalization of information received from others (teachers). That is, children need opportunities to explore and manipulate environmental objects in order to assign meaning to new information to then gain knowledge.

Piaget (1965) believed that children must have rudimentary knowledge about *relations* (comparisons among objects), *classification* (sorting skills), and *conservation* (constancy of quantity) before they are able to work with numbers and understand mathematical concepts and applications. These concepts form the basis for understanding number operations, mathematics symbols and language, and problem-solving strategies.

FIGURE 7-2 A Sequence for Teaching-Learning Whole Number Addition

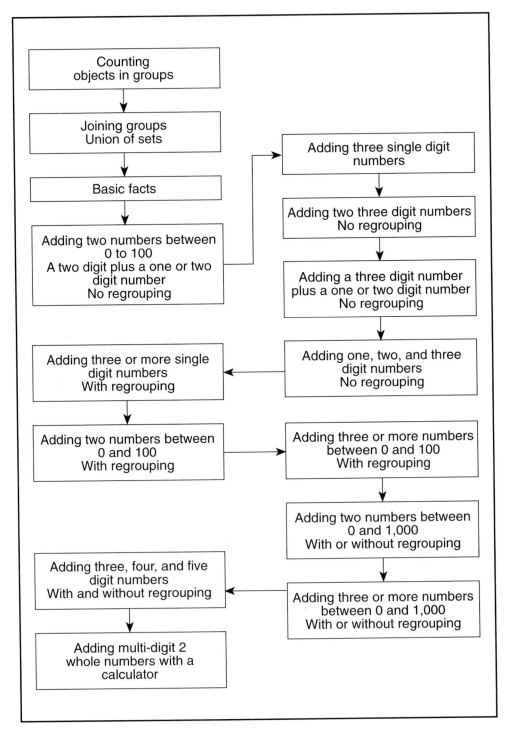

FIGURE 7-3 Piaget's Stages of Cognitive Development

Stages	Approximate Ages	Emergent Characteristics
Sensorimotor Infants, children develop concepts through interactions with physical environment.	Birth to 2 years	• Reflexive Behavior • Object Permanence • Goal-Directed Behavior • Rudimentary Problem-Solving
Preoperational Children begin to use language to express ideas; remain dependent upon perceptions.	2 years to 7 years	• Conservation Miscue • Centration • Perceived Appearances • Irreversibility (Operations) • Egocentricity
Concrete Operational Children develop concepts using concrete objects to explore relationships and model abstract ideas. Language gains importance for expressing and remembering concepts.	7 years to 12 years	• Inferred Reality • Transivity • Inclusion • Reversibility • Part-Whole Relationships
Formal Operational Children begin to think abstractly, are able to hypothesize from abstract possibilities to the real world; less dependent on concrete materials.	12 years to Adulthood	• Form and Content • Abstract Thought • Hypothesis Testing • Concept Formation

Relations refers to comparative concepts including bigger-smaller, same-different, fast-slow, yours-mine, and one-to-one correspondence.

Example: Associating a set of three items and the set of counting numbers 1, 2, 3.

Classification involves the ability to group items on the basis of a common characteristic or attribute; establishing sets.

Example: Sorting blocks by color or by shape; separating toy cars from toy trucks; grouping athletes by sports or positions played.

Conservation involves the ability to recognize that quantities do not change when the arrangement of the material is changed. Sequentially, number conservation precedes conservation of area and length. Conservation of volume typically emerges during adolescent years.

Example: Recognizing three blocks horizontally aligned represent the same number as three identical blocks vertically aligned. Recognizing that two squares of equal dimensions, one rotated to represent a diamond configuration remain congruent. Understanding that liquid poured from a small glass (full glass of liquid) into a large glass remains the same in volume (appears less as liquid only partially fills larger container).

A child's degree of competence with the three prerequisite concepts determines his or her readiness for more formal mathematics instruction; and may well determine the degree of success the child will experience in instructional settings. It is important for teachers, therefore, to assess and know each child's depth of understanding about relations, classification, and conservation to determine where instruction should begin.

MATURATION AND READINESS

All learners, including children with learning challenges, progress through Piaget's stages of development. The rate at which children progress varies according to many factors, including maturational readiness (mental maturity), affective readiness (attitudes toward learning and math), pedagogical readiness (understanding and using learning tools), content readiness (prerequisite skills and knowledge), and contextural readiness (global understanding of math uses and applications) (Underhill, 1976). In each Piagetian developmental stage, children experience some degree of learning readiness associated with the five domains described by Underhill. Gradually, as children developmentally mature, they become ready to learn increasingly more sophisticated increments of knowledge. Consider the college freshman who struggled with high school algebra, and now finds college algebra quite simple and even marvels at her previous difficulty.

Math readiness can be described as a continuous, cumulative process; new information eventually becomes part of the knowledge base (prior knowledge) that readies the learner for subsequent, more complex math concepts and principles.

Readiness levels are defined somewhat differently for each individual; essentially, students can only learn what they are ready to learn, when each is individually ready. Although this may seem a trite observation, it is an important concept for teachers of students with mild disabilities to consider.

Figure 7–3 presents Piaget's stages of cognitive development and includes the general age ranges Piaget associated with each stage. Figure 7–4 depicts the complement of mathematical concepts associated with these stages. Many teachers can attest to classroom based evidence that children acquire skills and described characteristics over time periods that exceed Piaget's timelines. Recent research suggests that some individuals, even persons without obvious learning handicaps, may never actualize skills associated with formal operations, for example, abstract thinking, even as adults. Yet, instruction in mathematics relies on abstract and symbolic thinking (using numeric symbols and language) almost from the very first introduction to numbers.

FIGURE 7-4 The Emergence of Mathematical Concepts: Readiness and Piagetian Theory

Age	Concepts
Three to five years (3-5)	• Rudimentary concepts such as more, bigger, smaller • One-to-one correspondence
Six to seven years (6-7)	• Cardinality • Ordinality • Conceptualization of a set • Joining sets • Place value • Addition • Equivalency concept • Conservation of numbers • Reversibility • Rational counting • Transivity • Subtraction • Part-to-whole fractions • Multiplicative relationships • General geometric forms, shapes
Eight to nine years (8-9)	• Parallelism • Three or more attribute classifications • Associative property of addition; $(a + b) = (b + a)$ • Distributive property of multiplication; $a(b + c) = ab + ac$ • Cummutative property of addition; $a + (b + c) = (a + b) + c$ • Fractions
Ten to twelve years (10-12)	• Percentages • Proportions • Probability • Conservation of weight and volume • Geometry

At the Institute for Research in Learning Disabilities at the University of Kansas, Skrtic (1978) became intrigued by the impact of telescoped math curricula on school-aged children, particularly on their readiness for learning math skills and concepts, and thus their learning efficiency. Skrtic believed that the telescoping effect created a severe discrepancy between the nature of the curricular demands—for example, symbolic learning—and children's ability to understand and therefore learn abstract material—readiness. He hypothesized that instruction based on symbolic learning contributed to difficulties children with learning disabilities experienced in math. Further, that symbolic teaching-learning may, in fact, cause some students to appear to be math disabled due to task demands beyond their developmental readiness capabilities.

In his research, Skrtic utilized *Lawson's Test of Formal Operations* (Piagetian tasks) to examine the developmental sophistication of thirteen- to fourteen-year-old males. Both learning disabled and nonlearning disabled students were included in the sample. Piaget's schema would suggest these students should be developing skills associated with formal operations stage; the level at which most math instruction occurs. However, Skrtic found that ninety-two percent of the learning disabled adolescents in the sample were functioning at the concrete stage of development, eight percent were able to solve problems when provided graphic aids (pictures), and zero percent were able to perform formal operational tasks. What was surprising, however, was that sixty-nine percent of the nondisabled sample also were at a concrete level of functioning, twenty-eight percent needed graphic assistance, and a mere three percent were able to function at the abstract, symbolic level. Subsequently, Skrtic, Kvam, and Beals (1983) determined that students' learning problems in mathematics may not be exclusively due to learning disabilities but may, in fact, be due to instructional disabilities.

Pupils with mild learning difficulties characteristically experience difficulty with abstract thinking (Skrtic *et al.*, 1983). Still, the mathematics textbooks and accompanying methods of instruction designed for children with learning difficulties typically emphasize abstract-symbolic processes. Instead, instruction for these (perhaps all) children should parallel the individual student's developmental learning capabilities, learning characteristics and needs. This would necessitate the inclusion of concrete, graphic, and symbolic instructional presentations.

Assessment

Assessment can be defined as a systematic process used to determine information about an individual's acquired knowledge, skills, and general levels of functioning. Information obtained through assessment processes—tests, observations, and interviews—provide the basis for nearly all decisions made regarding a child's school program. Promotions across grade levels, classroom placements, and referrals for remedial and special education programs are among the decisions that are affected by assessment procedures and outcomes.

Specific mathematics skills and knowledge are assessed for two primary reasons: 1. to determine eligibility for special education services, and 2. for the purpose of planning individualized instruction.

SEQUENCES OF THE ASSESSMENT PROCESS

Figure 7–5 (on page 252) depicts the assessment sequence most facilitative to determining a child's strengths and concerns (weaknesses) in mathematics knowledge (Skrtic *et al.*, 1983; Love & McGuire, 1985). Included in the assessment process are standardized achievement tests, individually administered diagnostic tests and initial error analyses, teacher-constructed tests, the clinical math interview, and a detailed error analysis. The outcomes derived from following this sequence permit teachers to identify a child's entry level, specific areas of successful and faulty learning, and, therefore, the remedial or compensatory instruction needed.

STANDARDIZED ASSESSMENTS

Standardized tests yield scores that can be interpreted on a relative measurement scale, for instance, a norm-referenced measure. Raw scores are converted to derived or standard scores to permit comparisons with a selected, clearly defined referent group. Scores obtained can include age and grade equivalents, standard or scaled scores, percentile ranks, and stanines.

Group Achievement Tests

Group achievement tests provide an initial level of academic screening that is both economical and easy to administer. School districts frequently use group achievement tests to identify children at risk for school failure, children of exceptionally advanced ability, and to provide a gross measure of program effectiveness (for example, relative standing in comparison to state and national scores). A selection of instruments commonly used in screening/assessing mathematics skills are described in Figure 7–6 (on page 253).

Because the results of testing hold potentially significant consequences for students, screening measures are not adequate for use as the sole evidence in making educational decisions. Screening instruments provide a global sampling of relative strengths and concerns in academic areas. Such tests generally do not include a sufficient number of items for each skill assessed to determine specific levels of proficiency or error patterns and acquisition deficits. However, results can assist educators in identifying children who may benefit from further, more specific evaluations of their skills.

Individually Administered Diagnostic Tests

In mathematics, as in other content areas, individually administered diagnostic tests assist teachers in clarifying relative strengths and concerns across content-specific domains. Figure 7–6 includes a list of diagnostic tests that are frequently used in schools. The results of such assessments are often a substantial factor in special education referral and placement decisions and subsequent IEP determinations.

Information obtained from diagnostic tests assists in the development of long-term instructional objectives and as a guide for general instructional planning. However, teachers often find that commercial diagnostic tests are not adequate for isolating information about an individual child's specific skill acquisitions and deficits in order to then determine instructional needs. Planning for individualized instruction requires more meticulous and precise diagnostic analyses.

FIGURE 7–5 The Assessment Sequence for Individualized Instructional Planning

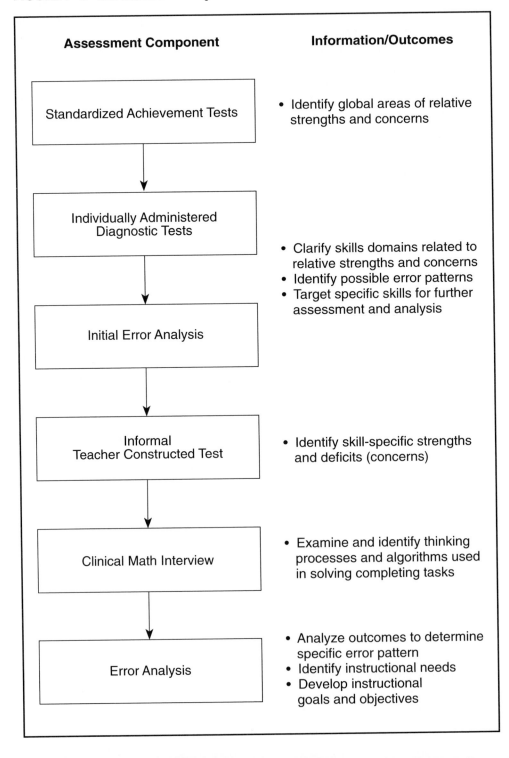

FIGURE 7-6 Commercially Available Assessment Instruments

Achievements/Screening Tests
_____

Title: *California Achievement Tests*
    Publisher/Author: California Test Bureau-McGraw Hill, 1977
    Grade Levels: K-12.9
    Areas Assessed [Math]: Computation, concepts, and applications

Title: *Iowa Test of Basic Skills*
    Publisher/Author: Riverside Publishing; Hieronymous, Lindquist, & Hoover, 1982
    Grade Levels: K-9
    Areas Assessed [Math]: Computation, concepts, and applications

Title: *Metropolitan Achievement Test: Sixth Edition (MAT6)-Survey Battery*
    Publisher/Author: Psychological Corporation; Prescott, Balow, Hogan, & Farr, 1985
    Grade Levels: K-12.9
    Areas Assessed [Math]: Numeration, geometry, measurement, problems
        solving, and operations

Title: *Science Research Associates Achievement Series, 7th ed.*
    Publisher/Author: Science Research Associates (SRA); Gardner, Rudman,
        Karlsen, & Merwin, 1986
    Grade Levels: K-12
    Areas Assessed [Math]: Concepts, computation, and problem solving

Title: *Stanford Diagnostic Mathematics Tests, 3rd ed.*
    Publisher/Author: Psychological Corporation; Beatty, Gardner, & Karlsen, 1984
    Grade Levels: 1.5-12
    Areas Assessed [Math]: Number system, numeration, computation, and
        applications

Individually Administered Diagnostic Tests
_____

Title: *Kaufman Test of Educational Achievement*
    Publisher/Author: American Guidance Services, Inc. (AGS); Kaufman &
        Kaufman, 1983
    Grade Levels: 1-12
    Areas Assessed [Math]: Computation and applications

Title: *KeyMath – Revised*
    Publisher/Author: American Guidance Services, Inc. (AGS); Connolly, 1988
    Grade Levels: K-9
    Areas Assessed [Math]: Basic concepts, operations, and applications

Title: *Sequential Assessment of Mathematics Inventory (SAMI)*
    Publisher/Author: Merrill; Reisman, 1984
    Grade Levels: K-8
    Areas Assessed [Math]: Mathematics language, ordinality, number/numeration,
        measurement, geometry, computation, word problems, and applications

Title: *Test of Early Mathematics Ability (TEMA)*
    Publisher/Author: PRO-ED; Brown & McEntire, 1984
    Age Levels: 4-9 years
    Areas Assessed [Math]: Number concepts, counting, basic calculations, and
        base-ten concepts

ASSESSMENT FOR INSTRUCTIONAL PLANNING

When programming for students with mild learning difficulties, knowing where to begin instruction is crucial. It is important that students who have mastered a skill are not subject to boredom from tedious repetitions, and that students who are lacking the prerequisite skills to learn new material are not pushed into anxiety and discouragement. Either scenario results in negative responses to mathematics (Tobias, 1981).

Assessment is a critical, continuous component in the diagnostic-prescriptive-instruction process when implementing mathematics programs for pupils with mild learning difficulties. The goal of assessment, from this perspective, is to determine 1. diagnostic information about the student's learning style and patterns; 2. the level of content knowledge already within the child's repertoire (strengths); and 3. areas of specific skills deficits (concerns). Based on this information, instructional goals and objectives can be developed and a personalized instructional plan can be devised. In the case where a student has been placed in a special education classroom, information obtained forms the basis for developing short-term instructional objectives in the Individualized Education Plan that are used to guide instructional planning.

Curriculum Based/Informal Assessment

Educators tend to rely heavily on the results of diagnostic assessments when programming for children with special learning needs. Many teachers have realized the frustration associated with attempts to devise individual instructional programs based on diagnostic results alone. Typically, the information is too global to provide specific clues about where to begin instruction, as well as how to best teach a particular child.

Informal assessment procedures are used to personalize the testing process. That is, the procedures involved in informal assessments are tailored to the individual child; therefore, the outcome provides teachers with child-specific information. For assessing mathematics skills and knowledge, teacher-constructed tests, interviews, and error analysis procedures combine to provide a sound information base upon which to develop short-term instructional objectives and implementation strategies.

Teacher-Constructed Tests   Diagnostic instruments provide a cursory description of troublesome mathematics content domains. Based on this information, teachers can target probable skills deficits to then devise informal, curriculum-relevant tests. Teacher-constructed tests, in conjunction with subsequent interviews and error analyses, can provide the type of diagnostic information needed to 1. pinpoint skill deficits or faulty learning sequences, 2. determine where instruction should begin, 3. determine how instruction should be delivered, and 4. identify skills the child has successfully learned.

The informal assessment-instruction goal is to pursue a comprehensive diagnosis of a particular concept, rather than merely focus on the obvious deficit skill. Constructing an effective instrument, therefore, requires careful attention to logical sequences and skills hierarchies. Knowing the sequence of skills that gradually leads to more advanced concepts enables a teacher to retroactively assess prerequisite skills acquisition and learning. For example, suppose a child, on a diagnostic test, missed computation items that require regrouping. Based on this evidence, it is difficult to ascertain whether the child simply has not yet learned the regrouping principle, or has an inadequate prerequisite knowledge base, such as place value. The teacher, based on knowledge of skills hierarchies, can "test down" to determine which prerequisite skills the child does and does not have in his repertoire; thus, determine where instruction or remedial intervention should begin.

Mathematics texts, standardized and diagnostic tests, and curriculum outlines provide excellent resources for developing an item bank of skill-specific test items. In addition, for teachers who choose to create items, these resources can be consulted to determine the proper format for individual problem types. In either case, the following guidelines are useful when preparing teacher-constructed tests: 1. isolate the deficit skill and prerequisite skills; 2. determine the individual's learning level—concrete, graphic, or symbolic; and 3. develop items that adequately assess selected skills (Reisman, 1982; Love & McGuire, 1985).

It is recommended that at least three items are included for each skill assessed to better ensure valid results. Several researchers who have studied the frequency of error pattern occurrence suggest an error is not "systematic" unless it occurs at least three times (Ashlock, 1990, p. 5). Further, the inclusion of at least three items reduces the probability of making a diagnostic error (Love & McGuire, 1985). That is, when the item pool includes three or more items, careless errors are more obvious and less likely to be interpreted as faulty learning or procedural error patterns. Consider Example A:

$$
\begin{array}{r}
\overset{2}{45} \\
+\ 37 \\
\hline
91
\end{array}
$$

A cursory error analysis suggests the child (1) "carried" the wrong digit when adding 5 + 7 as a careless mistake, or (2) might routinely use this incorrect algorithm. In the absence of sufficient evidence, however, the nature of the child's error is, at best, a guess. Even when given two problems of the same type, a child may compute one incorrectly and the second correctly, as demonstrated by the first two problems in Example B. In fact, the child may have used the same faulty algorithm in the second problem, but the nature of the problem (a sum of 11 in the addition of "ones" column digits) provides no additional clues. By presenting at least three problems, the pattern of the child's thinking begins to emerge.

Example B:

$$
\begin{array}{r}
\overset{2}{45} \\
+\ 37 \\
\hline
91
\end{array}
\qquad
\begin{array}{r}
\overset{1}{56} \\
+\ 25 \\
\hline
81
\end{array}
\qquad
\begin{array}{r}
\overset{2}{38} \\
+\ 14 \\
\hline
61
\end{array}
$$

Ashlock (1990) suggests the use of error pattern-based multiple-choice items as a means to gain insight to a child's mathematical thought processes. In this method, answer choices (distractors) are developed through the use of faulty algorithms commonly used by students. The student who has learned an erroneous process will systematically choose answers derived from using that process. Ashlock (p. 11) offers the following example:

$$\begin{array}{r} 4372 \\ -\ 2858 \\ \hline \end{array}$$

The answer is: a. 2526
b. 1514
c. 524
d. 2524

Analyzing a child's responses, both oral and written, provides valuable insight into the mathematical thinking processes the child applies when completing tasks. And Ashlock's multiple choice model can assist teachers in devising a more rapid route to isolating learned errors (see Chapter 4 in Ashlock, 1990, for an extensive list of sample error pattern distractors). Nonetheless, the analysis of written products has limitations. To most accurately understand a child's mathematical thinking, it is necessary to interview or simply ask the child to explain the processes used in completing selected items.

Levels of Assessment   Most teachers assess math skills at the abstract level—through the use of mental and written computations. Essentially, children are asked to compute problems, presented numerically and as story (word) problems, using numeral symbols or abstractions of real objects. However, several mathematics researchers believe assessment, and subsequent instruction, should be conducted at several levels of representations: concrete, graphic, and symbolic (Piaget, 1965; Skrtic, 1978; Reisman, 1982; Love & McGuire, 1985; Kamii, 1990). Using multiple levels of presentation permits an analysis of the level of readiness at which a child is functioning, thus the level at which mathematical understanding and instruction can efficiently occur.

Children, particularly children with learning problems, (and even some adults) routinely use concrete methods, such as finger counting strategies for completing computations. Concrete assessment involves the student's manipulation of objects to demonstrate a procedure. For example, a child may be presented the problem 6 - 2 = ? The child counts six apples; counts two that will be given to the teacher; then counts the apples he has retained to find the number remaining. Love and McGuire (1985, 1990) found that even at this earliest level of learning, as well as with graphic levels of representation, it is important to pair the symbolic representation of the problem with the manipulation task. The pairing process helps students recognize and eventually understand the relationship between the task, the numeral representation, and the computation. In addition, Love and McGuire found that the use of story problems added a functional dimension to the computation process, and assisted the students in learning essential mathematics language. In the example 6 - 2 = ?, such a story might simply be "You have six apples and you decide to share two with me [the teacher]. When you take away two, how many are left?"

Graphic procedures involve the use of pictures, tally marks, or similar pictorial representations of the number values to be manipulated. Using the same problem, 6 - 2 = ?, the story would be presented orally, paired with the symbolic computation, and the child would solve the problem using a picture. The task would involve counting the items pictured, then counting the two to be taken away, circling the two, and counting the remaining items.

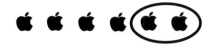

The symbolic or abstract level involves purely the manipulation of numerals to solve problems and computations. The task demand requires that students either write or verbally state the answer to problems presented.

When assessing a child's performance, even during the completion of written assignments, observing how a child solves a problem provides clues to the level at which the child is most comfortable in understanding the task. When a child uses a finger counting strategy or draws tally marks on her paper, the child is using a personally meaningful representation to picture the task; thus, is sending a valuable diagnostic message to the teacher.

The Clinical Math Interview (CMI)   Interviews offer a format for gaining diagnostic information that is both qualitative and quantitative. The purpose of the interview is to determine how the child approaches tasks, what thought processes are used, and whether or not learning has been effective and meaningful (Ashlock, 1990; Love & McGuire, 1990).

Interviews should not be confused with oral examinations; rather, the interview provides an opportunity to observe a child's behavior in response to different types of tasks (anxiety, confidence, sequential approach versus random) as well as in response to computational errors she independently detects. Further, it is a forum for the student to freely express the thinking and problem-solving strategies employed in completing their written tasks. Therefore, examiner behavior is crucial to the success of the interview. It is not a time for correcting, expressing opinions, or otherwise sending verbal and nonverbal messages to a child. Figure 7–7 (on page 258) outlines the procedures involved in conducting clinical math interviews. Included in the outline are suggestions for effective examiner/teacher interview behaviors, and an overview of positive outcomes or benefits to be realized through interview procedures.

The interview process is a highly effective procedure for identifying skill-specific strengths and concerns and can serve as an instructional interaction as well. When students verbalize their thoughts, many become more aware of the cognitive processes they have used and some even realize the errors they have routinely committed. Questions asked during the interview can encourage this level of awareness—or clue the teacher that the child is not particularly *metacognitively* aware. Garofalo (1987) recently addressed the effects of metacognition in mathematics learning and suggested several interview questions that benefit both the teacher and student in examining students' math behaviors. The following questions are excerpted from Garofalo's article and are suggested for use during interviews.

Think of everything you do when you practice solving mathematics problems. Why do you do these things?

What kinds of errors do you usually make? Why do you think you make these errors? What can you do about them?

Name some things you do when you are stuck on a problem. Do these things always help?

Tell when it's useful to check your work. Why? Is that the only time?

What kinds of problems are you best at? Why? The worst at? Why? (pp. 22–23)

Interviews and Error Analysis   The value of interviews cannot be overemphasized. While initial analyses of written work provide insight, it is through the interview that a child's actual thought processes become evident. In their research, Love and McGuire (1985) conducted initial analyses of mathematics problems completed by middle school students, followed by individual interviews with each. Initial error patterns Love and

FIGURE 7–7 The Clinical Math Interview (CMI)

I. PROCEDURE
  A. Computation
    1. Based on identified concerns, develop a set of representative problems for the student to complete; generally three problems per problem type.
    2. Give problem set to student to complete; allow reasonable amount of time for student to complete as many problems as possible (generally 40-50 minutes).
    3. Encourage student to work at a comfortable pace.
    4. Allow student to work uninterrupted.
    5. Tell student to cross out problems with errors and to begin again (vs. erasing).
  B. Teacher Check
    1. Make a photocopy of the student's computation paper(s).
    2. Check problems on the photocopy; do not mark on the student's original paper.
    3. Tally and note errors on the teacher's copy.
    4. Conduct preliminary error analysis; code errors in pencil.
  C. Student Verbal Analysis/Interview
    1. Tape record the session and take anecdotal notes.
    2. Conduct the interview in private.
    3. Use all incorrect problems/computations for verbal analysis and selected correct computations; particularly when responses to similar items are not consistent (i.e., when items within the set of three are neither all correct nor all incorrect).
    4. Analyze/work through one problem at a time.
      a. Have the student read the problem.
      b. Instruct the student to explain how he solved, computed the problem (e.g., Point to the problem and say, *"Tell me how you solved this one, number four."*).
    5. Code error analyses; record anecdotal notes.
  D. Teacher/Examiner Behavior Suggestions
    1. Tell student you want to learn more about the problem solving techniques she uses in computing math problems (when given original problem set and again when beginning the interview).
      a. Explain that you are interested in *how* the student completes the problems, rather than whether the answers are correct or incorrect.
      b. Explain that you, at the present time, will be unable to reveal whether problems are correctly or incorrectly solved.
    2. Allow student to talk without corrections and without interruptions.
    3. Create and maintain an enthusiastic, nonjudgmental atmosphere.
    4. Provide encouragement, positive reinforcement for efforts (e.g., *"Thank you, Joe, I appreciate how hard you are working."*).
II. OUTCOMES/BENEFITS
  A. Provides information about the student's:
    1. Current mathematics knowledge;
    2. Current level of mathematics functioning;
    3. Use/dependence on faulty or incorrect algorithms (paper and pencil procedures);
    4. Level of awareness regarding correct/incorrect results;
    5. Use of logic or faulty logic in problem solving.
  B. Provides specific information relevant to instructional planning; planning that is individualized and personalized for a particular student.

Source: Skrtic, 1978; Love & McGuire, 1985, 1987, 1990.

McGuire identified were not always the patterns explained by students. The following problem was completed by an eighth grade boy receiving math instruction in a resource room for students with learning disabilities. "Ray" shared that math was his "best and favorite" subject in school.

$$\begin{array}{r} 305 \\ 3\overline{)9015} \end{array}$$

Based on the initial analysis, it was believed that Ray began the division at the left, looked for combinations divisible by 3, then proceeded to divide 3 into 9, into 0, and finally into 15. When interviewed, Ray described the process in the following manner:

I looked for combinations that could be divided by 3. Then I divided up the problem in my head . . . 9 and 15. I know that 5 times 3 is 15 so I put the 5 on top. Then I did 3 times 3 is 9 and put the 3 on top. Zero doesn't mean anything so I didn't divide it . . . I just brought it up. It [the answer] didn't look right anyway with that big space between the 3 and the 5.

Ray was also asked to explain the process used in solving problems he seemed to have computed correctly. However, his explanation verified that even erroneous procedures can result in correct responses. Consider the following computation:

$$\begin{array}{r} 407 \\ 2\overline{)814} \end{array}$$

Ray explained that he ". . . looked for combinations that could be divided by 2 . . . knew that 2 times 7 is 14 . . . put the 7 on top . . . did 2 times 4 is 8 and put the 4 on top. This one looked funny with the space, too, so I put a 0 in the middle to make it look right."

In the absence of an interview, Ray's right-left error would have been overlooked, as would his conceptual confusion concerning the value of zero—and would have been neglected in remedial instruction. Consequently, the erroneous algorithm would have remained an error in his skill usage.

Interviews permit a glimpse into ways in which students perceive and mentally represent math problems. For teachers of children with learning difficulties this information can be especially helpful. The interview enables a teacher to *listen* to an individual student's pattern of thinking and problem solving to uncover patterns of faulty logic and learning (Skrtic, 1978; Ashlock, 1990).

In the preceding example, it eventually became clear that Ray cognitively understood computations as isolated parts that he perceived as logical, with no concern for or awareness of the problem as a whole. By testing-down through the skills hierarchy, it was determined that Ray routinely viewed problems as individual units; for example, when adding multidigit numbers, he added each column as a separate addition problem. Further, regardless of the operation he was using, Ray always began computations with the digits farthest to the right (appropriate except in division). When queried, he responded that his second grade teacher had told him to ". . . always start on the same side as the hand that you write with." From his perspective, he had mastered a complex rule!

It is important to note that this type of diagnostic assessment is a continuous and integral part of an effective mathematics program. Assessing students' academic progress, assessing instructional (teacher) effectiveness, and evaluating, creating, and modifying instructional plans are essential to a successful learner-focused program. The daily written work students produce provides the ongoing data base needed for formulating such diagnostic information. Thus, teacher-constructed tests plus the analysis of daily written work samples offer teachers powerful tools for developing individualized instructional programs.

Error Analysis

Examining work samples and written tests only to determine the number correct and incorrect eliminates opportunities to learn why and how children arrive at incorrect solutions (Ashlock, 1990). Instead, each written product can be approached as a diagnostic map of a child's thinking and learning processes. Diagnostically examining written samples creates possibilities to explore probable sources of error, test hypotheses about errors, and then construct a specific instructional plan.

Ray, the eighth grade student, shared that teachers had shown him " . . . different ways to divide . . . but . . . my way is easier for me . . . I'm used to it and I get a lot of them right." Essentially, children with learning problems, as do all children, typically believe their methods and strategies are logical and make sense. They tend to systematically apply procedures they have learned, whether correct or incorrect. It is the diagnostic examination of work samples plus interviews, therefore, that will reveal error patterns in a child's thinking, problem-attack, and procedural problem solving.

Written Computation Errors   Roberts (1968), Ashlock (1986, 1990) and others have extensively studied the phenomenon of written computation errors in relationship to intellectual ability and maturity. Roberts found that careless errors and a poor acquisition of addition and multiplication knowledge were relatively consistent difficulties across all grade and ability levels. Perhaps the most interesting finding was that for all ability groups, except the lowest quartile, errors due to erroneous algorithm techniques (for example, following incorrect procedures) occurred more frequently than any other type of error. Even among students in the highest quartile, such errors accounted for thirty-nine percent of the errors observed.

Researchers have identified various systems for classifying students' mathematical errors. Based on this research, five primary "failure strategies" or sources of students' computational errors consistently are reported.

1. *Lack of prerequisite skills*   The student has not integrated skills or has deficits in prior learning of skills needed to learn and use contingent skills.

2. *Wrong operation*   The student selects the incorrect operation for solving the problem type presented and may "force" the problem into the format selected.

3. *Obvious computational error*   The correct operation is applied, but poor recall or inefficient learning of number facts results in errors.

4. *Defective algorithm*   An algorithm is the step-by-step or pencil-and-paper procedure used to determine the result of an arithmetic operation. A defective algorithm is when the student attempts to use the correct operation but has difficulty in following or carrying out the steps involved in the problem-solving process.

5. *Random response*   The response provided has no apparent or identifiable relationship to the problem.

Diagnosing Errors   Much has been written about the analysis and diagnosis of mathematical errors; and many of the guiding principles are based on common sense, effective teaching practices. Perhaps the most extensive yet succinct resource for diagnostic analyses is the work of Robert B. Ashlock. His most recent text, *Error Patterns in Computation: A Semiprogrammed Approach (5th Edition)* (1990) provides numerous examples of error patterns, methods for diagnostic analysis, and methods for remedial instruction. In his text, Ashlock also suggests a coding system for teachers to use during the student interview. As teachers become more comfortable with and sophisticated in interviewing, many choose to develop personalized coding procedures to facilitate the recording process. A sample of common error patterns discussed by Ashlock are presented in Figure 7–8 (on page 262).

Ashlock condensed his procedures for diagnostically assessing written products into four general principles: 1. be accepting, 2. collect data—do not instruct, 3. be thorough, and 4. look for patterns (pp. 14–16). The first principle, be accepting, refers to the attitudes teachers convey to students during assessment, interviews, and overall instructional interactions. Students need to believe their teachers are genuinely interested in and respect them, are willing and want to help them learn, and will be accepting even when students' efforts yield incorrect results.

As difficult as it may be for many teachers, it is important during diagnostic assessment and interviews to listen to the student without offering correction. Students are more likely to share extensive information when they are able to freely express their thoughts in a judgment-free interaction. When teachers interrupt to provide correction, students are less likely to further discuss an "inadequate" performance. The purpose is to collect data for diagnostic and instructional planning and not for immediate instructional intervention.

Thoroughness addresses the belief that diagnostic assessment is a continuous process, rather than an isolated event. Daily work samples provide one source of continuous assessment data. In addition, diagnostic probes are an essential component of effective teaching. During instructional periods, teachers can observe students' behaviors and ask diagnostic questions. Questions such as "That's interesting . . . tell me how you decided that" and "Have I made that [this] clear? (versus "Do you understand?") offer a nonthreatening vehicle for students to provide informational feedback. This not only provides immediate clues to areas of potential difficulty, but provides an ongoing assessment of students' mathematical growth and skill acquisition.

Looking for patterns in a student's performance is an exciting problem-solving challenge. As noted previously, students systematically use procedures they are able to remember whether or not those procedures yield successful outcomes. To identify systematic applications of procedures, therefore, it is important to study both correct and incorrect computations. Once an error pattern has been determined, the teacher will know what instruction is needed to correct or remediate the error. In occasional instances, no apparent pattern will emerge. Under such circumstances, further diagnostic inquiry is likely to reveal that either the child has not learned or remembered a procedure, for instance, he does not know where or how to begin the problem; or the child, in fact, may never have been taught the target skill or prerequisite skills.

FIGURE 7–8 Common Error Patterns in Computation

Defective Algorithm	Example
Adds from left to right.	$\begin{array}{r} {}^{2\,3} \\ 524 \\ +\ 791 \\ \hline 118 \end{array}$
Adds all digits together.	$\begin{array}{r} 34 \\ +\ 5 \\ \hline 12 \end{array}$
Treats each digit's place as units (ones).	$\begin{array}{r} 467 \\ +\ 528 \\ \hline 9815 \end{array}$
Subtracts smaller digit from larger, regardless of placement.	$\begin{array}{r} 632 \\ -\ 287 \\ \hline 455 \end{array}$
Regroups in all multidigit subtractions.	$\begin{array}{r} {}^{\not{1}\not{1}} \\ {}^{4}\,524 \\ -\ 13 \\ \hline 118 \end{array}$
Adds regrouped number to multiplicand before multiplying.	$\begin{array}{r} {}^{1} \\ 24 \\ \times\ 3 \\ \hline 92 \end{array}$
Divides from right to left; remainder is placed to left of answer.	$\begin{array}{r} 2113 \\ 3\overline{)\,539} \end{array}$

Source: Adapted from Ashlock, 1990.

Instructional Techniques

Mathematics difficulties experienced by pupils with mild disabilities are often due to instructional factors rather than actual learning ability (Skrtic, 1978; Kennedy & Tipps, 1991). Regardless of the source of students' difficulties, however, teachers must responsibly provide appropriate, effective educational programs. Such programs systematically include opportunities for students to explore or, in the case of remedial instruction, re-explore concepts and skills toward establishing a meaningful mathematics knowledge base. This type of exploration is promoted through the use of concrete activities that are followed by practice with graphic representations (both levels paired with symbolic representations), and eventual use of symbolic or abstract problems (Piaget, 1952, 1965; Skrtic *et al.* 1983; Love & McGuire, 1985, 1990).

Teachers have considerable autonomy in determining instructional methods used in their classrooms. Nonetheless, there are general guidelines to follow when planning remedial or initial instruction. Many of these have been addressed in previous sections of this chapter. In the present discussion, instructional sequences, presentation techniques, and general curriculum content will be presented. Information about math games and activities, commercial programs, and computer software packages is included at the end of the chapter.

INSTRUCTION AND SEQUENCES

Sequencing refers to both the hierarchical structure of skills (overall curriculum plan) and the specific structural aspects of each skill introduced. The majority of pupils with mild disabilities usually can and should be taught mathematics concepts, skills, and algorithms in the same sequence used in regular mathematics classrooms. For the purposes of remedial instruction, CMI and error analysis results can be compared to instruction-learning sequences to determine where initial instruction should be focused. A checklist of the mathematical concepts included in comprehensive instructional programs is provided in Figure 7–9 (on page 264) (Kennedy & Tipps, 1988).

Sequencing Guidelines

Carnine *et al.* (1990) suggest three guidelines for establishing an instructural sequence: "1. preskills of a strategy are taught before the strategy; 2. easy skills are taught before more difficult ones; and 3. strategies and [concepts] that are likely to be confused are not introduced consecutively" (p. 5). As simplistic as this seems, teachers often begin instruction without sufficient diagnostic information to determine a student's relative standing in terms of these three instructional guidelines. Regardless of the student's age or grade placement, the preskills that are not in his repertoire, aspects of a new skill that are likely to present particular difficulty, and which strategies and concepts the student has learned and which may have been learned in faulty patterns all form the basis for determining the instructional program.

In both initial and remedial instruction, analyzing and sequencing different problem types subsumed under each skill, in terms of relative difficulty, enables teachers to anticipate

FIGURE 7-9 Checklist of Mathematical Concepts

A. Relationships
1. Size
2. Position
3. Comparison of two or more quantities
4. Measurement-comparisons
   a. Capacity/volume
   b. Linear/length
   c. Temperature
   d. Weight/mass
   e. Time
   f. Money
5. Geometric figures and shapes
6. Awareness of similarities and differences; categories; sets
7. Patterns

B. Readiness-Operations with Whole Numbers
1. Numberness/quantity; 0-9
2. Counting (1-100)
   a. Counting by ones
   b. Counting by twos
   c. Counting by tens
   d. Counting by fives
3. Place Value

C. Addition and Subtraction of Whole Numbers
1. Addition
   a. Signs
   b. Doubles
   c. 100 Basic addition facts (0-18)
   d. Single digit addition without regrouping
   e. Two digit addition without regrouping
   f. Single digit addition with regrouping
   g. Two digit addition with regrouping
2. Subtraction
   a. Signs
   b. Taking away; reducing
   c. Directional representations on number line
   d. Basic subtraction facts; opposite of addition facts
   e. Single digit subtraction
   f. Two digit subtraction without regrouping
   g. Two digit subtraction with regrouping

D. Multiplication and Division of Whole Numbers
1. Multiplication
   a. Signs
   b. Rapid addition
   c. Basic facts
   d. Regrouping
2. Division
   a. Signs
   b. Separating, reducing set size
   c. Opposite of multiplication
   d. Basic facts
   e. Regrouping

E. Measurement-Conducting/Computing Measurements
1. Capacity/volume
2. Linear/length
3. Temperature
4. Weight/mass
5. Time
6. Money

F. Rational Numbers
1. Numbers expressed as Fractions
2. Numbers expressed as Decimals

Source: Adapted from Kennedy & Tipps, 1988.

potential "trouble spots." Further, separating similar skills and strategies for instructional purposes significantly reduces the probability that students will later confuse concepts and rules.

Anticipating potentially difficult concepts is often more challenging than it would first appear. For example, one likely would assume that a child who is able to count numbers beyond the teen values would have little difficulty learning the symbols associated with the teen numerals. Yet, the teen numerals, especially 11, 12, 13, and 15, are particularly troublesome for many young children with learning problems (Carnine *et al.*, 1990). Irregularity of the numeral names and the reading direction are cited as two primary, probable sources of difficulty. First, numerals are typically read from left to right while teen numerals are read right to left. Further, not all teen numerals retain the units digit name; for example, 17 is read *seven*teen while 15 is read *fif*teen, rather than *five*teen, and 11 is completely unique. Skill analysis, in this case, indicates that instruction in symbol identification would be facilitated when the easier numerals are taught first (Carnine *et al.*, 1990).

A further example can be found in research conducted with the *DISTAR Arithmetic* programs. The authors found that in the initial program, students with learning problems regularly seemed to confuse the numbers 4 and 5. Through extensive analyses, the authors determined that it was the initial letter source (*four* and *five*) that created confusion for the children. When introductions of 4 and 5 were separated in revised editions of the program, the number of students confusing the 4 and 5 numerals significantly decreased (Engelmann & Carnine, 1989).

Task Analysis and Concept Analysis

Gagné (1977) proposed that learning improves when subskills needed to master a more complex task are identified and sequenced for instructional purposes. Task analysis and concept analysis procedures clarify the teaching-learning sequence needed to understand more complex tasks. Figure 7-10 (on page 266) provides the steps to follow in completing each type of analysis. Figures 7-2 (task analysis: addition) and 7-11 (concept analysis: circle) (on page 267) offer sample analyses as exemplars of analysis procedures and content.

Once a skill or concept analysis has been completed, and before it is used in instruction, the established sequence should be examined against several criteria. The analysis should first be reviewed in terms of the relevance of each component step. This includes an examination of identified subskills to determine whether each is a necessity for achieving the terminal performance task or whether included subtasks are trivial and unnecessary. A holistic evaluation of the overall sequence will reveal any redundancies in subtasks as well as signal any omissions; thus establishing the completeness of the sequence. A final check includes following the sequence as it has been written to determine whether the steps efficiently lead to accomplishing the terminal performance objective.

Instructional Implications

Identifying the subskills or components of more complex tasks serves many purposes. First, a clear diagram of the component skills provides an instructional map for introducing or remediating learning of the more complex concept. Second, students' appropriate usage and faulty patterns are more clearly defined. Third, teachers can better demonstrate the functional relationships among skill components and in relationship to the larger, more sophisticated skill or concept. Finally, the teacher will know what information the child does and does not know, thus permitting instruction to focus on the skills the child has yet to learn.

FIGURE 7-10 Guidelines for Conducting Task Analysis and Concept Analysis

Task Analysis

1. Define the terminal task: clarify the student performance objective.
2. Identify the subtasks and performance criteria needed to execute the terminal task: isolate each step required to reach the performance objective.
3. Prioritize the subtasks: establish the appropriate sequence of subtasks to follow in completing the performance task/objective.
4. Analyze subtasks for prerequisite skills: identify competencies needed to complete steps in the task sequence.
5. Establish task hierarchy: sequence prerequisite skills and subtask components needed to achieve task mastery.
6. Review analysis: evaluate for thoroughness, relevance, and efficiency.

Concept Analysis

1. Identify concept attributes: describe the characteristics of a concept representation.
2. Classify the attributes: isolate each as *critical* or *irrelevant*.
3. Select instructional examples and nonexamples: determine representations of what the concept includes and what the concept does not include.
4. Prioritize teaching examples and nonexamples: classify each in terms of concrete, graphic, and symbolic/abstract representations.
5. Select testing examples and nonexamples: classify each in terms of concrete, graphic, and symbolic/abstract representations.
6. Match testing examples/nonexamples to teaching examples/ nonexamples.
7. Review analysis: evaluate for thoroughness, relevance, and efficiency.

Source: Adapted from McGuire, 1985.

FIGURE 7-11 A Concept Anaylsis for Teaching-Learning the Concept of Circle

Attributes	Critical	Irrelevant
1. Closed geometric figure	X	
2. One continuous line (absence of angles)	X	
3. All points of line are equidistant from the center	X	
4. Orientation of position		X
5. Size: small, medium, large		X
6. Color		X
7. Texture: smooth, rough		X

Teaching Examples	Rationale
1. Red paper circle, 12" diameter	4, 5, 6, 7
2. Green cloth circle, 4" diameter	4, 5, 6, 7
3. Orange wood circle, 1" diameter	4, 5, 6, 7
4. Sandpaper circle, 2" diameter	4, 5, 6, 7
5. Circles drawn on paper, multiple sizes	1, 2, 3, 4, 5, 6, 7

Teaching Nonexamples	Rationale
1. Red paper square, 12" sides	lacks 2, 3
2. Green cloth rectangle, 4" x 2"	lacks 2, 3
3. Blue wood triangle, 1" sides	lacks 2, 3
4. Sandpaper oval	lacks 3
5. Curved lines drawn on paper, multiple sizes	lacks 1, 2, 3

Testing Examples	Rationale
1. Purple paper circle, 12" diameter	4, 5, 6, 7
2. Black plastic circle, 4" diameter	4, 5, 6, 7
3. Wood circle, 1" diameter	4, 5, 6, 7
4. Clear glass circle, 2" diameter	4, 5, 6, 7
5. Circles drawn on paper, multiple sizes	1, 2, 3, 4, 5, 6, 7

Testing Nonexamples	Rationale
1. Pink paper square	lacks 2, 3
2. Rectangle drawn on paper	lacks 2, 3
3. Red plastic triangle	lacks 2, 3
4. Green cloth oval	lacks 3
5. Curved lines drawn on paper, multiple sizes	lacks 1, 2, 3

Source: Adapted by McGuire, 1985.

TEACHING MATHEMATICS SKILLS

As previously discussed, instruction and assessment in mathematics are integrated processes. Throughout each instructional session, it is important to observe students' behaviors and to ask probing questions. This information provides feedback on the effectiveness of the instructional plan, signals the need to alter the instructional plan or use alternative methods, and guides future planning.

A major component in mathematics instruction to pupils with mild disabilities is the teaching-learning of basic concepts toward the acquisition of problem-solving skills. Because many of these students experience difficulty with abstract material, it is important to initially present concepts through activities involving concrete materials. Opportunities to experiment, play, and discuss their experiences enable students to form the basis for building more complex, abstract ideas. Piaget (1952) identified several concepts that form the foundation for developing a functional understanding of numbers. These concepts and examples of associated instructional activities are listed and briefly described in Figure 7-12.

Manipulatives

The sequence for teaching concepts and computation skills/algorithms begins with the use of manipulatives. Concrete objects appeal to many of the senses; therefore they offer a natural vehicle for students to apply skills in a functional manner. Most children, in fact, arrive in classrooms with some level of informal knowledge about basic mathematical operations and principles as a result of experiences with concrete or manipulative objects—counting candles on a birthday cake, or dividing a candy bar to share with a friend. Using the informal knowledge children already possess in a format with which they are familiar encourages the development of a functional understanding of arithmetic operations (Ashlock, 1990; Kennedy & Tipps, 1991).

When selecting manipulatives it is important to utilize various items for demonstrating each concept. As previously discussed, students tend to make associations or draw conclusions based on similarities among items or isolated experiences. Using a variety of materials teaches the generalization of a concept. For example, when teaching basic addition, combining groups of blocks, then groups of sticks, and possibly even groups of students better explains the concept of combining and deemphasizes the isolated attributes of the individual item sets combined.

Typically, manipulatives are associated with instruction designed for very young children. However, concrete materials are highly effective with students across all grade levels and can encompass multiple topics. One example of an advanced concept is understanding the value of pi (π; 3.1415+). Using a concrete model to demonstrate the relationships among the radius (r), diameter (d), and pi (π) clarifies this mysterious value. Try this one yourself.

1. Use a protractor or compass to draw a circle. Draw the diameter.

2. Cover the circumference of the circle with a piece of string; cut the string to the exact length of the circumference.

3. Use the string to find how many times you can measure the length of the diameter . . . you should find that just over three "diameters" fit into the length described by the circumference.

4. Voila! Pi describes the relationship between the length of the diameter and the circumference of a circle!

Manipulatives enable students to experience concepts, thus they can be used for initial instruction as well as in remedial teaching. Although some students will pass through the concrete stages of learning more rapidly than others, the need for these basic experiences is essential (Piaget, 1952, 1965; Skrtic *et al.*, 1983; Kamii, 1990).

FIGURE 7-12 Piagetian Concepts and Related Instructional Activities

Concept	Representative Instructional Activity
1. *Classification* Grouping objects by attributes, unique characteristics.	• Group blocks by color, shape. • Name shapes, colors used to form groups.
2. *One-to-One Correspondence* Recognizing the relationship between sets that contain equal numbers of objects.	• Match a set of three children with a set of three Teddy bears. • Match a set of six objects with the counting numbers 1, 2, 3, 4, 5, 6.
3. *Seriation* Ordering objects on the basis of ordinal characteristics; e.g., length, size, rather than relative value.	• Arrange line of children in class from tallest to shortest. • Arrange a group of blocks from smallest to largest. • Arrange players on school football team from heaviest to lightest.
4. *Conservation* Recognizing that changing the arrangement or configuration of objects does not change number or quantity.	• Form two identical clay balls; roll one into pancake shape. Identify whether or not two objects contain equal amounts of clay. • Pour liquid from filled small glass into larger container. State whether or not amount of liquid has changed.
5. *Reversibility* Recognize that order in which objects are presented does not change the relationship between the objects, or the outcome for combining the objects.	• Combine a set of three books with set of two books; then two books with three. Determine that total does not change. • Use small items to represent number sentences, equations: 2 items + 3 items = 5 items $\quad a + b = c$ 3 items + 2 items = 5 items $\quad b + a = c$ 5 items − 3 items = 2 items $\quad c − b = a$
6. *Number Concepts* Recognizing the relationship between the number of objects and the corresponding numeral.	• Place numeral card beside the corresponding number of blocks. • Place correct number of plastic chips on numeral card.

Source: Adapted from Piaget, 1952, 1965.

Place Value

The concept of place value is basic to all mathematical operations and computations. While students may be able to read multidigit numbers, such as 57 as fifty-seven, or 121 as one hundred and twenty-one, the actual value of each digit in a numeral may not be known. Love and McGuire (1985), for example, found that adolescents were able to assign the place names to multidigit numbers (for example, units, tens, or hundreds "columns") yet were unable to explain what the column values meant.

Before teachers begin place value instruction, they must assure that students have mastered certain prerequisite skills. Students need to know the counting numbers 0-9 as units, and to be able to read and write those units (Kennedy & Tipps, 1991). They need to understand that values can be expressed in various ways and as combinations: for example 4 can be expressed as $3 + 1$, $4 + 0$, or $2 + 2$. This forms the basis for understanding how a number such as 12 can be expressed as 1 ten + 2 ones or $10 + 2$ (Kennedy & Tipps, 1991, p. 233).

Introducing place value via manipulatives is critical toward developing this concept; reintroducing place value during remedial instruction necessitates the use of manipulatives. Students need to see that units (ones) range from 0 (none) to 9; once 9 is exceeded, they have reached a "different" value (tens).

In their search, Love and McGuire discovered that students across all grades experienced considerable difficulty in effectively regrouping or borrowing values when working with multidigit numerals. Interviews revealed that nearly all of the students believed that the units (ones) column accommodated values 1 through 10, rather than 0 through 9. The students explained that when they reached a value of 10 or greater in the units column, they could trade the units for a "one" in the tens column; many even believed they could retain the 10 value as units. None of these students were able to explain that the digit 1 in the tens column was of equal value to 10 individual units. Essentially, though able to appropriately label the columns, they were unable to describe the relative value of digits within those columns; 1 held the value of 1 regardless of the place column in which it occurred.

What Love and McGuire learned led them to devise a system for place value instruction that emphasized the concept of 0 to 9 in the units column, 10 to 90 in the tens column, and so on across the graduated place values. The manipulatives developed provided space for only 0 to 9 "pegs" to be placed in the units column; only pegs in groups of ten—from one group of 10 "units" to 9 groups—in the tens columns (single pegs did not fit); and 9 tens of tens in the hundreds column. Essentially, students were able to test and visualize the relationships among place values and the respective numbers and numerals. For example, they learned that 10 units could not "fit" into the ones column and required a move to a larger column value. The process of physically moving grouped pegs from the ones column to the next led most of the students to independently understand relative values and to realize the concept and procedure underlying regrouping or carrying. Many self-corrected related errors when given written computations during later sessions.

Place value instruction should first focus on units, followed by instruction in the values to 19. Once students understand place value through 19, they should practice with manipulatives that demonstrate values through 99. When students begin to work with larger numbers—greater than 999—their basic understanding of place value likely will eliminate the need for continued counting of units. Nonetheless, place value materials will continue to be useful for illustrating relative values and learning and practicing operations (Kennedy & Tipps, 1991).

hundreds	tens	units (ones)
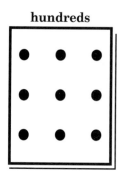	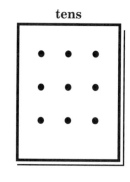	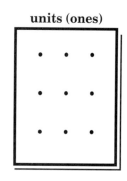

Estimation

Estimation skills are taught to help students judge the reasonableness of their responses; a critical component in problem-solving agility (Ashlock, 1990). In addition to use in completing classroom assignments, there are multiple functional aspects to learning this skill, for example, estimating the tab at the grocery store. Even when students are permitted to use calculators, judging the reasonableness of answers is important; that is, if data are incorrectly entered or the incorrect operations is selected, an unreasonable response probably will be obtained. Nevertheless, in the absence of estimation skills, students are likely to trust that calculator-derived answers are infallibly correct.

Estimation is a complex series of skills including rounding numbers; multiplying by 5s, 10s, 100s; addition and subtraction to appropriately round values; and, in measurement, understanding relative size or value. To practice estimating in computation, children can be presented a number of problems with multiple choice estimations as distractors. Also, students can be asked to provide an estimate of an answer rather than completing a computation, and to routinely provide estimates prior to completing calculations. Children enjoy activities such as "guessing" the number of beans in a jar, or how many students it would take to fill the space occupied by the football stadium.

The goal is to develop the habit of examining responses to determine whether or not each makes sense and is logically related to the problem solved. According to Ashlock, children who effectively learn to estimate and examine the reasonableness of responses are less likely to adopt incorrect computational procedures (1990, p. 20). Further, when students consider estimation a systematic part of the problem-solving process, they are more likely to use estimation skills for trial-and-error testing of potentially appropriate problem-solving strategies (Kennedy & Tipps, 1989).

Teaching Computation Skills

Remedial instruction should be based on and parallel the information obtained about individual students as a result of assessment procedures. Based on the assessment composite, teachers can prepare diverse, personalized presentation strategies and instructional modifications that will address multiple learning styles and needs.

The functional, meaningful aspects of computation should be paired with both initial and remedial instruction targeting the use of computational procedures (Ashlock, 1990; Kennedy & Tipps, 1991). Understanding the meaning of arithmetic operations enables children to determine when to select and use an appropriate algorithm. Further, students are better able to determine 1. what information is given, 2. what information is wanted, and

3. what information might be missing or needed, for example, fundamental skills in problem-solving procedures.

Students should first learn the underlying concepts plus the algorithms (paper-and-pencil procedures) for each of the four operations. Developing skills in computation helps students understand the logic in processes underlying operations, thus appropriate applications. One example is the association between counting and adding. Students with learning difficulties often will count the total number of objects in two groups of identified quantity to answer "how many?" With unequal groups of items, however, it is less time consuming to add the group [total] values; whereas in groups of equal size, multiplication is the better choice. When students understand the purpose and process of operations, they typically will choose the method that is least difficult and quickest toward determining a response (Kennedy & Tipps, 1991). Thus, when teaching students with mild disabilities the associations among procedures and operations must be clearly addressed.

Once students have adequately acquired computation skills, instruction in the use of calculators is appropriate. Calculators permit teachers and students to dedicate more instructional time to problem-solving activities, brain-storming sessions, and other, more functional activities. Essentially, less direct teaching time is consumed by completing routine computations.

Instruction in the use of calculators can and should be associated with daily life skills. Balancing a checkbook, determining grocery store costs, and computing gas mileage are simple yet realistic tasks that provide opportunities to practice calculator skills in a meaningful context.

Teaching Addition and Subtraction   Addition consists of one type of functional problem; the combination or joining of two or more groups. In contrast, subtraction problems can stem from four different situations: 1. take-away; how many are left? 2. comparison; how many more are in the second group? 3. completion; how many more does he have now than before? and 4. part-whole; if group A has x, and the total group is y, how many are in group B?

It is important to provide experiences and instruction with each of the possible problem types. During instructional sessions it is extremely important to point out and clarify the procedures associated with each problem type. This helps students learn the associations between the type of information sought in different problems (What is the problem asking?) and appropriate algorithms. Further, teachers must ensure that ample opportunities for students to practice and demonstrate acquisition of this knowledge are provided.

Multiplication   Most school programs emphasize three types of multiplication problems: repeated addition, arrays, and Cartesian products (Love, 1987; Kennedy & Tipps, 1991). When children have had adequate experiences with the principle of addition, familiar situations can be reused to introduce the concept of multiplication. Students, already familiar with the concept of combining or joining groups, can be presented a series of sets containing equal numbers of objects to be combined as a means to learn multiplication as a process of rapidly computing repeated additions. For example, a child might be given three sets of two objects each; the child can use counting skills to 1. determine how many are in each group and 2. how many groups. Children can use prior knowledge to determine the math sentence as described:

(objects)	ΔΔ		ΔΔ		ΔΔ	=	?
(symbols)	2	+	2	+	2	=	6

Following this step, children can be asked how many *times* they are adding the numeral 2. The teacher, while verbalizing this question should write the value and symbol 2 ×, drawing a clear association between the symbol × and the term *times*. (The quantity 2 occurs how many times? . . .) 3. Although learning handicapped children may require repeated trials with this process (some may need repeated trials with concrete, graphic, and symbolic representations), most children will see and understand that the multiple additions are the same as the multiplication process, and therefore are two ways to represent the same problem.

$$
\begin{array}{ccccccccc}
\triangle\triangle & & \triangle\triangle & & \triangle\triangle & = & ? \\
2 & + & 2 & + & 2 & = & 6 \\
 & & 2 & \times & 3 & = & 6
\end{array}
$$

An array is a configuration or arrangement of objects in rows of equal size. A simple classroom example would be a bookcase with three shelves, ten books on each shelf. For instructional purposes, arrays help students learn such concepts as the number of rows times the number in each row produces the total number in the array (the product). Further, this method helps students integrate the concept that even with different arrangements, for instance, 4 by 3 or 3 by 4, will produce the same results. Students can experiment with classroom desks, garden rows, or even plastic chips to test this concept:

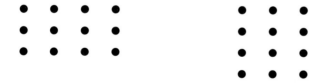

Again, teachers will need to point out and teach the association between the configuration and the operation pictured (4 *by* 3 and 4 × 3), as well as the relationship between 4 × 3 and 3 × 4 configurations. Clarifying the relationships among procedural products (outcomes), symbols, and terms is essential. Learning the array process is an important component in understanding various aspects of the multiplication operation (conservation, reversibility, transivity). Further, knowledge of array patterns provides the foundation for learning and understanding more complex skills, including measurement principles for determining area and volume.

Cartesian products are used to determine the number of possible combinations that can be made across two or more groups. The concept of Cartesian products can be informally introduced through common situations. For example, students might be given three different toppings for pizza and four pizzas and they are to determine the number of pizza combinations possible. Or, they might be asked to determine the number of team combinations (small groups) possible among students in the classroom.

Using the Cartesian product process can help clarify multiplications with values of one and zero. Students can be given a group with four options, such as ice cream flavors, and a second group with one option, chocolate sauce. The number of combinations is equal to the number of flavors; 1 choice × 4 options. Using the same example, if 4 ice cream flavors were offered, but there were no toppings (zero) available, there are zero combinations possible.

Division In multiplication, two factors are manipulated to determine a product. In division, the product and one factor are known and the task is to find the second factor. There are two types of division situations: measurement, determining the number of groups; and partitive, finding the number in each group. While the process is the same for each, understanding the type of problem, thus the information to be determined, enables children to identify what their answers mean.

Either division situation can be introduced first. However, most mathematicians suggest introducing division with measurement tasks because students are better able to understand the association between division and repeated subtractions (Kennedy & Tipps, 1991). Measurement tasks involve the repeated removal of equal size groups from an original quantity. For example, a student can be given ten cookies and asked to distribute them, two at a time, to determine how many children could be served. In this example, the original amount is known, the group or serving size is known (groups of two), and the question is to find the number of groups (servings) possible. The original question would be framed, "How many servings of cookies can we get from ten cookies when each serving has two cookies?"

In partitive division, the size of the original set (amount to be divided) is known, the number of servings needed would be given, and the question would be to determine how many items would be in each serving. Using the same cookies example, a student would be given the ten cookies to share equally among the group of five children. Distributing the cookies one at a time until all were shared answers the question, "How many cookies will each child receive if we have ten cookies and there are five children?"

As children become more comfortable with division processes, the associated terms should be introduced (Ashlock, 1990; Kennedy & Tipps, 1991). The meaning of the *dividend*, the size of the original group or quantity, never changes in division situations. In contrast, the meaning of the terms *divisor* and *quotient* are interchangeable and are determined by the problem type or division situation. In measurement, the divisor indicates the size of each group, and the quotient yields the number in each group; while in partitive division, the divisor and quotient meanings are reversed.

$$\text{divisor } \overline{\smash{)}\text{ dividend}}^{\textstyle \text{quotient}}$$

Teaching Mastery of the Basic Facts

Many children with mild disabilities experience difficulty in recalling basic math facts. This difficulty is compounded when children are learning to compute, particularly when computations become more complex. Typically, children who have not mastered basic facts resort to time consuming strategies, such as counting fingers or tally marks, to find basic computation results. Such processes are not only time consuming, but can be highly distracting. As a result, children often become "lost" in the process, become uncertain about the procedures attempted or even the original problem question, and proceed in a random approach.

Memorization or mastery of basic facts should begin after students have adequately demonstrated understanding of the concepts prerequisite to and underlying the operations. Once children understand how solutions are determined, the facts become more logical, meaningful, and useful pieces of information (Kennedy & Tipps, 1991). Further, the probability that students with mild learning difficulties will learn the basic math facts is significantly increased when instruction is personalized to each student's learning style and rate, and current levels of achievement.

Learning the basic math facts requires instruction followed by sufficient opportunities to practice recalling numbers. For pupils with mild disabilities, sufficient opportunities will be determined by several factors. First, it is important to know which facts the child has already mastered to permit instruction in new rather than repetitive material. Second, each child's learning rate should be accommodated; one child be able to learn five or more facts per lesson, while another may need several trials for each basic fact. Further, different facts may influence different rates for each child; teachers know that students' learning behavior can vary from day to day, and even, at times, within a single class period.

A third consideration is the way in which mastery is encouraged. Paper-and-pencil tasks are not necessarily the most effective method for encouraging fact recall. Rather, math games that incorporate mental arithmetic or a combination of task demands provide an environment conducive to practicing recall agility. Ashlock (1991) cautions against the use of games that involve elimination, such as in the spelling bee format. Rather, in appropriate games, incorrect responses are acceptable and the format incorporates multiple opportunities for students to suggest answers.

When working individually with a child, it is often helpful to deemphasize the correctness of responses and to encourage the child to offer the first response or answer that she considers. Frequently, the child's initial response will be correct! However, it is often the case that children do not trust their initial responses, especially when answers are not derived from using elaborate procedures. Consequently, these children "second guess" their responses, invest time in an extensive procedure and may often arrive at an erroneous response. The individualized interaction permits a child to practice recall safely with the teacher, and knowledge and confidence are gained as a bonus.

Some children, particularly upper elementary and secondary school students, have been subjected to years of monotony in attempts to learn the basic facts. For some of these children, manipulations and explorations with concepts, specific direct instruction, and all other available instructional options have been exhausted, yet the basic facts alone remain elusive and a mystery. In these rare situations, children may need the assistance of facts grids, calculators, or computers. These assistive aids should be used only after a child has demonstrated conceptual understanding, but continues to experience intolerable difficulty with facts recall. It is important, therefore, for teachers to ensure they have exhausted all instructional opportunities and not rush to supplemental "crutches" as substitutes for effective teaching.

Teaching Problem Solving

Verbal problem solving should be integrated with instruction from the student's first introduction to mathematics. Using real-world situations to explain concepts, calculations, and higher level complex skills creates a mind set that mathematics is a functional way of thinking about and organizing life activities. Students learn that mathematics skills are tools for problem-solving activities; further, the process of learning mathematics becomes a more meaningful and holistic problem-solving experience. There are limitless life situations to draw upon in teaching problem-solving skills: arranging classroom objects; sorting various items; shopping; purchasing books, materials for school; buying that first automobile; drawing, art activities; even maintaining a "bank account" of points earned in classes.

Kennedy and Tipps (1991) discuss three approaches to teaching problem solving: 1. teaching students about problem solving; 2. teaching for problem solving; and 3. teaching via problem solving. Each approach is conducive to learning-instruction in individualized, small group, and, under certain circumstances, large group configurations (p. 124).

In the first approach, children are taught a methodical process for problem attack and appropriate solving strategies. In recent years, several such procedures have been proposed. For example, a four step process includes 1. understanding the problem (What does it mean? What is the problem asking?); 2. devising a plan (What might be a way to find the answer? Are there any other possibilities?); 3. selecting and implementing a plan; and 4. reviewing the process (Did it work? Should another solution be tried?).

The second method, teaching for problem solving, involves the continual association of real-life situations with the mathematical concept or skill at the focus of instruction. In this model, applications to life-situations are emphasized throughout introductions to new concepts and skills, practice exercises, and the integration of material with new or more complex learning. For example, a multitude of problem-solving tasks can be associated with an assignment to build a birdhouse. Even the Pythagorean theorem ($a^2 + b^2 = c^2$) might gain practical value when students are challenged to determine roof-lines and gable dimensions!

The final approach, teaching via problem solving, uses real-life problems as the vehicle for teaching mathematics skills and concepts. Instruction begins with a problem situation, various skills and strategies are introduced as reasonable, logical methods to solve the situation. In this model, instruction emphasizes the gradual shift from concrete-to-graphic-to-symbolic representations. Teachers must activate creative processes to generate as many problem situations as possible that are relevant to the age, grade, and socio-cultural characteristics of their students; in fact, the students provide a most remarkable resource for generating a continuous pool of problem-solving challenges.

The National Council of Teachers of Mathematics (1989) has proposed instructional guidelines for teaching problem-solving skills. Essentially, these guidelines are:

1. Mathematics must be applied to solving real-world problems.

2. Problem solving should include methods of collecting, organizing, and interpreting information; drawing and testing inferences from data; and communicating results.

3. The use of computers should be taught and encouraged as a means to extend traditional means for problem solving and to implement new interaction and simulation strategies.

4. Problem-solving instruction should encourage the use of imagery, visualization, and spatial concepts.

Instructional Materials

Special education curricula tend to overemphasize methods, materials, and media and are often age-inappropriate, particularly when used with secondary level students

(Katsiyannis & Prillaman, 1990). In fact, many effective materials will be found in children's homes, in the classroom, or are teacher-constructed. The selection of materials is largely determined by the individual needs of the students and their learning styles, the mathematics material to be taught, and the teacher's personal teaching style. Nonetheless, there are commercially available curriculum materials and computer software that are beneficial both as instructional aids and as teaching resources. A sampling of these materials has been compiled and is provided in Figure 7–13 (on pages 278–279).

SUMMARY

This chapter has provided an introduction to teaching mathematics to children with mild disabilities and learning difficulties. Discussions focused on the integration of structural knowledge, skills, and the functional aspects of mathematics as a means to help teachers meet the instructional challenge posed by mathematics. The key points addressed are summarized for review and emphasis.

Although it is commonly assumed that children with mild learning disabilities experience difficulty when learning mathematics, research suggests that the use of effective teaching practices will enable most children to learn and apply math skills. Learning efficiency is determined by several critical factors: 1. each teacher's level of understanding about a given child's math knowledge including the way in which previously learned skills are understood—both effective and faulty patterns; 2. the nature and levels of math anxiety present and experienced by both the teacher and students, as well as efforts to reduce or counteract such anxiety; 3. the use of diverse instructional practices devised to meet individualized learning needs; 4. the manner in which the child uses acquired skills and knowledge—appropriate and inappropriate uses; and 5. the relationship of classroom instruction to the overall curriculum design and functional life skills. Thus, teachers must be creative. They must teach and accept strategies that include nontraditional constructions of mathematics to then emphasize math skills as tools for solving problems and daily life challenges.

The purpose in the mathematics assessment process is to clarify crucial instructional information to formulate a personalized intervention plan. Identifying the content within a child's mathematics knowledge base, the child's efficiency in problem-solving and computational tasks, and the child's cognitive readiness/learning level form the basis for making instructional decisions. Interviews and subsequent error analyses are critical components in this practice. Essentially, where and how instruction should be delivered is more clearly identified through the process of examining a child's acquired knowledge while isolating the types of errors systematically applied, such as faulty procedures or errors due to deficits in prerequisite skills.

Learning mathematics is a developmental process involving the continued use of concrete, graphic, and symbolic representations of problems. Effective instruction includes activities that range from the exploration of environmental objects and events, to learning skills needed to organize and understand environmental factors, to ultimately understanding and accepting math as a problem-solving life skill. For pupils with mild disabilities, the problem-solving emphasis in mathematics introduces a meaningful, realistic function to learning mathematics that will have benefits beyond the classroom.

FIGURE 7-13 Curriculum Materials, Resources, and Software

INSTRUCTIONAL MATERIALS/PACKAGES

Computational Arithmetic Program
    Smith & Lovitt, 1982
    Publisher: Pro-Ed
For students grades 1-6; provides 314 sequenced problems for all four operations; emphasizes basic computational sklls with whole numbers.

Corrective Mathematics Program
    Engelmann & Carnine, 1982
    Publisher: Science Research Associates
A remedial series for students grades 3-12 and adults who have not mastered basic skills. Includes 65 lessons in each of the operations; teacher-directed and independent practice activities.

Cuisenaire Rods
    Davidson, 1969
    Publisher: Cuisenaire Company of America
Cuisenaire rods are instructional aids to supplement teaching of concepts. Usually used in grades K-3, used in remedial instruction through grade 6.

Direct Instruction Mathematics (Second Edition)
    Silbert, Carnine, & Stein, 1990
    Publisher: Merrill Publishing Company
A structured, comprehensive instuctional program using direct instruction techniques. Appropriate for all grade levels, particularly for remedial instruction. Includes information for organizing instructional program, planning, instructional procedures. Instructional content covers skills, concepts, symbol identification, place value, operations, story problems, fractions, decimals, time, money, measurement, study skills, and geometry.

DISTAR Arithmetic Kits
    Engelmann & Carnine, 1972, 1975, 1976, 1989
    Publisher: Science Research Associates
A highly structured instructional program; uses direct instruction methodology. Includes operations, algebra, geometry, measurement, fractions, time, and money. Generally used in grades K-6; can be usd in remedial instruction for older students.

KeyMath Early Steps
    Connolly, 1982
    Publisher: American Guidance Service
Designed for K-1, also appropriate for remedial instruction. Includes 55 lessons with various activities to address multiple learning levels and styles. Includes units in geometry, numeration, addition and subtraction, measurement, time, money, and fractions.

Project MATH
    Cawley, Goodstein, Fitzmaurice, Lepore, Sedlak, & Althaus, 1976
    Publisher: Educational Development Corporation
Designed for preschool-6; can be used with secondary students for remedial instruction. Deemphasizes reading skills; focuses on varied learning styles, levels, and needs. Includes patterns, operations, sets, geometry, measurement, fractions, and life-skills.

FIGURE 7-13 Curriculum Materials, Resources, and Software (cont'd.)

PUBLISHERS OF MATHEMATICS LEARNING AIDS AND SOFTWARE

Creative Publications
5040 West 111the Street
Oak Lawn, IL 60453
1-800-624-0822

Delta Education
P.O. Box 915
Hudson, NH 03051
1-800-258-1302

DLM
One DLM Park
P.O. Box 4000
Allen, TX 75002
1-800-527-4747
1-800-442-4711 (TX)

Educational Activities, Inc.
P.O. Box 392
Freeport, NY 11520
1-800-645-3739
1-516-223-4666 (NY)

Hartley Courseware, Inc.
Box 419
Dimondale, MI 48821
1-800-247-1380
1-517-646-6458 (MI)

Houghton Mifflin
One Beacon Street
Boston, MA 02108

IBM Educational Systems
Dept. PC
4111 Northside Parkway
Atlanta, GA 30327

The Learning Company
6493 Kaiser Drive
Fremont, CA 94555
1-800-852-2255

MECC
3490 Lexington Avenue North
St. Paul, MN 55126
1-800-228-3504, ext. 527
1-800-782-0032, ext. 527 (MN)

Midwest Publications
P.O. Box 448
Pacific Grove, CA 93950
1-800-458-4849

Milliken Publishing Company
1100 Research Boulevard
P.O. Box 21579
St. Louis, MO 63132-0579
1-800-325-4136

Mindscape Inc.
3444 Dundee Road
Northbrook, IL 60062
1-800-221-9884

Random House Media
Dept. 517
400 Hahn Road
Westminster, MD 21157
1-800-638-6460
1-516-492-0782 (MD)

Scholastic Inc.
2931 East McCarty Street
P.O. Box 7502
Jefferson City, MO 65102
1-800-541-5513
1-800-392-2179 (MO)

Scott, Foresman and Company
1900 East Lake Avenue
Glenview, IL 60025
1-800-554-4411

Spinnaker Software Corp.
One Kendall Square
Cambridge, MA 02139
1-800-323-8088

Sunburst Communications
39 Washington Avenue
Pleasantville, NY 10570-2898
1-800-431-1934
1-800-321-7511 (NY)

Tandy Corporation
1700 One Tandy Center
Fort Worth, TX 76102

REFERENCES

Ashlock, R.B. (1986) *Error patterns in computation: A semi-programmed approach*, 4th Ed. New York, NY: Macmillan Publishing Company.

Ashlock, R.B. (1990). *Error patterns in computation: A semi-programmed approach*, 5th Ed. New York, NY: Macmillan Publishing Company.

Brown, S. (1990). Integrating manipulatives and computers in problem-solving experiences. *Arithmetic Teacher, 38*, 8–10.

Brownell, W.A. (1986). The revolution in arithmetic. *Arithmetic Teacher, 34*(2), 38–42. (Reprinted from *Arithmetic Teacher, 1*, 1954).

Brownell, W.A. (1987). Meaning and skill: Maintaining the balance. *Arithmetic Teacher, 34*, 18–25. (Reprinted from *Arithmetic Teacher*, 1956).

Bruner, J.S. (1966). *Studies in cognitive growth.* New York, NY: John Wiley & Sons, Inc.

Carl, I. M. (1989). Essential mathematics for the twenty-first century. *The Education Digest, 55*, 40–42.

Cawley, J.F. (1984). *Developmental teaching of mathematics for the learning disabled.* Rockville, MD: Aspen.

Cawley, J.F., Miller, D., & Carr, S. (1988). Mathematics. In G. Robinson, J.R. Patton, E.A. Polloway, & L.R. Sargent (Eds.), *Best Practices in Mental Disabilities*, Vol. 2.

Cawley, J.F., & Parmar, R.S. (1990). Issues in mathematics curriculum for handicapped students. *Academic Therapy, 25*, 507–521.

Education for All Handicapped Children Act, 20 U.S.C. 1401 et. seq.; 34 C.F.R. Part 300.

Engelmann, S.E., & Carnine, D.W. (1989). *Distar arithmetic III*, 2nd Ed. Chicago, IL: Science Research Associates.

Fleischner, J.E., Nuzum, M.B., & Mazzola, E.S. (1987). Devising an instructional program to teach arithmetic problem-solving skills to students with learning disabilities. *Journal of Learning Disabilities, 20*, 214–217.

Frank, M.L. (1990). What myths about mathematics are held and conveyed by teachers? *Arithmetic Teacher, 37*, 10–12.

Gagné, R.M. (1977). *The conditions of learning*, 3rd Ed. New York, NY: Holt, Rinehart and Winston.

Garofalo, J. (1987). Metacognition and school mathematics. *Arithmetic Teacher, 34*, 22–23.

Herold, P.J. (1979). Reasons for failure (From: *The math teaching handbook*). *The Exceptional Parent, 2*, 49–53.

Kamii, C. (1990). Constructivism and beginning arithmetic (K–2). In T.J. Cooney (Ed.), *Teaching and learning mathematics in the 1990s*. Reston, VA: National Council of Teachers of Mathematics.

Katsiyannis, A., & Prillaman, D. (1990). Teaching math using regular curricula. *Teaching Exceptional Children, 23*, 26–29.

Kennedy, L.M., & Tipps, S. (1988). *Guiding children's learning of mathematics*, 5th Ed. Belmont, CA: Wadsworth Publishing Company.

Kennedy, L.M., & Tipps, S. (1991). *Guiding children's learning of mathematics*, 6th Ed. Belmont, CA: Wadsworth Publishing Company.

Kogelman, S., & Warren, J. (1978). *Mind over math.* New York, NY: Dial Press.

Love, L.D. (1987). An evaluation of the effectiveness of a concrete, graphic, and symbolic approach to teaching place value on the acquisition of computation skills. *Dissertation Abstracts International*, 47.

Love, L.D., & McGuire, M.D. (1985). [Error patterns in student acquisition of math skills: Issues in instruction.] Unpublished data.

Love, L.D., & McGuire, M.D. (1990). *Evaluation alternatives: Diagnosis with an individual math interview.* Manuscript submitted for publication.

McGuire, M.D. (1985, February). *Direct instruction in mathematics for learning disabled students.* Paper presented at the meeting of Council for Exceptional Children, Kansas City, KS.

McKnight, C.C., Travers, K.J., Crosswhite, F.J., & Swafford, J.D. (1985). Eighth-grade mathematics in U.S. schools: A report from the second international mathematics study. *Arithmetic Teacher, 8,* 20–26.

National Commission on Excellence in Education. (1983). *A nation at risk.* Washington, DC: U.S. Government Printing Office.

National Council for Teachers of Mathematics. (1989). *Curriculum and evaluation standards for school mathematics.* Reston, VA: Author.

Patton, J.R., & Polloway, E.A. (1988). Curricular orientations for students with mental disabilities. In G. Robinson, J.R. Patton, E.A. Polloway, & L.R. Sargent (Eds.), *Best Practices in Mental Disabilities,* Vol. 2. Des Moines, IA: Department of Special Education, Bureau of Special Education.

Piaget, J. (1952). *The child's conception of number.* New York, NY: Humanities Press.

Piaget, J. (1965). *The child's conception of number.* New York, NY: W.W. Norton Company.

Polloway, E.A., Patton, J.R., Payne, J.S., & Payne, R.A. (1989). *Strategies for teaching learners with special needs,* 4th Ed. Columbus, OH: Merrill Publishing Company.

Reisman, F.K. (1982). *A guide to the diagnostic teaching of arithmetic.* Columbus, OH: Charles E. Merrill.

Roberts, G.H. (1968). The failure strategies of third grade arithmetic pupils. *Arithmetic Teacher, 15,* 442–446.

Silbert, J., Carnine, D., & Stein, M. (1990). *Direct instruction mathematics,* 2nd Ed. Columbus, OH: Merrill Publishing Company.

Skrtic, T.M. (1978). [Developmental readiness for learning math skills: Adolescent learning.] Unpublished data.

Skrtic, T.M., Kvam, N.E., & Beals, V.L. (1983). Identifying and remediating the subtraction errors of learning disabled adolescents. *The Pointer, 27,* 32–38.

Smith, T.E.C. (1990). *Introduction to education,* 2nd Ed. St. Paul, MN: West Publishing Company.

Tobias, S. (1981). Stress in the math classroom. *Learning, 9*(6), 38.

Underhill, R.B. (1976). Classroom diagnosis. In J.L. Higgins and J.W. Heddens (Eds.). *Remedial mathematics: Diagnostic and prescriptive approaches* (pp. 33–35). Columbus, OH: ERIC Center for Science, Mathematics, and Environmental Education.

U.S. Department of Education. (1980). *Second annual report to Congress on the implementation of P.L. 94-142: The Education for All Handicapped Children Act.* Washington, DC: U.S. Government Printing Office.

Wilson, J.W. (1990). Concerning this book. In R.B. Ashlock, *Error patterns in computation: A semi-programmed approach,* 5th Ed. (p. viii). New York, NY: Macmillan Publishing Company. (Reprinted from *Error patterns in computation: A semi-programmed approach,* 2nd Ed., 1980).

Wilson, R., & Majsterek, D. (1990). Mathematics instruction. In P.J. Schloss, M.A. Smith, & C.N. Schloss (Eds.), *Instructional Methods for Adolescents with Learning and Behavior Problems.* Needham Heights, MA: Allyn and Bacon.

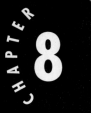

Supporting Students in the Mainstream

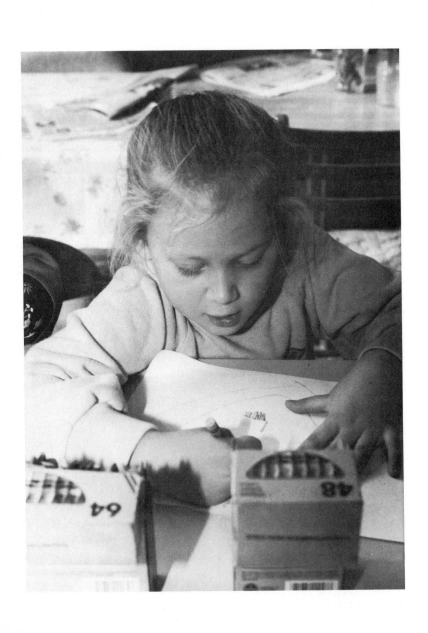

Outline

OBJECTIVES

After reading this chapter, you will be able to:

- define study skills;

- list and describe specific study skills;

- describe the nature of study skills;

- describe how study skills can be used with students with disabilities;

- discuss how to assess study skills;

- describe various methods to teach study skills;

- define accommodations;

- describe the role of special education teachers in accommodations by regular classroom teachers;

- describe the various types of accommodations used in regular classrooms.

Introduction

The way students with mild disabilities are educated has changed dramatically since the 1970s. As a result of students with mild disabilities receiving significant amounts of instruction in regular classrooms by regular teachers, an emphasis on their ability to succeed in this new environment has developed. No longer will these students succeed or fail based on their performance in special education classrooms; they will have to perform successfully in regular education programs (Smith & Dowdy, 1989). Also, their success or failure is no longer the sole responsibility of the special education teacher. Regular classroom teachers now play a major role in this outcome.

Without assistance, it is likely that many students with mild disabilities will be unsuccessful in mainstreamed settings. Simply integrating them into a "normalized" environment in no way means that they need fewer services than before. In order to facilitate the chances for these students to experience success in regular classroom environments, they need to have certain skills that will enable them to perform specific academic expectations. They need to have skills that will help them to study, remember, and respond in acceptable ways. In addition, regular classroom teachers need to be willing to make modifications in their requirements and teaching methods to give these students an opportunity to succeed.

Special education teachers can do several things to facilitate the success of students with disabilities in regular classrooms. First, they can teach students skills that will help them become successful in mainstream classrooms. Skills such as how to take notes, how to please regular teachers, and how to study for tests can greatly improve the chances of students being successful. In addition to teaching students with disabilities some of these skills, special education teachers can also help regular classroom teachers make accommodations for mainstreamed students. The use of study skills by students with disabilities and the implementation of accommodations by regular classroom teachers will both help students with disabilities succeed in their integrated placements.

Study Skills

Study skills include a wide variety of different skills that students can use to facilitate their success in academic and social settings. As a result, there are many different definitions of study skills. Hoover (1988a) defines study skills as "tools used to acquire, record, locate, organize, synthesize, and remember information effectively and efficiently" (p. 10). Study skills can also be defined as those skills and behaviors that facilitate academic and social success in and out of school situations. Study skills are techniques that help students learn how to learn as opposed to actually learning content (Locke & Abbey, 1989). Examples include skills that help students take in information properly, store information efficiently, retrieve information as needed, and express information in an understandable desireable manner.

Another term used to describe actions that students can take to improve their learning success is "strategies." Lenz and Deshler (1990) define a strategy as how an individual approaches a task, including the planning, executing, and evaluating of the performance of the task. There may be some confusion between study skills and strategies. We view both terms as describing techniques that students can use to improve their chances for achieving success in classroom situations. Therefore, the terms may be used interchangably in the remaining part of this chapter.

THE NATURE OF STUDY SKILLS

Study skills are definitely necessary for students to succeed in academic settings. They help students attend to auditory stimuli, comprehend what is read, take notes for later study, remember facts for tests, and express these facts as necessary. Without these kinds of skills students are at a significant disadvantage in schools. Unfortunately, some professionals consider study skills to be totally related to academic work in academic settings. As Polloway and Patton (1989) noted, this is a very "misguided notion" (p. 380). Study skills also help individuals succeed in settings outside the school. For example, adolescents must be able to manage their out-of-school time to balance work, social activities, and homework requirements. Also, young students need to be able to listen effectively in order to carry out the wishes of their parents. Time management and listening skills are examples of study skills that are used outside the school setting. The importance of study skills also goes beyond the school years. Adults need to have study skills for social and vocational activities. For example, many jobs require workers to read directions, follow specific instructions, manage time, and write legibly. With deficits in these areas, many jobs might be unobtainable. Study skills, although they suggest an association with academic work, are also related to social success. Adults unable to manage their time efficiently may have problems with social relationships. Never being on time, for example, can become such a bother for some people that it affects friendships.

Study skills, therefore, go well beyond helping students achieve academic success in a classroom. They impact on the abilities of children to succeed outside the classroom setting and in social situations; they are also related to the likelihood that adults will do well in jobs and social situations. Study skills simply help persons function in their environments, whether these environments are academic, social, or vocational.

In teaching study skills, teachers take on a role different from the traditional role of teaching content to students. By teaching study skills, teachers are helping students develop techniques for achieving success in other classes (Lenz & Deshler, 1990). For example, a traditional role has the teacher getting students to learn and remember facts simply for the sake of learning those facts. In study skills instruction, the teacher is arming students with skills that will enable them to learn their own facts.

There are numerous study skills. An example of a few include reading rate, listening skills, time management, notetaking, and test taking (Hoover 1988). There are several different ways these can be implemented. For example, there are numerous tips that help students successfully take tests. These might include looking for key words and phrases in questions and eliminating obvious wrong choices. For example, students could be taught to look for "always," "never," and "only" in true-false questions. These terms usually result in the statement being false. Students may also be taught to eliminate the obviously wrong answers in a multiple-choice test and focus on the remaining answers that could be accurate. By eliminating the obviously wrong answers, the odds of choosing the correct answer improve.

STUDY SKILLS AND STUDENTS WITH DISABILITIES

Many children simply learn ways to study that are effective without having anyone specifically teach them these skills. They learn by trial and error. Ways they try that are effective are repeated, while ways that are ineffective are deleted from their skill repertoire. They also learn by modeling the study skills used effectively by other students. And in some instances, students may set out to learn a particular study skill, such as increasing their reading rate. Think of your own evolution into your current study practices. Has anyone ever specifically taught you how to study? Why do you use the techniques you currently employ to take notes, study for tests, or manage your time? Most of us are fortunate in that we are able to develop these skills without a great deal of effort. We simply learn to use them.

Students with mild disabilities exhibit a variety of characteristics that may negatively impact on their studying skills (Gearheart, Weishahn, & Gearheart, 1988). These include memory deficits, problems in social skills, behavior control, reading comprehension problems, attention deficits, distractibility, and lack of organization. These characteristics can all result in problems with studying, with the end result being academic problems. In describing students without good study skills, Gleason (1988) notes that when given an assignment, these students "lack direction and the strategies needed for finding information in textbooks, looking up words in the glossary, interpreting maps, answering questions, or asking the teacher for help" (p. 52).

ASSESSMENT OF STUDY SKILLS

As with any skill, before developing and implementing intervention strategies with students, a comprehensive assessment should be completed to determine specific strengths and weaknesses (Smith, Price, & Marsh, 1986; Polloway & Smith, 1992). Some students with mild disabilities do not need instruction in study skills, whereas others do. While most of these students could benefit from this form of intervention, they do not all need the same programs. Therefore, assessing the study skills of students is an important first step before developing and implementing intervention programs in this area.

Formal Assessment of Study Skills

Formal assessment primarily includes standardized, norm-referenced tests administered in a structured manner. There are no formal, norm-referenced tests specifically designed to assess study skills; however, many of the areas that study skills address are evaluated as components of standardized tests. These include reading skills, memory skills, comprehension abilities, listening acuity and comprehension, and written language skills. Each chapter in the text has provided information regarding assessment of specific skills. Therefore, additional information will not be presented here. To determine which study

TABLE 8-1 Study Skills Questionnaire

STUDY SKILLS QUESTIONNAIRE

	Almost always	Sometimes	Very seldom
1. Do you listen to directions or instructions provided in class?	☐	☐	☐
2. Do you take notes regarding assignments?	☐	☐	☐
3. Do you ask questions when you don't understand?	☐	☐	☐
4. Do you pay attention to class lectures and discussions?	☐	☐	☐
5. Do you keep up with assigned readings?	☐	☐	☐
6. Do you feel disorganized most of the time?	☐	☐	☐
7. Do you participate in class discussions?	☐	☐	☐
8. Do you find it difficult to complete assignments in class?	☐	☐	☐
9. Do you feel adequately prepared most of the time?	☐	☐	☐
10. Do you find the vocabulary too difficult?	☐	☐	☐

Source: Gearheart, B.R., Weishahn, M.W., & Gearheart, C.J. (1988). *The Exceptional Student in the Regular Classroom,* 4th Ed. Columbus, OH: Merrill, p. 85. Used with permission.

skills are necessary, teachers need to analyze the results of specific diagnostic and achievement tests. By evaluating students' strengths and weaknesses, determinations can be made regarding needed study skills training.

Informal Assessment of Study Skills

Teachers can informally assess study skills using a variety of different methods. For the purposes of developing and implementing intervention programs, informal assessment probably works better than formal testing. The nature of informal assessment of study skills will vary with the study skill being assessed. Methods typically used include observations, interviews with students, interviews with parents, and checklists.

Table 8–1 presents an example of a questionnaire that could be used in an interview with students or modified and used with parents or teachers. The results of this type of questionnaire can help teachers determine general areas of strengths and weaknesses regarding study skills. An example of a checklist to evaluate a more specific study skill, notetaking, is in Table 8–2 (on page 288).

Using Assessment Data

Following the collection and analysis of assessment information, teachers should sit down and discuss the results with the students (Gearheart *et al.*, 1988). Students first of all should understand their deficiencies related to study skills and different ways they can help themselves become better students. Showing students that a few "tricks," or study skills, can result in positive academic outcomes may result in a motivation to learn and try these skills.

After evaluating a student's study skills and explaining strengths and weaknesses to the student, a plan to improve certain skills should be developed and implemented. For

TABLE 8-2 Questions to Assess Notetaking Skills

1. Can the student listen actively?
2. Can the student read actively?
3. Can the student use content-specific vocabulary?
4. Can the student locate the main ideas?
5. Can the student locate supporting details?
6. Can the student consolidate information?
7. Can the student organize information?
8. Can the student use abbreviations?
9. Can the student take notes legibly?
10. Can the student take notes from textbooks?
11. Can the student take notes from reference materials?
12. Can the student take notes from lectures?
13. Can the student take notes from multi-media sources?
14. Can the student reduce notes into concise statements?

Source: Beirne-Smith, M. (1989). A systematic approach for teaching notetaking skills to students with mild learning handicaps. *Academic Therapy, 24,* 425–437.

students with mild disabilities who exhibit deficiencies in study skills, programming can become a part of the individual education program (IEP). Examples of IEP objectives related to study skills include:

- Student will be able to identify and define major vocabulary words used in regular classes.

- Student will be able to identify major ideas presented in regular classroom textbooks.

- Student will be able to spell words presented in English class.

- Student will use the SQ3R study method in regular classes.

- Student will seek appropriate help from regular teachers.

- Student will seek assistance from special education personnel when necessary.

- Student will complete supplemental assignments (usually study guides).

- Student will be able to verbalize ideas from lecture notes.

- Student will demonstrate understanding of reading material (Smith & Dowdy, 1989, p. 484).

Although these only represent a small sampling of possible IEP goals and objectives related to study skills, they do indicate that some secondary special education teachers realize the importance of study skills and are including the instruction of study skills in students' programs.

METHODS TO TEACH STUDY SKILLS

For students with mild disabilities, formal instruction in study skills may be necessary to enhance the likelihood that these students will be successful in school. If these students are to be successful in mainstream classes, such as history, English, and science, they need to be able to take advantage of every strategy available; simply put, they need all the help they can get. Arming these students with a "bag" full of study skills will greatly increase their chances for being successful. There are a wide variety of study skills that can be taught to students to help them succeed in their classes. Table 8–3 (on page 290) lists several study skills and their significance to learning.

General Considerations in Teaching Study Skills

Study skills are already taught by many teachers, but not in an orderly manner. Often teachers tell students things like "make notes while you are reading a chapter," "use study cards when preparing for a test," and "use games (mnemonic devices) when trying to memorize certain facts." Teachers need to realize the broad range of study skills that are capable of being taught and develop an organized plan for teaching these skills to students who need them.

There are several general principles teachers should consider when teaching study skills. These include:

1. Discuss the importance of the study skill with students.

2. Describe how the particular study skill can benefit the student in a regular classroom situation.

3. Guide students through the steps necessary in using the study skill.

4. Provide ample opportunities for the student to practice the skill.

5. Alter the simulated situation so the student can understand how the study skill applies to similar but different situations.

6. Teach the student how to apply the study skill to new, different, and "real" situations (Gleason, 1988).

Simply learning study skills may not help students succeed in classrooms. After students have learned how to use specific study skills, they must learn how to transfer the skills to different situations, with different instructional personnel. Table 8–4 (on page 291) describes several ways to facilitate this transfer ability.

The ultimate success of students using study skills effectively is based on two factors: students' knowledge of skills and how they are related to a particular technique and students' motivation to use skills and learn (Ellis, Deshler, Lenz, Schumaker, & Clark, 1991).

TABLE 8-3 Study Skills and their Significance for Learning

STUDY SKILL	SIGNIFICANCE FOR LEARNING
Reading Rate	Rates vary with type and length of reading materials
Listening	Ability to listen is critical in most educational activities
Notetaking/Outlining	Ability to take notes and develop outlines is critical in content courses
Report Writing	Written reports are frequently required in content courses
Oral Presentations	Some teachers require extensive oral reporting
Graphic Aids	Visual aids can help students who have reading deficits
Test Taking	Students must be able to do well on tests if they are to succeed in content courses
Library Usage	Ability to find and use resource information from the library is critical in content courses
Reference Material/ Dictionary Usage	Using reference materials makes learners more independent
Time Management	Ability to manage and allocate time is critical for success in secondary settings
Self-Management of Behavior	Leads to independence

Source: Hoover, J. J. (1988). *Teaching handicapped students study skills,* 2nd Ed. Lindale, TX: Hamilton Publications.

Without these ingredients present, the effectiveness of study skills will be less than maximum. For example, it will be of little use if a student knows how to use a variety of study skills if there is no motivation to implement them and do well in classes. For example, if a student knows to look for certain words such as "always" and "never" as clues on a true-false test, but doesn't bother, the knowledge of the skill is of limited benefit. The following describes some specific study skills that teachers can use with students experiencing mild disabilities.

Study Skills Related to Reading Comprehension

The key to reading is comprehension. Indeed, some definitions of reading state that reading is comprehension (Smith, Graves, & Aldridge, in press). Reading fluently and rapidly

TABLE 8-4   Steps to Facilitate Generalization of Study Skills

- Tell students to try new skill in other settings.
- Discuss different settings skills could be used.
- Reinforce the importance of using specific study skills.
- Have students report on their attempts to use the skill.
- Discuss differences between special education classroom environment and regular classroom environment.
- Practice social skills with role-playing and coaching.
- Discuss with regular classroom teachers the study skills that students have learned.
- Suggest that the regular classroom teacher teach the entire class specific study skills.
- When students experience success with the study skill in the regular classroom, again discuss the importance of the skill.
- Provide continual review.

Source: Gleason, M. M. (1988). Teaching study strategies. *Teaching Exceptional Children, 20,* 52–53.

are desired reading characteristics; however, if the student cannot recall what was read, the reading will be of little use. There are many techniques that will help to improve students' comprehension skills; many students have validated their effectiveness (Rich & Pressley, 1990).

SQ3R   The SQ3R method is an example of ways to improve reading comprehension. It was described in detail in Chapter 5.

EVOKER   This is method for helping students read materials that require "close reading," such as prose, poetry, and drama. The steps in the method are:

1. *Explore*   The entire passage is read.

2. *Vocabulary*   During reading, make a note about words and places that are unfamiliar. Look these up after the first step.

3. *Oral Reading*   Read the passage out loud and with expression.

4. *Key Ideas*   Note the key ideas, including the main idea or theme.

5. *Evaluation*   Determine the importance of the key words and sentences to the overall passage.

6. *Recapitulation*   Reread the passage (Roe *et al.*, 1987).

PQRST   Still another example of reading for comprehension, or studying material for comprehension, is the PQSRT method. This approach was developed in the 1950s and has been successfully tested on numerous occasions. The research, which compared the effectiveness of studying using the PQRST method and a less specific method, revealed the advantages of the PQRST model (Staton, 1959).

Using this method, students first preview the material. This is accomplished by scanning the material to get a general idea of the content. Either during or after this preview stage, the reader formulates questions about what the content will likely contain. The third step is read. During the reading stage, the reading attempts to find the answer to the questions. In the fourth step, the reader states what has been read by paraphrasing the material. Finally, the fifth step is to test. This is when the student, as in the state stage, paraphrases the material. However, during this step, time has elapsed from the initial reading (Staton, 1959).

Each of these methods that use several distinct steps have commonalities. The primary link among the methods is the attempt of the reader to impose some structure and format to the reading activity. Reading becomes an activity with a purpose and method rather than simply a process where the words are "read" either orally or silently.

Summaries   Students who read for content can often improve their comprehension if they summarize, in writing, the content of a section of reading (Roe *et al.*, 1987). Gerr (1988) suggests that students be taught how to paraphrase their reading materials when writing summaries. Paraphrasing content can occur through the use of self-questioning, such as "What is this paragraph about?" and "Who were the key people in the story?"

Summaries can benefit students in several different ways. First they help students condense the reading material. Good summaries are much easier to study when preparing for tests than having to read the entire text. Summaries also help students understand how the content is organized. Finally, summaries require students to paraphrase the information; this requires that the student understand and comprehend the material.

Semantic Mapping   Another approach to help students comprehend their reading is semantic mapping. Semantic mapping is a graphic organizing strategy where students develop a visual organization of the story or content (Sinatra, Berg, & Dunn, 1985; Schewel, 1989). In some ways semantic mapping is similar to diagraming a sentence. Figure 8–1 depicts a semantic map of the familiar story, "The Three Little Pigs." By developing a visual display, students are able to see the relationships within stories and better remember the content. Research on the efficacy of using semantic mapping has concluded that it is an effective method for improving reading comprehension (Schewel, 1989).

Schewel (1989) suggests that teachers use the following general strategy for introducing the semantic mapping strategy.

1. The teacher presents a stimulus word or a core question related to the story to be read.

2. Students brainstorm to generate words related to the stimulus word or predict answers to the questions, which the teacher lists on the board.

3. Students, with the teacher, then put related words or answers in groups, drawing connecting lines between topics, thus forming a semantic map.

4. After reading the selection, students and teacher discuss the categories and rearrange or add to the map developed prior to the reading (p. 442).

Underlining   Teaching students how to underline important parts of the reading content can improve reading comprehension. Many students learn to underline on their own. This especially occurs in college when students may purchase their textbooks and can

FIGURE 8-1 Semantic Map of "The Three Little Pigs"

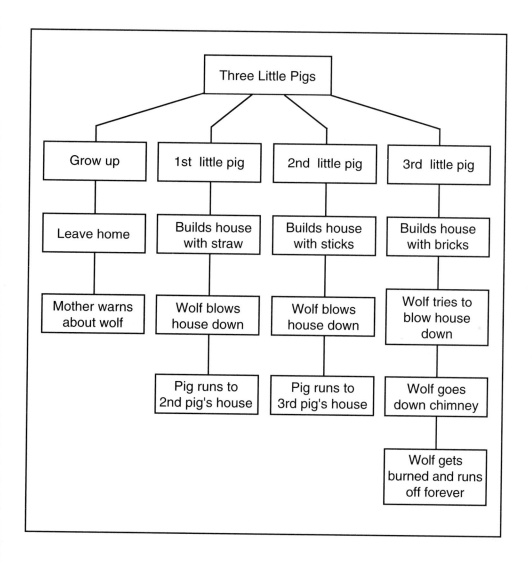

therefore write in them. Since textbooks used in public schools are state owned, students should not write in them. Therefore, teaching students how to use underlining and allowing them to write in their books may both be necessary.

Since students with mild disabilities have such difficulties reading, comprehending, and studying materials for tests, teachers should attempt to work out a way they can underline and make margin notes in their texts. Even if the few textbooks used by students in special education had to be bought each year out of special education supply funds, it would probably be worth the expense.

One way to teach underlining is to ask students to identify the three or four most important sentences in a paragraph that present most of the facts. Then go around to different students and ask them to give you one of the sentences they underlined. Write these sentences on the board and keep a record of the number of times sentences were chosen. Then lead a discussion about which sentences were the most important and why. This should help some students who had a difficult time determining which sentences were the most important and which ones should be underlined for later review.

Study Skills and Reading Rate

Students have to read more and more materials as they progress through the grades. In elementary grades, students first read in order to learn how to read. In upper elementary grades, they begin to read for content; they read history books, science books, and social studies books. This practice of reading for content only increases as the students matriculate through the school until the ability to read fairly quickly becomes a factor.

There are several study skills that relate to reading rate that can be taught to students. These include skimming, scanning, and rapid reading (Hoover, 1988). Since students with mild disabilities are frequently slow and poor readers, teaching them how to use these techniques will be very helpful to them in content courses. When teaching students to use a skimming technique, teachers need to focus on two different skimming techniques. When skimming for the main ideas in a passage, students should be taught to look for certain cues. These could include:

- key words in the passage;

- flow of thought used by the author;

- punctuation and other visual features.

Skimming for detail requires the reader to be looking for preselected words or phrases (Kaufman, 1980). For example, if the reader is skimming for facts about the reasons for the Civil War, words such as "reasons," "justifications," "purposes," and "slavery" may be targeted. Skimming techniques can greatly reduce the amount of time required to read several pages of text.

Young and Savage (1989) suggest several additional ways to help students improve their reading rate. Their first suggestion targets students who have a habit of vocalizing every word they read. By practicing reading in word groups, as well as holding a pencil between their teeth or chewing gum, students can often overcome this cumbersome, plodding style.

Students should be encouraged to read in word groups. Looking and verbalizing each word results in very slow, cumbersome reading (Smith *et al.*, in press). Show students that they have a wider eye-span than one word. One way to do this is to spontaneously cover the last part of a sentence a student is reading orally. Often the student has already seen the words and is therefore able to complete the sentence. Have students practice using their wider eye-span by looking up from time to time during oral reading and continuing to visualize the reading passage (Young & Savage, 1989).

Other suggestions to improve reading rate noted by Young and Savage (1989) include teaching students to read in phrases, skip over unimportant words, and practice timed readings. When teaching students to read phrases, have them practice recognizing phrases or words that fit together well in a group. For example:

The little boy/ opened the present/ and played with the new toy.

By visualizing words that fit together, students are better able to use their wide eye-span and read several words together.

Study Skills and Reading Vocabulary

Students can become better readers if they understand the words they read. A good reading vocabulary helps students read more efficiently and comprehend at a higher level. There are several different ways to enhance reading vocabulary. Dixon (1987) suggests teaching synonyms as a way to increase reading vocabulary. Using this method, students are taught the concept of a particular word and synonyms to that word.

Students can also be taught vocabulary through traditional, direct teaching methods, or the newer whole language approach. Regardless of the way vocabulary is taught, students with limited reading skills will benefit greatly if they are able to recognize words rather than having to decode them one at a time. Chapter 5 presents other techniques to improve reading vocabulary.

Study Skills and Memory

Memory deficits are frequently present in students with mild disabilities. (Pressley, Scruggs, & Mastropieri, 1989; Kaufman, 1989; Patton *et al.*, 1990; Colson & Mehring, 1990; Scruggs & Mastropieri, 1990; Swanson & Trahan, 1990). Being able to remember facts and figures is critical for success in regular classrooms. Without these skills, students have problems with remembering facts for tests, remembering rules for grammar, and remembering specific processes required to solve math problems. Teachers can facilitate the success of students with disabilities in integrated classrooms by helping them learn strategies to improve their memory deficits (Swanson & Trahan, 1990).

General Strategies

Vogel (1990) suggests the following strategies for helping students with learning disabilities remember facts. These suggestions should also work for other students with disabilities.

1. *Review regularly*   Since learning is synonymous with reviewing for many students, regular reviewing will help with remembering facts.

2. *Use various visual cues to highlight important facts*   Color code, underline, and use other highlighting methods to strengthen visual memory.

3. *Copy material*   Copy notes and important facts; the act of writing may improve memory.

4. *Read out loud*   Often, hearing the information will help students remember it better than simply seeing it.

5. *Tape record lectures*   Once lectures are tape recorded, students can study while doing other activities, such as driving.

6. *Rehearse material*   Read notes out loud, write important facts, read notes silently, and paraphrase information.

7. *Review frequently*   When reviewing materials, use various strategies that facilitate recall, such as listing and categorizing.

Mnemonics

In addition to these skills, students can use other methods to help them remember information. One commonly used approach is to use mnemonic devices. Mnemonic devices are associations that can be made between what needs to be remembered and some common fact. A mnemonic can be defined as "a specific reconstruction of target content intended to tie new information more closely to the learner's existing knowledge base and, therefore, facilitate retrieval." (Scruggs & Mastropieri, 1990, pp. 271–272). There are several different types of mnemonic strategies. These include the keyword method, pegword method, acronyms, reconstructive elaborations, phonic mnemonics, spelling mnemonics, number-sound mnemonics, and "Yodai" methods (Scruggs & Mastropieri, 1990). Gfeller (1986) even suggests using musical mnemonics for students with disabilities. Table 8–5 describes each of these methods.

Often individuals use first letter associations to remember things. This method is the acronyms model and is perhaps the most common form of mnemonics (Scruggs & Mastropieri, 1990). For example, *Every Good Boy Deserves Fudge* is a common phrase that helps music students remember the line notes on the treble clef (Colson & Mehring, 1990). Often, these letter associations can be nonsensical and still be effective. For example, *A Rat Of Exceptional Status Made As*. This particular mnemonic helped one of the authors remember the seven stages of learning used by Hewett (1969) of 1. attention, 2. response, 3. order, 4. exploratory, 5. social, 6. mastery, and 7. attention more than twenty years ago; the mnemonic still works.

Although there has been debate over the use of mnemonics, research supports its effectiveness. After reviewing the research literature on mnemonics, Scruggs and Mastropieri (1990) concluded that these approaches have resulted in positive memory gains and furthermore "impacts greatly on recall, comprehension, and effective outcomes" (p. 279).

Study Skills and Test Taking

Giving tests is one thing that teachers do at all grade levels in all subject areas. Until a better method of evaluating students is developed, giving tests will likely continue to be the primary method of assessing competence (Scruggs & Mastropieri, 1986). Many students are good test takers. They understand the general, common-sense rules regarding taking tests. However, for many students with disabilities, these common sense test taking skills are not present. As early as the 1950s it was recognized that some students needed help in learning how to take tests. Staton (1959) provided several tips for students when preparing for tests. These included things like review but do not cram, simulate questions and their answers during study, and attend to material that was emphasized in class. These are general suggestions, but they are quite effective for many students. Studies have shown that students with disabilities can be trained in test taking skills (Scruggs & Mastropieri, 1986). Therefore, special education teachers may need to spend time helping their students learn how to take tests. Gearheart *et al.* (1988) list the following suggested methods.

TABLE 8–5 Description of Mnemonic Strategies

STRATEGY	DESCRIPTION
Keyword Method	■ pairs new word with previously learned words
	■ employs acoustically similar key words as meaningful proxies
	■ key words presented in pictures
Pegword Method	■ used to recall a specific list of words
	■ pegwords are rhymed with numbers
	■ numbers related to key words
Acronyms	■ most familiar mnemonic strategy
	■ first letter in words strung together in a phrase cue key words
	■ phrase can be nonsensical
Phonic mnemonics	■ letters associated with pictures using appropriate phonetic sound
	■ used extensively to teach initial phonetic/letter associations
Spelling Mnemonics	■ cues to help spelling skills
	■ example: She screamed E-E-E when she was in the cemetery (3 Es in cemetery)
Number-Sound Mnemonics	■ used to recall strings of numbers
	■ learn number-sound relationships
	■ develop words to reflect numbers, such as dates
"Yodai" Methods	■ mathematical procedures using rhymes and visual imagery
	■ used mainly in Japan
Musical Mnemonics	■ uses music as memory aid

Source: Gfeller, 1986; Ellis & Lenz, 1990; Scruggs & Mastropieri, 1990.

1. Help students understand examination directions and terms, such as "define," "list," "compare," "contrast," and "defend."

2. Teach students to watch for cue words such as "never," "all," and "always."

3. Tell students what you expect. Is the emphasis on content, organization, spelling, grammar, mechanics, or creative expression?

4. Provide students with a copy of a previous test, talk about it, and use it as a teaching tool.

5. With objective tests, encourage students to read all questions carefully and answer first those questions whose answers they know immediately. They may then consider more carefully the remaining questions.

6. With essay examinations, encourage students to outline their answers before writing.

7. Encourage students to answer all questions unless there is a penalty for incorrect answers.

8. Encourage students to write clearly and distinctly.

9. Encourage students to leave sufficient time to reread their answers, paying attention to such things as punctuation and spelling (p. 84).

Study Skills and Listening

As was noted in Chapter 6, which focused on receptive language, listening is a complex skill that is vitally important to students. Without attending to auditory stimuli and processing it properly, students miss out on a significant portion of the information that is transmitted in a classroom. As students get older, the amount of auditory information presented in classrooms compared to visual information only increases (Herr, 1988). Therefore, without the ability to listen and comprehend auditory signals, students with disabilities will be at a major disadvantage in mainstream classes (Bauwens & Hourcade, 1989).

Students can be taught to listen using a variety of study skills. Chapter 6 pointed out one method for helping students learn to listen. This approach, developed by Forster and Doyle (1989), helped students listen through the use of auditory advanced organizers. By knowing what they are listening for, students are better able to focus their auditory attention.

Mandlebaum and Wilson (1989) describe a five step process to teach listening skills. In step one, teachers assess students to determine their optimal listening comprehension skills. This is accomplished through informal listening inventories, formal listening comprehension tests, or simple observations. After the listening comprehension level of the student is determined, the teacher develops 400 to 500 word stories, at appropriate grade levels, with comprehension questions. In step three, the teacher reads the stories to students and asks the comprehension questions. Steps four and five include evaluating the results of the comprehensive questioning and analyzing the results for instructional purposes.

In another listening strategy, students are taught to listen by the teacher using a series of verbal prompts. This method, called the LISTEN strategy, lists six LISTEN instructions on a 3×5 card, which is on each student's desk. The instructions are:

1. *Look;*

2. *Idle your motor;*

3. *Sit up straight;*

4. *T*urn to me;

5. *E*ngage your brain;

6. *N*ow.

These verbal prompts are later only used as visual prompts and help students to focus on the auditory stimuli.

Study Skills and Notetaking

Being able to listen in classrooms is important, but the ability to make notes for later study is also important. Taking good notes that facilitate later review of the material adds to the importance of listening. Whereas many students learn to take notes and to refine their notetaking skills by simply doing it, students with disabilities often do not develop this skill without assistance. The inability to take good, comprehensive notes that help with later studying can result in failure for students.

Notetaking is not a simple skill. It includes "skill in selecting, organizing, manipulating, and recording information from a variety of sources including lectures, textbooks, supplementary readings, and reference materials" (Beirne-Smith, 1989, p. 425). Students can be taught how to take notes. Beirne-Smith (1989) suggests a five step process for teaching students how to take notes. These steps are 1. evaluate current notetaking skills, 2. teach necessary preskills, 3. teach the system of notetaking, 4. facilitate notetaking practice, and 5. provide for generalizations. Table 8–6 (on page 300) describes this five step process.

Kaufman (1980) suggests teaching students to take notes by using an outline format. Using this system, students learn the traditional method of indenting and numbering used in outlining. This helps students organize auditory information by listing major headings, then using the outline model to place less important, but related content, under the major headings. Outlines can be organized around various formats, including time order, causes, problems, results, likenesses, differences, and characteristics (Young & Savage, 1989).

For example, an outline for taking notes in a classroom lecture on Chapter 5 of this textbook could include heads and subheads found in the chapter. By setting up the outline for notetaking, the notes will likely be more organized and complete. The page for notes for Chapter 5 might look like Figure 8–2 (on page 301).

Study Skills and Outlining

As noted above, outlining content is important for students when they are preparing for studying. Outlines are a method of organizing materials in a related manner. Students can use outlines to organize information in notes, as well as when outlining material for reviewing. For example, rather than making notes from a written text in a random fashion, the use of an outline format using chapter heads and subheads will assist students in visualizing the overall relationships among various components (Kaufman, 1980).

Study Skills and Writing Reports

Students are often required to write reports and papers for outside assignments. Written expression is very important in our society, especially for students who often have to complete written academic assignments. Hoover (1988b) lists several ways that teachers can help students learn how to write reports successfully. These include:

TABLE 8-6 Steps to Teach Notetaking Skills

STEP	DESCRIPTION
Evaluate Current Performance	■ evaluate using notetaking checklist
	■ examine student's notes
Teach Preskills	■ teach active listening/reading
	■ teach content-specific vocabulary
	■ teach consolidation and organizing skills
	■ teach abbreviations and codes
	■ teach legibility
Teach the Notetaking System	■ teach notetaking from textbooks
	■ teach notetaking from reference materials
	■ teach notetaking from lectures
	■ teach notetaking from multimedia
	■ teach making concise statements for study and review
Provide for Practice	■ practice single skills daily
	■ add skills after one has been learned
Provide for Generalization	■ use multiple trainers
	■ train in multiple settings
	■ train with all student's teachers

Source: Beirne-Smith, M. (1989). A systematic approach for teaching notetaking skills to students with mild learning handicaps. *Academic Therapy, 25,* 425–437.

1. Teachers can teach students to understand the purpose of the writing assignment. Different purposes require different writing styles and levels.

2. Teachers can help students learn to organize their ideas. Learning how to outline makes report writing more efficient.

3. Students need to learn to write simple, short reports before longer, more complex efforts.

4. Teachers need to teach students the importance of proofreading and different strategies for proofreading.

5. Students need to learn the how and when to use the dictionary and other reference materials.

FIGURE 8-2 Example of an Outline

I. **Introduction**

II. **Teaching Reading**

   A. **Nature of Reading**

   B. **Reading Process**

   C. **Status of Reading in Today's Schools**

   D. **Reading and Students with Mild Disabilities**

   E. **Methods to Teach Reading**

   F. **Remedial Reading Approaches**

   G. **Grouping for Reading Instruction**

III. **Teaching Listening Skills**

   A. **Nature of Listening**

   B. **Methods to Teach Listening Skills**

When writing reports, students must be aware that teachers often prejudge the content of papers by their appearance. While this is an unfortunate reality for students with sloppy handwriting and poor organizational skills, it can work to the students' advantage if they are taught how to make their written work look good. Archer (1988) suggests that teachers instruct students in making their written work look good through examples. This can be accomplished by showing students examples of papers that look good, and examples of papers that have a negative appearance. The teacher and students discuss each example and what makes the papers good or bad.

Study Skills and Oral Reports

Occasionally students are required to give oral reports to classes. If they have problems with oral expression they may have a difficult time performing well with oral reports. Some regular classroom teachers put a lot of emphasis on oral reports, such as book reports, science project reports, and activity reports. Therefore, special education teachers need to ensure that their students develop sound oral reporting skills.

Many of the skills necessary to write good reports are the same skills necessary to give reports orally (Hoover, 1988a). Therefore, teachers may want to teach study skills related to oral reports in conjunction with teaching students how to complete written reports.

Reliance on an outlining system, as previously noted, can facilitate the completion of both oral and written report writing. For students to do their best in oral reporting, they need to practice. Therefore, teachers should arrange for practice opportunities, with "dress rehearsals" being the last step before the report is given in the content classroom. During oral reporting by some students, other students have the opportunity to observe appropriate oral reporting skills, and can therefore model good oral reporting.

Time Management

Remember your first semester as a college freshman? It may have been the first time you were on your own and solely responsible for your time management. Most college students do well with time management; they may not have good time management skills in the beginning, but they develop them quickly in order to achieve success. Time management is also important for students in grades K through twelve, especially in the upper elementary and secondary levels. Students who are good readers, good listeners, and generally good students may not have the same time pressures as students who experience problems. Therefore, time management for students with disabilities is an even more critical skill than for their nondisabled peers.

Unfortunately, many students with disabilities do not manage their time effectively. Therefore, they must be taught various time management skills. Teachers can help students develop these skills by 1. teaching them to develop and use time schedules, 2. teaching students to identify their best times and environmental conditions for studying, and 3. showing students how to divide large segments of study time into manageable, shorter periods with breaks and self-reinforcing systems (Gartland, 1989).

One technique might be to have students keep a daily log of how they spend the majority of their school and postschool day. After the log is completed, the teacher and students can discuss how time is spent and better ways to use the time. Often students can better manage their time if they can realize how they spend their time during the day. Another simple time management technique is for the teacher to set a timer to go off every five or ten minutes. Each time the timer goes off students record what they are doing. At the end of the class period, the teacher and students discuss the findings.

Dictionary and Reference Materials Usage

Students need to be able to use dictionaries and other reference materials for completion of oral and written reports, studying particular topics, and looking up words for meanings and correct spelling. For students with disabilities, these skills are very critical because of their typical problems in content courses and frequent deficits in spelling and vocabulary (Polloway & Smith, 1992). To help students learn how to use these materials, teachers need to ensure that they have several basic skills, including understanding alphabetical order, using cross referencing, and determining key words in context (Roe *et al.*, 1987). Table 8–7 lists several additional skills that are prerequisite to effective use of dictionaries and other reference materials.

Library Skills

In order for students to be successful in upper elementary and secondary grades, they need to be able to use the library. Most students learn how to use the library with minimal instruction from librarians and teachers, as well as modeling the library skills of other

TABLE 8–7   Skills Necessary to Use Reference Books

1.   Ability to alphabetize words

2.   Knowledge about the organizational structure of dictionaries, encyclopedias, atlases

3.   Ability to use guide words to locate specific words

4.   Ability to use cross-referencing to locate information

5.   Understanding of how to use pronunciation guides

6.   Ability to discriminate among several different definitions for the same word

7.   Understanding and ability to use map symbols and keys

8.   Ability to use map scale for realistic distances and sizes

9.   Ability to determine directions from maps

10.   Ability to use appropriate volume to find specific information

11.   Ability to determine key words for reference purposes

Source: Roe, B. D., Stoodt, B. D., & Burns, P. C. (1987). *Secondary school reading instruction: The content areas.* Boston: Houghton-Mifflin.

students. Students with disabilities may need extra help in learning how to use the library. For this group of students, the ability to use the library effectively may be more important than for nondisabled students. This is because the library is an easy place for these students to be integrated with nondisabled peers, and these students may need all the resources they can get to help them succeed in regular classes (Wesson & Keefe, 1989).

There is a hierarchy of library skills necessary for optimal usage of library resources. Teachers and librarians need to determine where along this sequence students are functioning and develop training opportunities for students to facilitate their mastering of the hierarchy. The following is an example of a library skill hierarchy, ranging from lowest skill level to highest.

1.   The student demonstrates appropriate behavior in the library media center (LMC).

2.   The student can locate age- or ability-appropriate books, material, and equipment.

3.   The student handles books properly.

4.   The student can follow procedures for checking out a book.

5.   The student returns books undamaged by the due date.

6.   The student can properly use LMC equipment, (cassette player, computer, filmstrip viewer).

7.   The student can state the definitions of and differentiate between fiction and nonfiction books.

8. The student knows how the fiction section is organized and can locate a specific book given the author and title.

9. The student knows how the nonfiction materials are organized and can locate a specific book given the Dewey Decimal number.

10. The student can differentiate reference materials from fiction and nonfiction materials.

11. The student can locate reference materials.

12. The student can label, define, and locate parts of a book including the title page, table of contents, index, glossary, bibliography, and appendixes.

13. The student knows how the card catalog is organized and can locate specific card catalog information on request.

14. The student can accurately record card catalog information and use the information to locate a specific book.

15. The student can use parts of a book (table of contents, glossary, index) to locate specific information.

16. The student can use dictionaries, encyclopedias, atlases, and almanacs to find specific information.

17. The student can identify which reference materials are appropriate for locating various types of information.

18. The student can use reference materials to obtain topical information useful in writing a report. (Wesson & Keefe, 1989, p. 29)

Accommodations

Helping students with disabilities learn skills to aid them in regular classrooms may not be enough to ensure their success. In addition to their having skills, they often need the assistance of regular classroom personnel to experience success. Accommodations are various strategies that teachers can employ to give students with disabilities an equal opportunity to succeed. They include a variety of methods of adapting and adjusting school organization, curricula, or instructional methods to the learner that is part of a circumventive effort for students. As such, they do not form a particular approach, but a collection of strategies to help students with disabilities cope in content-oriented classes. Providing accommodations is the most likely method that regular classroom teachers get involved with intervention programs for these students (Gearheart *et al.*, 1988). Accommodations are not "give-aways" where teachers simply enable disabled students to pass their courses. Rather, accommodations are modifications that teachers can make that give these students an equal chance to succeed.

There are many different accommodations that teachers can employ to help students with disabilities. The exact nature of the accommodations is related to the extent of a student's disability. Providing accommodations should be based on the individual needs of the child. In other words, teachers should not simply apply the same accommodations to all students with disabilities and expect them to be equally successful. As a result, specific accommodations necessary for a student with a disability may be noted in the student's individual education program. This will make it more likely that the accommodations will actually be implemented.

TYPES OF ACCOMMODATIONS

Accommodations can be applied at the administrative level as well as in regular classrooms. At the administrative level, accommodations include various administrative controls that can affect students with disabilities. An example is the curricular variations that are available for students. In regular classrooms, there are many accommodations that can be made that will improve the chances for students with disabilities to experience success. For instance, an accommodation that can be implemented in a regular classroom is adapting the way students are required to respond on tests. Figure 8–3 depicts the various accommodations possible in regular classrooms.

The variety of modifications that regular classroom teachers can make in their classrooms to facilitate the success of mainstreamed disabled students is endless. The only factor that limits these accommodations is the creativity of the teacher. The following describes several accommodations that have been used successfully by regular classroom teachers with students with mild disabilities. As noted in Figure 8–3, there are seven major components of accommodations that can be implemented in regular classrooms. These are 1. teacher controlled variables, 2. milieu, 3. curricular variations, 4. materials, 5. classroom management, 6. time and space, and 7. parental interactions.

FIGURE 8-3 Components of Accommodation

Regular Class Techniques	Administrative Options
Teacher Variables	Personnal Development
Milieu	Curricular Variations
Curricular Variations	Enrollment
Materials	Student Progress
Classroom Management	
Time and Space	

Teacher Controlled Variables

Regular classroom teachers control many variables that can make academic success likely or unlikely for students with disabilities. The primary role of regular classroom teachers is to teach subject matter or basic skills. Each secondary teacher is trained in a discipline, while elementary teachers are trained in teaching basic skills. The state's curriculum guide, course syllabus, and commercial materials are uniformly tied to the framework of each course topic presented in the classroom. The following general observations may be made about regular classes.

1. Although the nature of learning activities may vary from class to class, the knowledge content of similar courses is based on invariant key concepts and principles.

2. Each discipline contains several broad concepts linked together to form the structure of the discipline.

3. This structure contains subordinate concepts and facts that comprise the substance of lectures and reading or other assignments.

By extracting key concepts and principles from courses, regular classroom teachers can identify precise targets for course work, the general structure and format of content, and the relationship of units, lectures, and assignments. The different accommodations included under the rubric, teacher-controlled variables, deal with ways to accommodate for various manifestations of disabilities.

Topical or Course Outlines   Topical outlines, also called course outlines, are nothing more than an enhanced course outline that presents the flow of the class. Key concepts and principles, as well as expected accomplishments of students as determined by the local curriculum guide are included. Topical outlines benefit all students by visually depicting the general outline of the course. The major advantage of the topical outline is that it assists upper elementary and secondary students in their attempts to organize thoughts, notes, and information into a meaningful record to be used in directing them to the acquisition of course outcomes. A simple outline on the blackboard is a simplified version of a topical outline. The outlines at the beginning of each chapter in this textbook help the reader focus on the nature of the content included.

Study Guides   Study guides are a more formalized and demanding procedure than a topical outline. They are designed with specific objectives, assignments, and evaluative criteria. They can be used by teachers to help students determine key information while studying content subject areas, such as history and science. Study guides generally are a set of written questions that help students look for certain information (Horton, Lovitt, Givens, & Nelson, 1989). They can also include many different components, including outline of the material, study questions, definitions of key terms, and outlines designed to be completed while reviewing materials (Salend, 1990).

Study guides might include the following sections.

1. Specific objectives to be accomplished

2. Period of time during which the learning activities will be completed

3. Specific products of study such as book reports and experiments

4. Specific reading assignments and other learning activities

5. Evaluative criteria

Several studies have found study guides to be effective in improving comprehension skills of students with disabilities (Swafford & Alvermann, 1989; Ellis & Lenz, 1990).

In addition to teacher-developed, traditional study guides, these aids can also be developed for use on microcomputers. Computerized study guides are used in conjunction with computer-assisted instruction (CAI) (Ellis & Lenz, 1990). In one study, it was determined that computerized study guides helped remedial students and students with learning disabilities achieve academic success in social studies classes (Horton *et al.*, 1989). The group using CAI and computerized study guides performed significantly higher on tests than similar students who did not have access to the CAI study guides. A description of CAI will be presented in Chapter 12.

Technical Vocabularies and Glossaries   Being able to understand the words in reading assignments can be a major hurdle for students with disabilities. Since reading is a deficit area for many of these students (Polloway & Smith, 1992; Smith *et al.*, in press), their ability to understand the technical vocabulary used in content reading materials is essential. Lists of terms and concepts that may be unfamiliar to students can be included in a technical vocabulary list or glossary. The skills necessary for using a vocabulary list or glossary are the same as those for dictionary use (Kaufman, 1980). For students whose reading is a major problem, these terms and concepts can be put on a tape recorder for student use.

Advance Organizers   Advance organizers are prereading questions that are designed to help the reader focus on the material that is about to be read. They "provide a structured framework that assists students in learning new content." (Putnam & Wesson, 1990, p. 57) By reading these questions and keeping them in mind during the content reading, students are able to "look" for specific facts in the material. The questions simply "cue" the reader for information. Advance organizers at the beginning of each chapter in a textbook help the reader focus on the important material in the chapter.

The use of advance organizers in a unit of study is incredibly simple and can be related to traditional reading assignments, compressed reading matter, or even tape-recorded passages. An example of advance organizers related to an upper elementary science class might include the following.

1. What is electricity?

2. How is electricity important to us?

3. How is electricity made?

4. How is electricity carried from its original source to our homes?

Advanced organizers have been studied extensively with mixed results regarding their effectiveness in improving reading comprehension (Swafford & Alvermann, 1989). However, they are an excellent accommodative strategy that do provide some students with an advantage when reading for content.

Graphic Organizers   Graphic organizers are written and spatial representations of key vocabulary or content found in content reading materials. They provide a supplement to textbooks with graphics, such as charts and diagrams (Ellis & Lenz, 1990). Several studies have determined their effectiveness with students who experience reading problems (Swafford & Alvermann, 1989; Ellis & Lenz, 1990). Since students with disabilities have such difficulty reading and understanding content in textbooks, graphic organizers are designed as a way of helping them understand what they read. Graphic organizers are similar to semantic maps, but are developed by teachers.

Horton and Lovitt (1989) describe a four step process for developing graphic organizers. In step one, the teacher organizes the reading materials into sections of about 1,500 words. This number of words allows most students to read the materials, complete a graphic organizer, and complete an examination. Step two is when the teacher develops an outline of the main ideas in the reading. These main ideas become major sections in the graphic organizer. In step three, the teacher selects a format for the graphic organizer that fits the content. Different reading materials suggest different organizations. Finally, in step four, the teacher prepares a teacher-version and student-version of the graphic organizer. Developing the teacher-version first enables the developer to determine what needs to be included in the student-version for best results.

Audio-Visual Aids   Audio-visual aids provide teachers with an excellent teaching method. Almost without exception, schools have a wide variety of audio-visual equipment that can be used in the teaching-learning process. This ranges from a simple piece of chalk and a chalkboard, to a complex computer terminal with color graphics and technical software. Other commonly used audio-visual aids include slide projectors, overhead projectors, movie projectors, video-cassette recorders, and televisions (Smith, 1990).

Smith and Ingersoll (1984) conducted a survey of schools to determine the extent the schools used audio-visual materials. Their findings revealed that more than thirty percent of all teachers in the survey used audio-visual kits on a weekly basis. One of the newest entries into the audio-visual educational market is video-cassette technology. Since the first VCRs were initially marketed in the early 1970s, their growth in our society and schools has been phenomenal (Smith, 1990). Reasons for the widespread adoption of VCRs in schools include their being a conventional form of media available at a reasonable cost. Also, VCRs are easily controlled by teachers rather than big corporations determining what type of materials will be available for use (Reider, 1984). Computer technology is also a form of audio-visual equipment that enhances educational opportunities for students with mild disabilities. Chapter 12 focuses entirely on technology, with a heavy emphasis on microcomputers.

Curricular Variations

While regular classroom teachers must ensure that the content of their classes coincides with the curricular expectations of the district, they still have some latitude in how they implement the curriculum. Some of the variations that can be controlled by teachers include 1. alternative modes of expression, 2. methods of testing students, 3. course descriptions, and 4. instructional modes used. By varying these components of the curriculum, regular classroom teachers are able to accommodate for certain needs of students.

Alternative Modes of Expression   Some students have acceptable skills in oral expression but have serious problems with written expression. For these students, teachers need to make provisions that enable oral responses to questions, homework assignments, and reports. In contrast to these students, some students have written language strengths but deficits in oral language. Again, in this situation, teachers need to deemphasize oral expression and allow students to respond in writing.

Methods of Testing Students   Related to alternative modes of expression is the way teachers administer tests to students. Obviously, if students cannot respond orally or in writing, the teacher will need to alter various testing procedures to avoid requiring students to use their weak response mode. Therefore, teachers may need to have various forms of the same test in order to allow students with disabilities to complete the test in a fair manner.

Another way regular classroom teachers can modify testing is through the use of special education teachers. Special education teachers can administer the test orally and provide other accommodations during the testing, such as giving extra time, to ensure that students with disabilities have a fair chance for success. An obvious concern of many regular classroom teachers is that the special education teacher will not maintain the integrity of the examination process. Therefore, if special education teachers become involved in alternative testing they must assure teachers that the test will be administered fairly and that the test itself will be maintained without compromise.

Two important aspects of teacher-developed tests include "format" and "content." The following should be considered when developing the format of a classroom test.

1. Spacing of items on the pages

2. Space allowed for responses

3. Margins

4. Readability of the test

5. Test length

6. Test organization

7. Test instructional

8. Item type

For content, teachers need to consider the clarity of the vocabulary used and the level of responses required from students.

Vogel (1990) summarized several different ways teachers can accommodate students with disabilities during testing. These include:

- allow students more time;

- allow readers or taped exams;

- provide alternative forms of the exam (for example, objective and essay);

- permit students to take the exam in a separate room free from distractions;

- let students use various response modes, such as word processors or oral;

- allow students to rephrase questions to ensure they understand the intent of the question;

- permit students to use alternative ways to exhibit mastery, such as a paper or term project rather than a formal exam;

- allow the use of computational aids, such as calculators;

- do not use double negatives or other wording sequences that could confuse students with reading comprehension problems;

- provide adequate scratch paper, lined paper, or other aids for students with poor written expression skills;

- let students answer directly on exam rather than on computer answer sheets;

- do not count spelling or grammar errors when testing for content.

Course Descriptions   A very simple accommodation that can be used by secondary teachers and teachers in upper elementary grades in subjects areas, such as social studies, is the preparation of a course description. The general goals of the course and particular topics to be covered in the course are included. Similar to course outlines and study guides, course descriptions help students understand the course content and course requirements at the beginning of the class period.

Materials Development and Modification

An extremely important consideration for students with disabilities integrated into regular classrooms is the nature of the materials used in instruction (Hoover, 1990). For example, if the materials have a reading level too difficult for a student, or if the materials are too long for students whose reading rate is extremely slow, then the student may become frustrated and not learn the material. There are ways teachers can modify materials to help students with disabilities learn the material in the course. These include:

- taped lessons;

- compressed texts;

- games;

- learning packets;

- talking books.

Taped Lessons   For students with significant visual losses, teachers secure reading materials that are presented on audio tape, or they allow students to use tape recorders in lectures or discussions to acquire information. Students with significant reading problems can also benefit from taped lessons. Although the research into the effectiveness of audio taped textbooks is limited, results indicate that some students with disabilities can benefit from the format. The success when using taped lessons can be enhanced significantly when certain cues are presented on the taped materials (Ellis & Lenz, 1990).

Compressed Texts   Reducing the amount of reading content is a method of adapting the content (Hoover, 1988b). Often students with mild disabilities are capable of reading and comprehending the materials; however, due to their slow reading rates, they get significantly behind in their reading assignments. This can have a very detrimental effect on their success in classes. By compressing the amount of reading material, students are able to keep up with their assignments.

Most textbooks include a lot of information that is not critically important to students acquiring the important concepts. Textbooks can be compressed by eliminating much of the information that is not critical to students. One way to accomplish this is to read a passage and paraphrase the information. This usually results in significantly less reading materials, but with critical facts left intact.

Games Games can be used effectively with all students in the teaching and learning process. For students with limited reading abilities, games provide an opportunity for learning basic concepts without a heavy emphasis on reading. Special education teachers and regular classroom teachers can collaborate on the development of games for teaching content that would be enjoyable and motivating for all students.

The types of games used in teaching students with mild disabilities are endless. Games can be used to teach math facts, spelling facts, and facts about content subjects. For example, the spelling bee format can be used to ask factual questions in math or content subjects. Also, variations of Bingo can be used to help students learn spelling skills, as well as number recognition and basic computation skills. Examples of games to teach skills can be found in many professional journals. *Teaching Exceptional Children* is an excellent resource for games and other "fun" techniques to teach skills. Additional journals that frequently describe games in teaching include *Intervention, Academic Therapy, The Reading Teacher*, and *Journal of Reading*. Many books also focus on the use of games to teach students various skills and content information.

Learning Packets To facilitate individualized, self-paced learning, teachers may want to develop learning packets. These can take the form of different materials combined to teach a particular unit or topic. For example, teachers wanting students to learn about Colonial America could develop a learning packet with specific information about this period of time, various activities that would require the student to become actively involved in learning, and games to provide motivation. Worksheets, advance organizers, outlines for completion, and other aids can be included to facilitate learning.

Talking Books Students with visual impairments have long used talking books to supplement their Braille or large print materials. Talking books, actually books that have been taped, can be "read" by listening. For students with significant reading deficits, this could be an important means for acquiring knowledge.

Some teachers may not like the availability of talking, or taped books for students with disabilities. They may feel that it is unfair that students with disabilities listen to a chapter while other students have to read the material. Taped readings should be placed in a central location, such as the library, and made available for all students. Many students without disabilities may try the taped materials once, however, if they are capable of reading for content it is unlikely that they will choose listening over reading for themselves. Listening to a recording of a textbook can be very boring; students will likely not choose this means of obtaining information unless they truly are unable to read the materials.

Milieu

Milieu is a variable in learning that interacts with other facets of teaching, making it difficult to measure its importance and effect in isolation. Milieu means all of the factors that are interacting in a classroom. Milieu should be viewed as interwoven with teacher attitude, techniques, curriculum, teacher training, and teacher personality. Factors included in milieu include 1. the teacher's definition of a "good" student, 2. student-teacher interactions, and 3. student interactions.

Definition of a Good Student   How teachers define a "good" student has implications for the successful integration of students with disabilities in regular classrooms. The values and expectations of the teacher set the tone for the classroom. Some teachers may like students who sit quietly, rarely ask questions, and complete their assignments with limited discussion and interactions. On the other hand, some teachers like students who are energetic, questioning, and constantly actively involved in learning. Students need to be able to fit the teacher's expectations as closely as possible.

Student-Teacher Interaction   The milieu will in some ways dictate student-teacher interactions. Some teachers want learners to be self-motivated and self-reinforcing. They want limited interactions. Others want a great deal of interaction with students. Again, students need to be able to fit into the teacher's expectations for interaction.

Student Interaction   The way students interact with each other is a key element in milieu. Some teachers encourage interaction among students while others discourage it. For students who need to work collaboratively with their peers to maximize their learning opportunities, the type of student interaction encouraged and reinforced by teachers is important.

Time and Space Modifications

Adopting instructional settings may be required as a result of certain problems exhibited by some students. For example, some students may need specialized seating arrangements, may work better in groups than individually, and may prefer a structured time schedule.

Learning Centers   Learning centers can greatly accommodate some students in regular classrooms. They can facilitate learning by providing interesting, motivating activities for students in a less structured environment than one that only has traditional rows of desks. Learning centers can facilitate accommodation of students with mild disabilities in the following ways.

1. Allowance for individual rates and levels of performance is more easily maintained.

2. Student differences in performance are much less noticeable to peers.

3. A wider variety of activities are employed without drawing attention to individual students.

4. Opportunity for the occurrence of peer learning is increased.

5. Interactional learning models are used more effectively.

6. Responsibility of the teacher to be a "ringmaster" is eliminated.

7. The environment imposes a natural control on behavioral problems because students are actively engaged in learning activities.

Modular or Flexible Scheduling   Some students do not perform well in highly structured settings; they need periodic change. Modular and flexible scheduling allows for modifying the learning environment for differences often found in students with disabilities. Varying schedules can help meet the unique needs of students and offer variety for students.

Alternative Seating Arrangements The physical location of a student in a classroom often is related to the student's success. For example, a highly distractible student may need to be seated close to the teacher and away from obvious distractions, such as the door, windows, near a "busy" bulletin board, or other students. A consideration with seating arrangements is whether to change seating from time to time or leave students in the same seats for the entire school year. Some students actually become bored with their seating and need a change. Possible seating alternatives include small mats on the floor, going outside in pretty weather, or taking students to the library for the class period (Wood, 1984).

SUMMARY

This chapter has focused on ways to support students with disabilities in regular classrooms. As a result of Public Law 94-142, which requires schools to provide services to students with disabilities in the least restrictive environment, and subsequent service models, such as the regular education initiative, more students with disabilities are receiving a larger portion of their educational programs in regular classrooms. Without some support services, these students will likely fail in these "normalized" settings.

Two ways are presented that can facilitate the success of students with disabilities in regular classes. These include study skills and accommodations. Study skills are strategies that students can be taught to use that will improve their chances for doing well in regular classes. There are many different strategies; a few examples include ways to comprehend reading materials, techniques to increase reading rate, strategies to help with memory deficits, and ways to organize materials, take notes, and use references. These methods, along with others, were discussed in the chapter. It was pointed out that before students are taught specific study skills, they need to be evaluated to determine the specific skills they need in order to be successful in mainstream classes.

The second major method to help students with disabilities succeed in regular classrooms that was discussed was accommodations. Accommodations are modifications that teachers can implement that will facilitate success for students. Many different accommodative strategies were presented. Some examples include administrative accommodations, such as scheduling and teacher training, and a variety of different modifications that can be made in regular classes by regular classroom teachers.

Some of the accommodations suggested for teachers include compressing texts, enabling students to use tape recorders, using audio-visual materials, using advance organizers and study guides, and making accommodations for the way students complete examinations. These accommodative strategies, along with others, were presented. In addition, ways to develop and implement the accommodations were presented.

REFERENCES

Archer, A.L. (1988). Strategies for responding to information. *Teaching Exceptional Children, 20,* 55–57.

Beirne-Smith, M. (1989). A systematic approach for teaching notetaking skills to students with mild learning handicaps. *Academic Therapy, 24,* 425–437.

Bauwens, J., & Hourcade, J.J. (1989). Hey, would you just listen. *Teaching Exceptional Children, 21*, 61.

Cohen, S.B., & Hart-Hester, S. (1987). Time management strategies. *Teaching Exceptional Children, 20*, 56–57.

Colson, S.E., & Mehring, T.A. (1990). Facilitating memory in students with learning disabilities. *LD Forum, 16*, 75–79.

Dixon, R. (1987). Strategies for vocabulary instruction. *Teaching Exceptional Children, 19*, 61–63.

Dunlap, L.K., Dunlap, G., Koegel, L.K., & Koegel, R.L. (1991). Using self-monitoring to increase independence. *Teaching Exceptional Children, 23*, 17–22.

Ellis, E.S., Deshler, D.D., Lenz, B.K., Schumaker, J.B. & Clark, F.L. (1991). An instructional model for teaching learning strategies. *Focus on Exceptional Children, 23*, 1–24.

Ellis, E.S., & Lenz, B.K. (1990). Techniques for mediating content-area learning: Issues and research. *Focus on Exceptional Children, 22*, 1–16.

Forster, P., & Doyle, B.A. (1989). Teaching listening skills to students with attention deficit disorders. *Teaching Exceptinal Children, 21*, 20–22.

Gartland, D. (1989). Study-skills instruction for students with learning disabilities. *LD Forum, 15*, 11–13.

Gearheart, B.R., Weishahn, M.W., & Gearheart, C.J. (1988). *The exceptional student in the regular classroom*, 4th Ed. Columbus, OH: Merrill.

Gfeller, K.E. (1986). Musical mnemonics for learning disabled children. *Teaching Exceptional Children, 19*, 28–30.

Gleason, M.M. (1988). Teaching study strategies. *Teaching Exceptional Children, 20*, 52–53.

Herr, C.M. (1988). Strategies for gaining information. *Teaching Exceptional Children, 20*, 53–55.

Hewett, F.M. (1969). *The engineered classroom*. Boston: Allyn & Bacon.

Hoover, J.J. (1990). Curriculum adaption: A five-step process for classroom implementation. *Academic Therapy, 25*, 407–416.

Hoover, J.J. (1988a). *Teaching handicapped students study skills*, 2nd Ed. Lindale, TX: Hamilton Publications.

Hoover, J.J. (1988b). Implementing a study skills program in the classroom. *Academic Therapy, 24*, 471–476.

Horton, S.V., & Lovitt, T.C. (1989). Construction and implementation of graphic organizers for academically handicapped and regular secondary students. *Academic Therapy, 24*, 625–640.

Horton, S.V., Lovitt, T.C., Givens, A., & Nelson, R. (1989). Teaching social studies to high school students with academic handicaps in a mainstreamed setting: Effects of a computerized study guide. *Journal of Learning Disabilites, 22*, 102–107.

Kauffman, J.M. (1989). *Characteristics of behavior disorders of children and youth*, 4th Ed. Columbus, OH: Merrill.

Kaufman, M. (1980). *Reading in content areas*. West Lafayette, Indiana: Kappa Delta Pi.

Lenz, B.K., & Deshler, D.D. (1990). Principles of strategies instruction as the basis of effective preservice teacher education. *Teacher Education and Special Education, 13*, 82–95.

Locke, E.T., & Abbey, D.E. (1989). A unique equation: Learning strategies + generalization = success. *Academic Therapy, 24*, 569–575.

McWhorter, K.T. (1987). *Efficient and flexible reading*, 2nd Ed. Boston: Little, Brown.

Mandlebaum, L.H., & Wilson, R. (1989). Teaching listening skills in the special education classroom. *Academic Therapy, 24*, 449–459.

Patton, J.R., Beirne-Smith, M., & Payne, J.S. (1986). *Mental retardation*, 2nd Ed., Columbus, OH: Merrill.

Podemski, R.S., Price, B.J., Smith, T.E.C., & Marsh, G.E., (1984). *Comprehensive adminstration of special education*. Rockville, Maryland: Aspen Systems.

Polloway, E.A., & Patton, J.R. (1989). Study Skills: Introduction to the special issue. *Academic Therapy, 24*, 379–381.

Polloway, E.A., & Smith, T.E.C. (1992). *Teaching language skills to students with mild disabilities,* 2nd Ed. Denver: Love Publishing.

Pressley, M., Scruggs, T.E., & Mastropieri, M.A. (1989). Memory strategy research in learning disabilities: Present and future directions. *Learning Disability Research, 4,* 68–77.

Putnam, M.L., & Wesson, C.L. (1990). The teacher's role in teaching content-area information. *LD Forum, 16,* 55–60.

Reider, W.L. (1984). Videocassette technology in education: A quiet revolution in progress. *Educational Technology, 24,* 12–15.

Rich, S., & Pressley, M. (1990). Is teaching reading comprehension strategies acceptable to teachers? *Teacher Education and Special Education, 13,* 126–132.

Roe, B.D., Stoodt, B.D., & Burns, P.C. (1987). *The content areas,* 3rd Ed. Boston: Houghton-Mifflin.

Salend, S.J. (1990). *Effective mainstreaming.* New York: MacMillan.

Scruggs, T.E., & Mastropieri, M.A. (1986). Improving the test taking skills of behaviorally disordered and learning disabled children. *Exceptional Children, 53,* 63–68.

Scruggs, T.E., & Mastropieri, M.A. (1990). Mnemonic instruction for students with learning disabilities: What it is and what it does. *Learning Disability Quarterly, 13,* 271–280.

Sinatra, R.C., Berg, D., & Dunn, R. (1985). Semantic mapping improves reading comprehension of learning disabled students. *Teaching Exceptional Children, 17,* 310–314.

Smith, G., & Smith, D. (1989). Schoolwide study skills program. The key to mainstreaming. *Teaching Exceptional Children, 21,* 20–23.

Smith, T.E.C. (1990). *Introduction to education,* 2nd Ed. St. Paul: West.

Smith, T.E.C., & Dowdy, C.A. (1989). The role of study skills in the secondary curriculum. *Academic Therapy, 24,* 479–490.

Smith, T.E.C., Price, B.J., & Marsh, G.E. (1986). *Mildly handicapped children and adults.* St. Paul: West Publishing.

Smith, T.E.C., Graves, S.A., & Aldridge, J.T. *Teaching reading,* in press. St. Paul: West Publishing.

Staton, T.F. (1959). *How to study.* Circle Pines, MN: American Guidance Service, Inc.

Swafford, J., & Alvermann, D.E. (1989). Postsecondary research base for content reading strategies. *Journal of Reading, 33,* 164–169.

Swanson, H.L., & Trahan, M. (1990). Naturalistic memory in learning disabled children. *Learning Disability Quarterly, 13,* 82–93.

Vogel, S.A. (1990). *College students with learning disabilities: A handbook,* 3rd Ed. Copyright: Vogel.

Wesson, C.L., & Keefe, M. (1989). Teaching library skills to students with mild and moderate handicaps. *Teaching Exceptional Children, 21,* 29–31.

Wood, J.W. (1984). *Adapting instruction for the mainstream.* Columbus, OH: Merrill.

Classroom Management

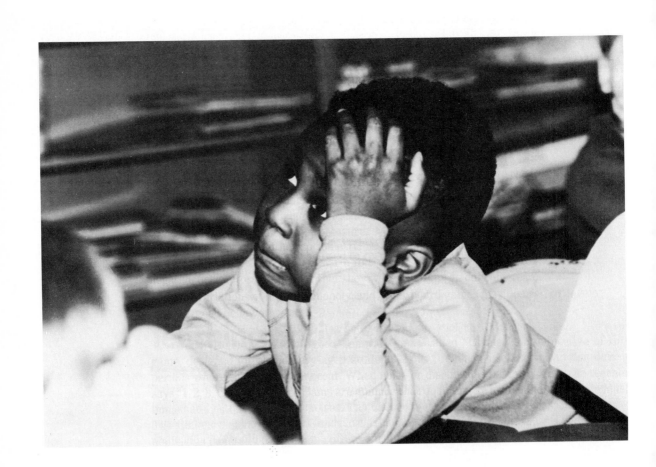

Outline

OBJECTIVES

After reading this chapter, you will be able to:

- discuss the importance of classroom management with students with disabilities;

- discuss the nature of classroom management;

- list the assumptions underlying classroom management;

- describe regular and special education classrooms;

- define engaged instructional time;

- discuss how room arrangement and scheduling relate to students' behaviors;

- state how to make classroom rules;

- discuss how teachers' behaviors affect students' behaviors;

- define behavior management;

- describe the key components of behavior management;

- define extinction;

- discuss behavior modification and how to implement it in a special education classroom;

- describe how to use time out, token economies, daily reports, card games, and contingency contracting;

- explain how to use time out procedures.

Introduction

A primary objective for special education teachers is to effectively implement the individual educational programs of students with disabilities. For most students with disabilities, teachers focus their instructional time on remediating academic and social skills to facilitate their success in schools and post-school environments. For example, teachers spend time on direct instruction, remediation, role playing, modeling, and other strategies that help students develop skills to succeed academically and socially. In order to effectively implement these instructional programs, teachers must ensure that order is maintained in their classrooms. Teachers can be more effective in their use of instructional time when students are acting appropriately and are attending to the learning tasks. Inappropriate, off-task behaviors only interrupt the learning process.

Another important reason for teachers to focus on students' behaviors is the welfare of other students. Appropriate behaviors facilitate the learning of students exhibiting the appropriate behaviors, as well as other students in the classroom. Likewise, inappropriate behaviors can interfere with the learning of all students. Therefore, teachers must maintain control of students' behaviors to facilitate the learning of all students in the classroom.

Classroom order and discipline are considered a primary role for teachers. The topic of discipline is consistently one of the most discussed topics related to public education in this country (Smith, 1990). Discipline is consistently rated as a leading problem in our schools by respondents to the annual Gallup poll on attitudes toward public schools (1988, 1989, 1990). For example, in the most recent poll, fifty-three percent of the respondents listed discipline as a key problem for schools (Gallup, 1990). As a result of the public's perception, teachers must address discipline in their classrooms.

For many teachers, managing the behaviors of their students represents a never-ending problem. They find that they can deal effectively with some students, while others seemingly "take them to task" on a daily basis. Often, teachers become very frustrated and may even quit teaching because of their inability to control behaviors in their classrooms. In a recent report published by the United States Department of Education, The National Center for Education Statistics (1988) stated that nearly forty percent of public school teachers believed that disciplinary problems resulted in difficulties in teaching.

For special education teachers of students with mild disabilities, managing classroom behaviors is even more important than for regular classroom teachers. Special education teachers usually have students in resource rooms for only a portion of the school day; when providing instruction in regular classrooms as part of a consultation/collaboration model, there may be even more limited individualized instructional time for these students. Therefore, teachers must take advantage of the time they have with these students. Maintaining appropriate behaviors in the classroom results in more on-task learning time.

Another reason classroom management is so critical for special education teachers is because special education teachers are attempting to facilitate the successful integration of their students into regular classrooms. Special education teachers need to help students with disabilities control their behaviors in both special education settings and regular classroom environments. Students with disabilities whose behaviors are in control and who are compliant with the rules of the regular classroom have a much greater chance of success than students whose behaviors cause problems. Many students with disabilities may experience failure in mainstreamed settings because of behavior problems, not because of poor academic skills.

Students with mild disabilities, therefore, need to be able to exhibit appropriate behaviors and follow classroom rules to facilitate their success in regular classrooms. This need for behavior control does not end when these students exit the school; after high school, persons with disabilities also need to exhibit positive behaviors. Inappropriate behaviors on job sites, in social situations, and in community settings can greatly impede the success of these individuals in becoming independent, contributing members of society. As with success in regular classrooms, exhibiting appropriate behaviors in the post-school environments is critical for success.

There are many different techniques that teachers can use to manage the behaviors of students in their classrooms. These range from highly behavioral methods, such as behavior modification, to group classroom management systems, such as assertive discipline. Examples of management strategies that have been used effectively with students with disabilities include:

- diagnostic procedures that pinpoint student entry-level behavior relative to appropriate instructional objectives,

- clearly stated and prominently displayed classroom rules and related consequences,

- an organized and predictable classroom,

- appropriate behavior acknowledged and intermittently reinforced,

- novelty and variety in instructional activities and models of appropriate behavior. (Feldman, Rosenberg, & Peer, 1984, p. 36)

Teachers use a wide variety of methods to deal with the behaviors of their students. Wolfgang and Glickman (1986) combine these methods into seven primary approaches.

1. *Silently Looking On*   Using this approach, teachers simply look at students who are behaving inappropriately. Often students will behave appropriately if they know that the teacher is paying attention to them.

2. *Nondirected Statements*   Nondirected statements, such as "I saw you throw that piece of paper," will alter the student's behavior. It reflects the behavior back on the student.

3. *Questions*   Often teachers use questions, such as "What do you think you are doing?" to get the student's attention. This frequently will result in appropriate behaviors.

4. *Directed Statements*   Directed statements may be required to help students behave appropriately. Statements such as "Get back in your seat" carry more emphasis than silently looking on or nondirected statements.

5. *Modeling*   Often teachers feel as if they have to help the student demonstrate appropriate behaviors. They may actually take the student's hand, open a book to the correct page, and put a pencil in the student's hand.

6. *Reinforcement*   A commonly used method to deal with students' behaviors is reinforcement. Students are rewarded with positive reinforcements when their behaviors are appropriate.

7. *Physical Intervention/Isolation*   The most dramatic behavioral intervention is physical intervention or isolation. Teachers may feel that other less intrusive methods have been ineffective and therefore use this method. With physical intervention, teachers actually remove students from their classes, send them to the principal's office, or some other overt action.

These seven strategies are used by teachers every day. The information presented in this chapter presents information regarding ways to manage the behaviors of students. The ways presented will generally fit into one of the seven primary approaches. Using these techniques will enable teachers to be successful working with students whose behavior controls are limited.

The Nature of Classroom Management

Classroom management is not a simple process of controlling behavior; it is a complex concept that includes numerous components. Classroom management can be defined as "the processes and provisions that are necessary to create and maintain environments in which teaching and learning can occur." (Duke & Meckel, 1984, p. 3) Not only does classroom management include the means to create situations where learning can occur, but it also means establishing environments where learning can be maximized, to a reasonable level. As such, classroom management is not a simple procedure that relies on only one approach, such as behavior modification or punishment to control students' behaviors. Rather, it includes a myriad of components, including:

- time allocation and management,

- space utilization,

- selection and use of materials,

- record keeping,

- management of students' behaviors (Duke & Meckel, 1984).

Classroom management, therefore, includes just about everything teachers can do to create the positive learning environment necessary for teachers to teach effectively and students to learn efficiently. Actions that affect the amount of time students spend on learning activities, the types of materials used, and controlling behaviors are all integral components of classroom management.

The effective management of behaviors is the component of classroom management that is the focus of most teacher education programs. Without the ability to manage the behaviors of students, teachers have difficulties in creating effective learning environments. Behavior management includes "all those actions (and conscious inactions) teachers and parents engage in to enhance the probability that children, individual and in groups, develop effective behaviors that are personally self-fulfilling, productive, and socially acceptable." (Walker & Shea, 1984, p. 4) As a result of the importance of behavior management in classroom management, a large portion of this chapter will focus on how to manage student behaviors.

When developing and implementing classroom management procedures, teachers and other school personnel need to keep in mind that caring and kindness often go a long way in helping maintain positive classroom environments. Students who believe that their teachers care about them and who receive appropriate recognition are more likely to exhibit appropriate behaviors than students who have different attitudes. Teachers need to exhibit a pleasant, positive attitude that can be modeled by their students. When talking about classroom management, it is easy to forget the humanistic factor involved in managing the behavior of students. We often get wrapped up in behavior charting, appropriate reinforcers, and frequency counts. Being flexible and using common sense often go further in classroom management than the most sophisticated management systems. Still, teachers need to understand various classroom management techniques, and use flexibility in their implementation.

Teachers who maintain positive control of their classrooms facilitate the learning of all students. If students are not disruptive, loud, and acting out, then all students are better able to concentrate and learn. When possible, teachers should focus their attentions on positive, appropriate behaviors, and reinforce those behaviors. This approach works better than attending only to inappropriate behaviors that may be motivated by simply needing the teacher's attention.

The consequences of teachers not being able to manage their students' behaviors are obvious. First, the students whose behaviors are out of control are not able to attend to a learning task and comprehend information. Secondly, other students in the classroom are likely affected negatively. If disruptive students create enough of a disturbance, the learning for all students is affected. Third, students who display significant behavior problems will likely have problems in post-school environments. On job sites, in social settings, and in activities that require various degrees of self-control, young adults who had difficulties managing their behaviors likely will be at a disadvantage.

ASSUMPTIONS UNDERLYING CLASSROOM MANAGEMENT

There are several assumptions that underlie classroom management. These include:

1. Classroom management is an integral part of teaching.

2. Teachers can be trained to handle behavior problems effectively.

3. Teachers are in the best position to determine how they most effectively can manage their classrooms.

4. Teachers often are so busy reacting to day-to-day problems that they fail to reflect on the purposes of classroom management.

5. Teaching is one of the most important, challenging, and frustrating occupations in contemporary society. (Duke & Meckel, 1984, pp. 4–8)

One of the most important assumptions underlying classroom management is that effective ways to manage the classroom behaviors of students can be learned by teachers. Although some adults may have better instincts regarding how to manage the behaviors of students and create an optimal learning environment than others, these skills can be learned. Therefore, teachers and prospective teachers need to study ways to manage the behaviors of students in classroom settings to maximize the learning activities presented by teachers. There are several different ways to learn classroom management activities. These include:

1. modeling effective classroom management procedures used by other teachers;

2. attending staff development activities regarding classroom management;

3. team teaching with teachers who are successful classroom managers;

4. attending formal training courses that focus on classroom management;

5. independent readings on classroom management; and

6. trying different classroom management techniques and determining which approaches are effective.

GOALS OF CLASSROOM MANAGEMENT

Aside from the general goal of classroom management being the facilitation of learning and teaching, there are several specific goals. These include 1. more time for learning, 2. access to learning, and 3. management for self-management (Woolfolk, 1990). Teachers who use effective classroom management principles have more time for instruction than teachers who are ineffective managers. If teachers do not have sufficient control of their students, they spend inordinate amounts of time trying to gain control; this cuts directly into instructional time. Another goal for classroom management is access to learning. Similar to the first goal, effective management of behaviors in the classroom means all students have more access to learning. Disruptive students can lead to the denial of instructional time for all students.

The final goal of classroom management is to help students develop self-management skills. After students leave structured school environments, they will not have teachers or overseers to help them manage their behaviors. In college or other post-secondary training sites, on jobs, and in social situations, young adults must be able to manage their own behaviors. Without this skill, these individuals will find themselves without jobs and friends; their success will be significantly limited. Therefore, students must learn self-management strategies if they are to have a chance for successful independent living. For this reason, the ultimate goal of classroom management programs is self management (Walker & Shea, 1984).

The Nature of Classrooms and Other Environments

Although classroom management suggests a school classroom setting, classroom management occurs in the context of the school, home, and community. Since this textbook focuses on teachers and students with mild disabilities, the emphasis will be classroom management in school-related environments. These include regular classrooms, special education classrooms, cafeteria, auditorium, playground, hallways, and school-related trips. Since classroom management focuses on the facilitation of instruction, the regular classroom and special education classroom are the focal points where teachers need to exercise most control over students' behaviors. Special education teachers should assist regular classroom teachers in the management of the behaviors of students with disabilities who are mainstreamed. In order to do this, special education teachers need to have a general understanding of the regular classroom environment.

REGULAR CLASSROOMS

While regular classrooms vary in many ways, there are some general characteristics that apply to most of these environments. These include the fact that classrooms have a lot of different kinds of students doing things at the same time and at a fast pace (Woolfolk, 1990). They are not static, quiet places. Rather, regular classrooms are busy, dynamic environments where a great deal takes place. Table 9–1 (on page 324) summarizes some common characteristics of most classrooms.

The majority of regular classrooms are staffed by one teacher. While some regular classrooms may also have a teacher's aide present part of the school day, the regular teacher is the person primarily responsible for the classroom environment and classroom management. Aides may assist in the implementation of classroom management principles, but the regular teacher determines which management system to use and how it should be implemented. The number of students in classrooms varies from district to district and state to state. In 1988, the average number of students in classrooms ranged from a low of 18.9 to a high of 28.6. Table 9–2 (on page 325) presents data summarizing the number of students found in most classrooms.

Organization of Regular Classrooms

Regular classrooms are organized in two different ways: vertically and horizontally. Vertical organization refers to how the school determines which students should enter school at a particular time, and how they progress through the school (Ragan & Shepherd, 1977). Without this form of organization, there would be no plan for students starting to school and moving through the grades. Most schools use a graded vertical organization. Using this approach, students move through the school's curriculum in steps, called grades. Although some schools use a nongraded organization, in which students progress at their own rates, the majority continue to use the graded model (Smith, 1990).

TABLE 9-1 General Characteristics of Classrooms

MAJOR AREA	CHARACTERISTICS
Multidimensional	■ Many students are coming and going. ■ Students have many different goals and abilities. ■ Students and teachers have to share limited resources. ■ Students with low abilities may slow down remainder of class.
Simultaneity	■ Many different things happen at the same time. ■ Teachers must determine if all students understand directions. ■ Most events are unpredictable.
Immediacy	■ The pace of classrooms is very fast. ■ Teachers enter into hundreds of verbal exchanges daily.
Unpredictable	■ Most classroom events cannot be predicted. ■ Often teachers' best plans go wrong and require on-the-spot solutions.

Source: Woolfolk, 1990.

Schools are also organized horizontally. This organization groups students for instructional purposes. The most commonly used horizontal organizations are self-contained and departmentalized. In the self-contained model, students stay in the same group and are taught by the same teacher most of the school day. Departmentalized programs require students to move from one teacher to another for various subjects. Lower elementary grades generally use a self-contained approach, while upper elementary and secondary grades are more likely to follow a departmentalized model (Smith, 1990).

Regular classroom teachers can help prevent inappropriate behaviors among students with disabilities by using appropriate classroom arrangements. For example, if students are easily distracted, they should not be seated near the door or open windows. A better location would be near the teacher's desk or in a corner without extreme visual or auditory distractions. Students with mild hearing losses need to be seated where they can take best advantage of the teacher's oral instructions and information; likewise, a student with a mild visual impairment needs to be seated in a location where maximum use can be made of visual information. If students are not able to participate in the classroom activities, as a result of distractibility, sensory impairments, or other disability, they are more likely to exhibit inappropriate behaviors; therefore, seating arrangements are important.

TABLE 9–2 Number of Students in Regular Classrooms

STATE	1982	1989	STATE	1982	1989
Alabama	20.7	18.7	Missouri	17.0	15.9
Alaska	17.0	16.0	Montana	16.5	15.8
Arizona	19.8	18.2	Nebraska	15.7	15.0
Arkansas	18.6	15.7	Nevada	21.2	20.3
California	23.1	22.7	New Hampshire	16.8	16.2
Colorado	18.7	17.8	New Jersey	15.9	13.6
Connecticut	15.0	13.1	New Mexico	18.8	18.5
Delaware	17.8	16.4	New York	17.6	14.9
Dist. of Col.	18.5	13.3	North Carolina	19.9	17.5
Florida	19.9	17.1	North Dakota	16.8	15.4
Georgia	18.8	18.5	Ohio	19.7	17.6
Hawaii	22.7	21.1	Oklahoma	17.2	16.5
Idaho	20.9	20.6	Oregon	20.3	18.4
Illinois	18.5	17.1	Pennsylvania	17.3	15.9
Indiana	20.0	17.8	Rhode Island	16.1	14.5
Iowa	16.5	15.8	South Carolina	19.0	17.2
Kansas	15.7	15.2	South Dakota	15.8	15.4
Kentucky	20.8	17.8	Tennessee	20.5	19.3
Louisiana	19.6	18.2	Texas	18.4	-
Maine	18.0	14.6	Utah	27.4	24.5
Maryland	18.5	16.8	Vermont	15.3	13.6
Massachusetts	15.2	13.7	Virginia	17.8	16.1
Michigan	22.9	19.8	Washington	21.7	20.4
Minnesota	17.1	17.0	Wisconsin	17.2	16.0
Mississippi	19.3	18.4	Wyoming	15.0	14.6
		U.S. Average	18.9	17.4	

Source: U.S. Department of Education, 1990

Characteristics of Students in Regular Classrooms

Regular classrooms usually contain students who are similar in age and are classified as nondisabled. While these students may present a wide range of characteristics, they are generally classified as average to above average in intelligence and do not display any deficiencies extensive enough to warrant classification as disabled. Still, in many ways nondisabled students are similar to those with disabilities. The key difference is that the learning and behavior problems are not significant enough to result in classification as disabled. While they are similar in age and general characteristics, the learning and behavior of these students varies a great deal.

SPECIAL EDUCATION CLASSROOMS

Students with disabilities are usually served in classrooms and programs specifically designed for special education. As noted in Chapter 4, these classrooms for students with mild disabilities are usually either self-contained classrooms or resource rooms. In self-contained special education classrooms, students stay with the same teacher for most of the school day. This is in contrast to special education resource rooms that are classrooms where students with disabilities go for part of the day for specialized interventions.

Special education classrooms differ from regular classrooms in several dimensions. First, they usually have smaller numbers of students. Chapter 4 described various special education settings and revealed that most states have maximum numbers of students that can be served in self-contained special education classrooms or resource rooms. Also, teacher's aides may be present in special education classrooms to reduce student-teacher ratios. Regardless of the student-teacher ratio, and whether or not aides are present, the special education teacher is responsible for implementing classroom management practices for all students served in the program.

Characteristics of Students Served in Special Education

Students served in special education programs are similar in that they all display some condition that results in their being classified "disabled". This could include deficits in cognitive skills, sensori-motor skills, physical abilities, or general learning skills. The one overall characteristic is that the disability exhibited by the student must adversely affect the student's educational performance. Beyond this similarity, there are significant differences among students classified as disabled. The population of students served, even in the same resource room or same self-contained classroom, presents a very heterogeneous population.

Some students served in special education programs have good control over their behaviors, while others display significant behavior problems that must be addressed by the special education teacher and regular school personnel. Those students who exhibit problem behaviors often require the most intervention time from the special education teacher. This results in students who are in control of their behaviors getting less of the teacher's time for assistance. The special education teacher, therefore, must manage the behaviors of all students so some students are not penalized by the misbehaviors of others and increase the learning opportunities for those with behavior problems.

Planning for Classroom Management

Teachers who implement sound classroom management principles must plan properly; they do not simply react to students' inappropriate behaviors successfully. In fact, reacting in knee-jerk fashion to specific behaviors will usually not result in appropriate behaviors. While it may appear that some teachers simply "do it," effective classroom managers have planned extensively. This planning for classroom management will include the consideration of what subjects are taught, what kinds of students are served, and the preferred management styles of the teacher. Parents and students themselves should be involved in planning specific classroom management interventions (Maher, 1987). By including parents in planning, they will more likely be consistent in carrying out the plan in the home setting. The involvement of students will only encourage them to achieve success with the plan.

Teachers should focus on the prevention of inappropriate behaviors. Keeping students occupied with meaningful activities that result in appropriate positive reinforcements is the best way to prevent inappropriate behaviors. Often students act inappropriately because they are bored or they feel they are not receiving adequate attention. All students need attention; all students need to be recognized. By arranging the classroom so that students receive attention and recognition for appropriate behavior teachers will eliminate a great deal of inappropriate behaviors.

Several components should be included in planning for classroom management. These include the amount of time students are engaged in learning activities and the general arrangement of the teaching day or period. Other components necessary for planning include 1. room arrangement, 2. display areas, 3. classroom rules, 4. schedules, and 5. grouping considerations (O'Melia & Rosenberg, 1989). By carefully considering these components, teachers are more likely to develop a classroom management plan that will result in permanent behavior improvement. Implementing classroom management plans without sufficient planning may result in interventions that are less than optimally effective.

ENGAGED INSTRUCTIONAL TIME

Engaged time is the time that students are on-task doing assigned work (Slavin, 1988). Engagement can be defined as "the amount of time a child spends in developmentally and contextually appropriate behavior." (McWilliam, 1991, p. 42) Engagement is important to instructional activities (Greenwood, 1991). For example, Jones and Warren (1991) note the relationship between engagement and language learning. Students who are not engaged in meaningful activities are likely to display behavior problems.

Teachers who succeed in keeping their students engaged in meaningful classroom activities are more likely than other teachers in getting their students to display appropriate behaviors with peers and adults. Teachers can facilitate engagement by considering the physical environment of the classroom, social dynamics of the classroom, and instructional practices. As noted by Whaley and Bennett (1991), "an attractive, interesting, and well-managed classroom will capture the interest of young children with disabilities" (p. 51).

There are several ways teachers can keep students engaged in meaningful classroom activities. Examples include:

- Use games and "fun" activities in learning as much as possible.

- Arrange learning activities so all students can experience some levels of success.

- Consistently reinforce appropriate behaviors with reinforcers that students consider positive.

- Use group classroom management practices (described later in chapter).

- Vary instructional format from large group to small group to one-on-one.

- Use a variety of audio-visual materials.

GENERAL ARRANGEMENT OF TEACHING DAY OR PERIOD

How teachers organize their student's time during the day or teaching period is an important consideration for classroom management. This is directly related to the amount of time students are actually engaged in meaningful activities. If teachers properly plan the day or teaching period, students will likely focus their attention on the learning activities. Olson (1989) noted that how teachers get the day or teaching period started sets the stage for on-task behaviors. The following activities are suggested to begin the day or period.

1. Assign an order task to begin the day, such as copying assignments or paragraphs from the board.

2. Establish a set routine for entering the class.

3. Take the first five or ten minutes to review the classroom rules.

4. Give the students time to write in a personal diary or log that the teacher and others may read only with permission.

5. Assign a fun ditto or a manipulative activity that can be done independently at students' desks—copying string designs on a geoboard or building a tower with straws.

6. Allow five minutes for students to talk to their friends.

7. Begin with a goal-setting activity.

8. Have older students who are on a token system plan a daily budget from the token salary they receive each week.

9. Write a fun or challenging question on the board reviewing something you have taught that, if completed correctly within about five or ten minutes, is worth extra credit. (pp. 546–547)

In addition to beginning activities, Olson (1989) notes the importance of planning activities to bring closure to the day or teaching period. Closure helps students understand the nature of the activities and helps them prepare for another follow-up activity. By starting the day or period off in a planned manner and ending the day or period with closure, teachers make maximum use of available instructional time; this in turn leads to less inappropriate behaviors in the classroom.

ROOM ARRANGEMENT

Special education classrooms are arranged in different ways, often depending on the space available, furnishings and materials present, and the preferences of the teacher. The way rooms are arranged can impact on students' behaviors. Often students simply refuse to engage in a particular behavior, or decrease a particular behavior, because they do not like the instructional setting. In these situations, teachers need to find an environment where the student will work on the targeted behavior (Spooner, Test, & Jolly, 1990).

There are several different physical arrangements possible in special education classrooms. These include areas for one-on-one instruction, small group instruction, and large group instruction. Space should also be allocated for learning centers, and possibly isolated study carrels for students who have problems with distractions. The physical arrangements of the rooms can facilitate behavior control. For example, using a variety of learning centers can help students with short attention spans by allowing them to complete short tasks at a center before moving on to another activity. Students do not have the opportunity to become bored, which often results in disruptive behaviors.

DISPLAY AREAS

Display areas present in classrooms can affect the behaviors of students. Display areas can be used to showcase the work of students, post rules, post announcements and other materials, and schedules (O'Melia & Rosenberg, 1989). They include bulletin boards, tables with students' materials, walls designated for posting students' work, and highlighted areas in the room. By using display areas, teachers can provide reinforcement to students as well as remind them about rules and procedures. For example, displaying a student's work that has received a high grade serves to positively reinforce that student's effort. Also, posting a list of students whose behaviors have been exemplary is a better technique than posting those whose behavior has been inappropriate.

CLASSROOM RULES

An important consideration when planning for classroom management is the set of general classroom rules that are adopted by the teacher. Classroom rules can be thought of as the "dos" and "don'ts" of the classroom. Without these general rules, teachers will find themselves constantly dealing with similar behaviors in different ways and having to answer the same questions repeatedly (Woolfolk, 1990). Classroom rules vary significantly from teacher to teacher. Some teachers have very strict, specific rules, while others have only a few, general, fairly permissive rules. A key when using classroom rules is that they are explained to students in ways that the students thoroughly understand them. If students do not understand the rules, then they should not be held accountable for abiding by them. One way to ensure that students understand classroom rules is to post them in a conspicuous location and to have students say them out loud at the beginning of the school day. Having students remember and report when they actually follow a rule is also a good way of ensuring that they know and understand them (Westling & Koorland, 1988).

Teachers can use role playing to help students understand rules. They could post classroom rules, discuss the rules, and then have students act out abiding by the rules, and receiving positive reinforcement, or breaking the rules, and receiving negative consequences. Role playing helps students understand, through actions, what is expected of them. This helps some students assimilate expectations. For some students, understanding through verbal discussions may be difficult; going through the motions of abiding by the rules and receiving positive reinforcement may be easier to understand.

Below is an example of role-playing classroom rules.

1. Teacher reviews rules for the entire classroom.

2. One student is designated to explicitly follow a particular rule, such as staying in his seat.

3. The teacher tells the entire class that the designated student is demonstrating staying in his seat and then verbally praises the student.

4. Another student is designated to leave his seat.

5. As the student leaves his seat, the teacher tells him to return to his seat and indicates which negative consequence will be applied.

6. The final part of the role play is a class discussion that summarizes the activity and describes why the first student was positively reinforced and the second student received negative consequences.

Another very important principle when dealing with classroom rules is that teachers implement and enforce them consistently. Enforcing rules for some students while ignoring them for others only creates a classroom climate of unknowns. And, unknowns about rules, consequences, and how rules will be implemented only create situations where inappropriate behaviors are likely. Students are unsure what rules they must follow and under what circumstances. Rules must be enforced uniformly.

Classroom rules differ between elementary and secondary classrooms. In general, classroom rules for elementary students are more basic and more specifically spelled out than rules for secondary students. Tables 9–3 and 9–4 provide examples of classroom rules found in an elementary classroom and a secondary classroom. When possible, classroom

TABLE 9-3 Examples of Elementary Classroom Rules

1. All students should stay in their seats unless there is a need to be other places.
2. Students should keep their hands and feet to themselves.
3. Students should always take turns when talking to others.
4. Students should always have paper and pencil with them.
5. Students should respect their classmates' space and work out disagreements without fighting.
6. Students should always take turns during group activities.

Source: Westling & Koorland, 1988.

rules should be stated positively (Westling & Koorland, 1988). Other general considerations when developing classroom rules include:

1. Select the fewest possible number of rules. Students should not be expected to remember a long list of rules. Keep the list short and limited to general, important rules.

2. State rules behaviorally. Make sure that students understand how rules are operationalized. A rule that is not stated in behavioral terms may be misunderstood by students.

3. Detail clear consequences for both compliance and noncompliance. A key in getting students to follow rules is that they understand the consequences. Students

need to know about positive consequences that result in abiding by the rules as well as the negative consequences if rules are broken.

4. Ensure that rules are situation-specific. Make sure that students understand specific situations where rules apply. Overly general rules may be difficult for some students to understand (O'Melia & Rosenberg, 1989).

TABLE 9–4 Examples of Secondary Classroom Rules

1. Students should respect their classmates space and not talk except in group activities.

2. Students should always bring paper, pencil, books, and class work to class.

3. Students should not eat or chew gum in class.

4. Students should not write notes to each other during class time.

5. Students should stay in their seats during class time unless teachers give them permission to move around.

SCHEDULES

A major consideration when providing educational services to students with disabilities is scheduling, especially for students who spend part of their day in the regular classroom and part in the resource room (Smith, 1990). There are some times that are better for students to leave their regular classrooms for resource room help than others. For example, students should not have to leave the regular classroom during activities they enjoy. Since these students have experienced a great deal of failure and have often developed a dislike for school, they need to be able to participate in activities they like. Students should also not be expected to leave their regular classroom during times they may miss out on important academic activities, such as reading, math, and written expression. A more appropriate time for their leaving the classroom might be during a reading period when the student's group is working on independent activities, or an enrichment period when the student will not benefit from the classroom interactions.

Students with disabilities also may react negatively to change. Changing their schedules, or having schedules that vary from day to day, may result in these students displaying inappropriate behaviors. Therefore, time spent developing sound schedules may result in fewer problems during the implementation of programs. Devoting more time at the beginning of the school year to scheduling may mean fewer problems because of fewer changes.

GROUPING CONSIDERATIONS

The arrangements used to group students with disabilities is also a consideration for classroom management. Students with disabilities are served in large groups, small groups, and one-on-one situations. Some students might be able to function very well in one setting, whereas another type of grouping may result in inappropriate behaviors. Just as there is no one best method to teach students with disabilities, there is also no one grouping model that is always effective. Therefore, teachers need to have a variety of grouping options available for students. Matching students with their preferred grouping arrangement may facilitate appropriate behaviors and therefore eliminate inappropriate behaviors.

Grouping can provide a nonintrusive intervention approach for use with students who have behavior problems. Groups enable teachers to use group dynamics to help shape behaviors (Salend, 1987). Students with disruptive behaviors can be grouped with those who display appropriate behaviors. In one case study, a student with a mild disability and behavior problems was placed in a group of students who displayed appropriate behaviors. Data collected on the disruptive student revealed that the group placement had a significant impact on his behaviors. During the time he was placed in the group, the student's inappropriate behaviors dropped significantly when compared to behaviors exhibited in a group of students with behavior problems. Therefore, rather than allowing students with behavior problems to assimilate into groups of children who typically exhibit inappropriate behaviors, teachers should group them with well-behaved students (Stainback, Stainback, Etscheidt, & Doud, 1987).

TEACHER BEHAVIORS

One factor in maintaining appropriate classroom behaviors that is often overlooked is the behaviors of teachers. Teachers represent critical elements in the classroom environment and are therefore an integral part of the dynamics of the classroom. The behaviors exhibited by teachers toward students has an impact on students' behaviors. DeLuke and Knoblock (1987) note that "problematic student behaviors often arise because teachers and students find it difficult to coexist peacefully in the classroom" (p.18). In order to help prevent inappropriate behaviors from students, they recommend the following.

1. *Communicate respect to each student.* Teachers need to let each student know that he or she is respected. This can be accomplished by teachers actively listening to students, responding to students' communication efforts, and accurately interpreting students' communication efforts.

2. *Seek out diverse sources of information.* Teachers need to understand their students. In order to do this, they have to rely on information from a variety of sources, including observations, interactions with students, and direct recordings of behaviors.

3. *Develop curricula that prevents behavior problems.* Using the appropriate curricula with students is vital in order to prevent inappropriate behaviors. Students who are not challenged by the curriculum, or who are incapable of experiencing success in a particular curriculum, will likely exhibit behavior problems. Therefore, teachers must determine a curriculum that meets individual needs of students.

4. *Use instructional procedures that minimize inappropriate behaviors.* Just as teachers need to determine appropriate curricula for students, they also must determine and implement instructional procedures that meet the unique needs of students. No two students are exactly alike; therefore, teachers need to have a full bag of tricks to use.

Teachers play a critical role in establishing an environment that is conducive to appropriate behaviors, or one that may result in a variety of inappropriate behaviors. Teachers need to use their influences to create the environment that is most likely to result in behaviors that facilitate learning.

Teachers may not be aware of their behaviors that result in students' inappropriate behaviors. One way teachers can determine if their behaviors are affecting students' behaviors is to do an analysis of their own behaviors in the classroom that preceeded certain students' behaviors. They should make a written note to themselves and analyze this information after several episodes of inappropriate behaviors. This type of analysis can help teachers understand what, if any role, their behaviors are having on students' behaviors.

Classroom management is the control teachers have over their classrooms. With good classroom management, teachers are able to spend quality time on instructional and other learning activities. When classroom management does not achieve its needed objectives, inappropriate behaviors may significantly interfere with learning. Therefore, teachers must use a variety of methods to manage the behaviors of their students to facilitate learning. By using such techniques as physical arrangement of the classroom, engaged time of students, and the development and implementation of sound classroom rules, teachers are capable of managing the behaviors of their students. However, there are times when teachers need to rely on more structured management techniques. Behavior management is a more formalized method of classroom management that teachers may have to implement.

CONSIDERATIONS BEFORE IMPLEMENTING A STRUCTURED PLAN

Prior to implementing a behavior management plan, teachers need to conclude that a formalized plan is necessary (Sulzer-Azaroff & Mayer, 1991). Teachers must ask specific questions to arrive at this conclusion. Figure 9–1 (on page 334) provides a checklist for teachers to use to help them arrive at this conclusion.

Behavior Management

Behavior management is one component of classroom management designed to encourage appropriate behaviors as well as deal with inappropriate behaviors. It is used to decrease behaviors that are undesirable, while increasing desirable behaviors. Behavior management includes using positive and negative reinforcers to either maintain or increase some behaviors; this in turn decreases inappropriate behaviors (Ellenwood & Felt, 1989). Behavior management is based on behavioral psychology and behavioral principles.

BEHAVIORAL PRINCIPLES

Behavioral learning theories are based on several specific principles. These include consequences, reinforcers, punishers, immediacy of feedback, shaping, extinction, and reinforcement schedules (Slavin, 1988). These principles govern the application of behaviorism to

FIGURE 9-1 Practical Considerations in Planning an Applied Behavior
Analysis Program

Directions: Circle either Y (yes) or N (no) for each question.

1. Does a problem merit a behavioral program?
   Y N   a. Has assistance been sought from several sources?
   Y N   b. Does the behavior of the person or group depart substantially
            from that "typical" of comparable people or groups?
   Y N   c. Have dramatic behavior changes recently occurred?

2. Have direct or informal solutions been attempted?
   Y N   a. Physical examination?
   Y N   b. Changes in assignments and responsibilities?
   Y N   c. Changes in physical or social environment?
   Y N   d. Direct requests for behavior change?

(If you answered *no* to any of these questions, consider informal methods
before you institute a systematic applied behavior analysis program; but if
answers are affirmative or not applicable, feel justified in proceeding.)

3. Does the proposed behavior analysis program have sufficiently
   high priority and level of support to justify proceeding?
   Y N   a. Is there sufficient evidence that is likely to succeed?
   Y N   b. Is the problem critical?
   Y N   c. Will the public support the program?
   Y N   d. Will the program receive supervisory support?
   Y N   e. Will the path toward attaining the goal be under the control of
            those involved?
   Y N   f. Is the behavior analyst competent to conduct the program
            successfully?
   Y N   g. Are resources adequate?
   Y N   h. Are different organizations unable to handle the problem
            adequately?

Source: Sulzer-Azaroff, B., & Mayer, G.R. (1991). *Behavior analysis for lasting change.* Fort Worth: Holt,
Rinehart and Winston, Inc., p. 23. Reprinted with Permission.

behavior management. They have been shown to be very effective in modifying behaviors
(Diebert & Harmon, 1973; Walker & Shea, 1984; Slavin, 1988; Woolfolk, 1990). When using a
behavioral approach to managing behaviors, teachers have to understand and implement
many of these principles.

Consequences

Probably the most important principle of behavioral learning theory is that behavior can be
changed due to the immediate consequences that follow that behavior. Consequences are

things that occur following a behavior. They can be positive, such as a teacher giving a student an *A* grade for good school work, or negative, such as a child getting "grounded" for fighting with a sibling. The systematic provisions of consequences by teachers have been shown to be a very powerful management tool (Brady & Taylor, 1989). Positive consequences make the behavior more likely to recur, while negative consequences make the behavior less likely to recur. Consequences that result in pleasures are considered reinforcers, while those that are unpleasant are considered punishers (Slavin, 1988). When at all possible, teachers should use positive reinforcement.

Reinforcers

Reinforcers are consequences that increase the likelihood that a behavior will occur in the future. Reinforcers can be of several different types—positive reinforcers, negative reinforcers, primary reinforcers, and secondary reinforcers (Slavin, 1988). A positive reinforcer is something that is considered as "good" by the student, such as candy. A negative reinforcer is when something negative is taken away as a consequence. An example would be to stop (remove) an ongoing loud noise when students sit in their chairs. Primary reinforcers are those that are directly given to students following behaviors. Reinforcers are considered secondary when they are paired with a primary reinforcer and eventually take the place of the primary reinforcer.

Reinforcers can also be intrinsic or extrinsic. Intrinsic reinforcers are internal; there is no overt rewarding of the behaviors. Extrinsic reinforcers are overt rewards, either tangible or intangible. Students will rarely respond to interventions based on intrinsic reinforcers as well as to extrinsic reinforcers. Adults similarly respond better to extrinsic than intrinsic reinforcers (Mehring & Colson, 1990). When using extrinsic reinforcers, it is critical that teachers select consequences that are deemed positive if students are expected to consider them as rewards. What teachers think of as a positive consequence may be thought of as negative by students. Table 9–5 (on page 336) summarizes the different types of reinforcers.

Punishers

As noted above, consequences that are negative or that are unpleasant are considered punishers. Most of you recall being punished when you did something wrong. Punishers can be very mild, such as having to stay in during recess, to very severe, such as corporal punishment. The obvious objective of punishment is to encourage students to stop doing certain things. Again, think of examples when you were punished for doing something wrong. Your parents or teachers may have punished you in hopes that you would stop doing something.

Punishment has been shown to improve the behaviors of students when used appropriately (Slavin, 1988). However, teachers need to be aware that positive reinforcement is considered to have longer lasting effects on behaviors than punishment. When using punishment, teachers should also use positive reinforcement to reward appropriate behaviors. This will result in a more permanent behavior change than simply using punishment alone. Punishment should not be used unless other forms of behavior management have failed.

Shaping

Shaping is the reinforcement of certain behaviors that are leading to the desired outcome. When students are expected to do certain things but are unable to achieve the objective at

TABLE 9–5 Summary of Different Types of Reinforcers

TYPE OF REINFORCER	DESCRIPTION
Primary Reinforcers	■ satisfy human needs
	■ examples: food, security
Secondary Reinforcers	■ acquire value by being associated with primary reinforcers
	■ examples: grades, money, praise, smiles, tokens
Positive Reinforcers	■ given to students following appropriate behaviors
	■ examples: candy, grades, stars, praise
Negative Reinforcers	■ taking away unpleasant situations when appropriate behaviors are elicited
	■ example: stop flicking the light when the talking stops

Source: Slavin, 1988.

once, they are reinforced for making gains in the desired direction. An example would be a student who is constantly out of his seat. The objective of not getting out of the seat might be achieved gradually, over a period of time. Reinforcement should be provided at various stages to reward the student for getting closer to achieving the goal. Shaping is also called "successive approximations" and implies that as long as the student is doing the kinds of things that are leading to the ultimate, desired behaviors, then the student should receive some reinforcement (Woolfolk, 1990).

Extinction

When undesired behaviors disappear, the process of "extinction" has occurred. Extinction is a very important component of a behavior management program when dealing with students' inappropriate behaviors (Slavin, 1988). Extinction is when certain behaviors, such as acting out behavior, ceases to be a problem. This can result from reinforcing some competing behavior or from withdrawing all reinforcements for the undesired behavior. For example, the teacher may want a student to stop talking to his "neighbors." In order to accomplish this goal, the teacher may reinforce the student for successfully completing a written assignment. Reinforcing the student's on-task behavior, makes it more likely to occur and therefore, makes the talking less likely to occur.

Extinction may also result from ignoring the inappropriate behaviors. Teachers need to realize that when reinforcements for the undesired behaviors are withdrawn, the

TABLE 9–6 Reinforcement Schedules

SCHEDULE	DEFINITION
Fixed Ratio	Students are reinforced after a specified number of correct responses.
Variable Ratio	Students are reinforced after a variable number of correct responses. The number varies each time.
Fixed Interval	Students are reinforced after a specified period of time has elapsed.
Variable Interval	Students are reinforced after a variable amount of time has elapsed. The amount of time varies for each reinforcement.

undesired behavior may actually increase. This is the natural reaction when the student is desperately seeking some reinforcement. However, if the behavior continues to go unreinforced, it likely will result in extinction. Extinction is a very important component of a behavior management program when dealing with students' inappropriate behaviors (Slavin, 1988).

Schedules of Reinforcement

Reinforcements can occur immediately after particular behaviors are displayed, every time they are displayed, or on some other schedule that is not so rigid. The reinforcement schedule, therefore, is the "pattern with which the reinforcer is presented (or not presented) in response to the exhibition of the target behavior." (Walker & Shea, 1984, p. 34) The interval between reinforcement may have an impact on the increase or decrease of the target behaviors (Repp, Felce, & Barton, 1991).

There are four general schedules for reinforcement. These include fixed ratio schedule, variable ratio schedule, fixed interval schedule, and variable interval schedule. They may result in the student being reinforced after a certain number of appropriate behaviors, or after a certain time interval. Teachers need to be aware of the characteristics of these different ratios and when they are most appropriate when attempting to manage behaviors. Table 9–6 summarizes each schedule.

BEHAVIOR MODIFICATION

Behavior modification is the most common classroom application of behavioral principles used in managing behaviors. Behavior modification can be defined as "techniques offering tools and systematic procedures that teachers may implement to change or modify unacceptable or defiant behavior and encourage more acceptable and appropriate behavior" (Gearheart, Weishahn, & Gearheart, 1988, p. 392). Behavior modification is the application of behavioral psychology to behavior management. It emphasizes using positive reinforcement to change behaviors. When using this model of behavior management, the teacher is the controlling agent; students and peers have limited control of the situation (D'Alonzo & Miller, 1977).

Before implementing a behavior modification approach, or any other behavior management method, teachers need to develop a specific behavior intervention plan for specific students. The following steps are included in developing this plan.

1. Define the exact problem behavior in observable, concrete terms.

2. Determine the severity and importance of the behavior.

3. Identify the frequency (per minute, day, etc.) of the target behavior.

4. Devise a plan for the target behavior. Determine which rewards could be given for improved performance.

5. Set modest goals and determine performance level required to receive reinforcement.

6. Evaluate the results of the intervention.

7. Determine if modifications are needed. (Ellenwood & Felt, 1989, p. 15)

A behavior management plan should be developed in conjunction with the IEP for students who need to have specific attention focused on their inappropriate behaviors. Parents, teachers, assessment personnel, and others who are involved with the student's educational program should be involved.

Positive Reinforcement

A key factor in the successful implementation of behavior modification is the selection of positive reinforcers. If the reinforcer used is not considered as a reward by the student, then positive reinforcement is not occurring. The result will likely be continued inappropriate behaviors, or a lack of the desired target behavior. There are several different ways teachers can ensure that the reinforcers they select are viewed as positive by students. Westling and Koorland (1988) suggest the following.

- Ask students what they like and record their answers.

- Have students complete written interest surveys. Ask them to write down what they like to eat, toys they prefer, games they enjoy, how they like to spend their free time, etc.

- Give students a chance to try out different reinforcing activities. Watch and record the toys, games, foods, materials, or activities they seem to enjoy the most.

- Ask previous teachers, parents, or other persons who know the student what activities are most desirable.

■ Note the effect of potential reinforcers on the student's work when they are presented following appropriate behavior or increased performance.

■ Note the things the student does best and frequently. In this category, even certain types of school work can be effective (p. 107).

There are several different kinds of positive reinforcers. These include 1. edible reinforcers, such as cookies; 2. tangible reinforcers, such as toys; 3. activity reinforcers, such as extra recess; and 4. social reinforcers, such as praise (Sulzer-Azaroff & Mayer, 1991). Social reinforcers have the advantage of being a natural part of the school environment. Examples of potential social reinforcers are listed in table 9–7 (on pages 340–341).

When using social reinforcers, teachers need to be aware of the differences in praise and encouragement. Praise focuses on the teacher being pleased with the student's performance, while encouragement focuses on the student and the process of the student's efforts. While praise may be needed with some students, a better approach is providing encouragement. Constant praise may condition the student to always look for a reward of some sort, even a social reward. Encouragement, on the other hand, will help students feel good about their efforts (Wolfgang & Glickman, 1986). Teachers may begin with praise and then replace the praise with encouragement in small segments.

The following demonstrates some of the differences between praise and encouragement (Wolfgang & Glickman, 1986).

Praise	Encouragement
1. "I (teacher) like what you have done."	1. "You're trying harder."
2. "Great job! What a smart person."	2. "You must be happy with (playing that game, being with others, and so on)."
3. "You get a star (token, free time) for doing that."	3. "It must be a good feeling to know you're doing well."
4. "I'm going to tell everyone how proud I am of you."	4. "You have every reason to be proud."

Behavior modification has been used effectively in classroom situations with all kinds of students (Walker & Shea, 1984; Slavin, 1988; Woolfolk, 1990). When using behavior modification to change behaviors, teachers must be consistent in providing the reinforcements on schedule. Consistency is a critical component to an effective behavior modification program.

Altering Preceding Stimulus

Another way of controlling behaviors using the behavior modification model is to alter the stimulus that occurs before the behavior. Behavior modification generally focuses on the stimulus of the behavior being the reinforcement that follows the behavior. The stimulus can also be a preceding event. Specific events may occur that result in behaviors, often inappropriate behaviors (Gardner, Cole, Davidson, & Karan, 1986). By determining which

TABLE 9–7 Potential Social Reinforcers for Children, Youth, and Adults

CHILDREN	YOUTH AND ADULTS
Nod	Nod
Smile	Smile
Tickle	Laugh (with, not at)
Pat on shoulder, head, back	Wink
Hug	Signal or gesture of approval
Wink	Orienting glance directly toward face
Kiss	Assistance when requested
Signal or gesture to signify approval	Positive comment on appearance
Swing around	Pat on the back
Touch on cheek	Handshake
Holding on lap	Asking client to discuss
Fulfillment of requests	something before group
Eating with children	Asking client about items of
Assistance	interest to individual
Joining class during recess	Asking client to demonstrate
Saying (adding reason)	something
yes	Saying (adding reason)
nice	very good
good	okay
great	beautiful
fine	good for you
very good	exactly
fantastic	thank you
very fine	that's interesting
excellent	_____ is excellent
unbelievable	that's great
marvelous	yeah
atta-girl, atta-boy	great
far out	right
I like that	I agree
right on	good job
right	good idea
that's right	fantastic
correct	fine
_____ is really paying attention	what a clever idea!
wonderful	unbelievable
you really pay attention well	you really are being
you do that well	creative, innovative . . .
I'm pleased with (proud of) you	see how you're improving
that was very nice of you	that looks better than
that's good; great	last time
wow	keep up the good work
oh boy	you've apparently got the idea
very nice	little by little we're getting there
good work	see how _____ has improved
good job	

continued

TABLE 9-7 Potential Social Reinforcers for Children, Youth, and Adults (cont'd.)

CHILDREN	YOUTH AND ADULTS

great going
good for you
_____ is a hard worker today; good for you
that's the way
that's interesting
much better
okay
you should show this to your parents
you're doing better
that's perfect
that's another one you got right
you're doing very well
see how well _____ is doing?
look how well he (she) did
_____ is really working
watch what he did; do it again
show the class your _____
_____ is really working hard; he is going to be able
  to _____
wow, look at _____ work
you look nice today
_____ is working nicely, keep up the good work
I can really tell _____ is thinking by what she just
  said
_____ is sitting quietly and doing his work; good
  for him/her
_____ is listening with such concentration; that's
  very polite, _____, thank you
you should be proud of the way you're sitting quietly
  and listening to me while I'm giving a lesson
_____ just earned another point by sitting quietly
  and listening while I was reading; good job _____
_____ walked quietly to her seat; thank you
good, you sharpened your pencil before class; now
  you're ready to go
_____ has all of her supplies on her desk and is
  ready to go; good!
_____ has gotten his materials and has started to
  work already; good!
it's nice to see the way _____ raises his hand when
  he wants to share
the whole class is really listening politely to one
  another
this whole row is sitting quietly with their chairs on
  the floor; great!

you're really becoming an expert at
  this
do you see what an effective job _____
  has done?
you are very patient
that shows a lot of work
you look great today
it really makes me feel good when I
  see so many of you hard at work
that's the best job I've seen today
you're paying attention so nicely
the interest you are showing is great
it makes me happy to see you
  working so well
that's a thoughtful (courteous) thing
  to do for _____
_____ has gotten his materials and
  has started to work already; good
  going!
_____ is ready to start
you're really very considerate of one
  another

Source: Sulzer-Azaroff, B., & Mayer, G.R. (1991). Behavior analysis for lasting change. Fort Worth: Holt,
Rinehart and Winston, Inc., pp. 162-163. Reprinted with Permission.

preceding event is related to the inappropriate behaviors, these stimuli can be changed with the result of altering the following behaviors.

There are several ways to determine which preceding stimuli result in inappropriate behaviors. One way is to anecdotally note what was occurring before the inappropriate behavior. The notation should include time, place, students and teachers involved, and specific behaviors that could have elicited the inappropriate behaviors. After determining the preceding stimuli, teachers should develop a plan to eliminate the specific activities that appear to result in the behaviors.

Sulzer-Azaroff and Mayer (1991) suggest that teachers keep a narrative recording and sequence analysis. This is a running description of behaviors that occur in a specified setting. Unlike logs or diaries, which are used to record behaviors after they occur, a narrative recording "involves writing down what is happening in the natural context" (p. 26). The teacher does not target a specific behavior, but keeps a record of behaviors that occur during different periods of time. Later analysis of this recording can help teachers determine not only the events that precede inappropriate behaviors, but those that result in appropriate behaviors. Table 9–8 provides an example of a narrative recording and sequence analysis.

A better method of dealing with inappropriate behaviors is to determine the preceding stimuli that result in appropriate behaviors. A similar method noted above for determining the stimuli that precede inappropriate behaviors can be used to determine preceding stimuli that results in positive behaviors. Once detected, teachers should facilitate the continuation of the stimuli to facilitate the likelihood of the appropriate behavior responses.

TABLE 9-8 Sample Behavior Sequence Analysis

ANTECEDENT EVENT	DEXTER'S BEHAVIOR	CONSEQUENT EVENT
Teacher asks, "Who will help find information on dinosaurs for a diorama for the science fair?"	Looks out window	Teacher shrugs shoulders and says, "I'll help you myself as long as no one volunteered."
Teacher says, "Dexter, I know that you have a special interest in dinosaurs. You'd probably be particularly interested in helping. I'd like to count on your participation; may I?"	Replies, "Sure, I have some models I can bring in to school tomorrow."	Teacher says, "Great." John smiles and nods approval.
John moans, scratches his head, and says, "I can't do this geometry problem."	Says, "You're dumb."	Teacher says, "You can hardly afford to call John anything when you don't complete your work either."
Jeanette moans, scratches her head, and says, "I can't do this geometry problem."	Says, "Here, let me help you. Remember the rule about right triangles?"	Teacher ignores Dexter; Jeanette smiles and gives Dexter a grateful "Thanks."

Source: Sulzer-Azaroff, B., & Mayer, G.R. (1991). *Behavior analysis for lasting change.* Fort Worth: Holt, Rinehart and Winston, Inc., p. 27. Reprinted with Permission.

Ecological View

That behaviors result from various stimuli in the environment is an ecological view of behaviorism. The basic assumption is that behaviors do not occur in isolation, but are a product of the environment. By determining which environmental factors may be leading to appropriate behaviors and which ones are resulting in inappropriate behaviors, teachers are able to impose some control over behaviors. A good way to determine which environmental events may lead to inappropriate behaviors is through a critical incidents log or an ecological survey (Sugai, 1986). Through such recording mechanisms, information is obtained regarding the student, behaviors, and environmental factors (Evans, Evans, & Gable, 1989). Figure 9–2 (on pages 344–345) presents an example of an ecological survey form.

OTHER BEHAVIORAL MANAGEMENT APPROACHES

As noted, behavior modification is the most likely intervention based on behavior management that is used. There are numerous ways to implement behavior modification and behavior management programs. These include:

- token economy,
- contingency contracting,
- good behavior games,
- daily report cards,
- limit setting (Ellenwood & Felt, 1989).

Some of these approaches are based strictly on the principles of behaviorism, previously described, while others reflect a more general inclusion of behavioristic principles. When reading the following descriptions of these approaches, keep in mind that teachers can implement them in a variety of different ways. Teachers that are flexible in their implementation will be more successful than teachers who attempt to use these techniques rigidly.

Token Economy

A token economy system to positively reinforce students has been used effectively in many classrooms. When using a token economy system, students are given tokens as positive reinforcers when they display appropriate behaviors or perform in certain ways academically. Tokens can be anything that enable teachers to give students credits. Some teachers have used poker chips, pennies, check marks, stars, stickers, coupons, or any other item that can be accumulated by students. After acquiring these tokens, students redeem them for specific reinforcers, such as small toys, time on the playground, free time, special class jobs, money, or other privileges (Woolfolk, 1990).

Maher (1989) describes a behavior management system that uses a punch out card as a token reinforcer. Students are allowed to use a hole puncher to punch holes in a punchcard (a 3×5 card with a picture of graph configuration) as reinforcement. When the card is all punched out, the student receives some surprise tangible reinforcement. Regardless of how the token reinforcement system is used, several general guidelines should be considered (Westling & Koorland, 1988). Table 9–9 (on page 346) presents examples of these guidelines.

FIGURE 9–2 Ecological Survey Form

Name of person(s) completing form _____ Date(s) _____

I. General Information
Name of child _____ Address _____
Telephone number _____ Date of birth _____ Age ____ Sex ____
School _____ Teacher _____ Grade _____
Who does the child live with and for how long? (List parent, siblings, others.) _____
_____
Mother's and/or father's place of employment: _____
Mother _____ Father _____
Language spoken in the home _____
What present problems (academic and/or social) does the child have? _____
What do you think is causing these problems? _____
What expectations do you have of your child? _____

II. Educational Information
Previous psychological and/or educational testing:
Test _____ Date _____ Results _____
Educational history: preschool _____
                  elementary _____
                  secondary _____
Does the child enjoy reading? _____
Does the child read at home? ____ If yes, list types of materials read at home _____
What academic areas does the child like? _____ dislike _____
How well does the child adjust to school situations? ____ very well ____ fairly well ____ poorly
How would you describe the child's performance in school? (In terms of grades earned and behavior.) _____
How would you describe the conditions in the classroom and school that could influence this child? (e.g., classroom discipline, size of classes, and instructional factors.) _____
Does the child regularly complete homework? _____
Has the child ever been retained? _____ What grade? _____
Is the child absent or tardy frequently? _____
Has the child ever been suspended? _____ Explain _____
Has the child ever been in or referred to a special education classroom? _____
What type? _____
Has the child ever had special reading instruction or any special adaptations in instruction? ____
What grade? _____ Explain _____
Have any of the child's brothers or sisters had problems in school? ____ Explain _____

III. Home/Community Information
How would you describe the conditions in the home and community that might affect this child? (Adequacy of housing, basic needs, significant events such as divorce, etc.) _____
_____
Is the child involved in regular activities in the community? (Recreational, religious, etc.) __
Does the child interact regularly with peers? _____ Explain _____
How many hours of TV does the child watch each day? _____
What programs does the child enjoy watching? _____
Is the child always supervised by an adult at home? _____ yes _____ no
If not, how much time does the child spend unsupervised daily? _____

Source: Evans, Evans, & Gable (1989). An ecological survey of student behavior. *Teaching Exceptional Children*, *21*, pp. 14–15. Used with permission.

FIGURE 9-2 Ecological Survey Form (cont'd)

IV. Medical History and Early Development

Health of mother during pregnancy: ____good ____fair ____poor
Explain: _____
Condition of child at birth: ____good ____fair ____poor
Explain: _____

Infant and preschool development:

Motor development:	good	fair	poor
Language development:	good	fair	poor
Social development:	good	fair	poor
Cognitive development:	good	fair	poor

Please provide any other information about infant/prechool development that might be helpful _____
List any childhood diseases, significant illnesses, major injuries, or hospitalizations your child has had _____
List any physical impairments, conditions, allergies, physical complaints, frequent minor injuries your child has _____
List any medications your child has taken or is currently taking _____
Date of child's last physical examination _____Physician who has primary care of child __
_____Address _____
Has the child had a vision screening? ___Hearing evaluation? ___Findings_____
Has the child had any special medical examinations? (Neurological etc.) _____
Please indicate the type of examination, date, and findings: _____
Does the child regularly engage in some form of exercise? ___Explain _____

V. Behavioral Information

For his/her age, do you consider your child to be socially _mature _average or _immature?
Explain: _____
Who disciplines the child? _____What form of discipline is used? _____
Does the child exhibit any behaviors that you find annoying or unacceptable? _____
List behaviors _____
For each behavior listed above, indicate the following:
 Describe the specific behavior: _____
 How often does the child exhibit this behavior? (e.g., daily, weekly?)
 How would you rate the behavior? ____mild ____moderate ____severe
 Where does the behavior take place? _____
 Who is present when the behavior occurs? _____
 Does the behavior occur during any particular activity? _____
 What happens immediately before the behavior occurs? _____
 What happens and what does your child do immediately after the behavior occurs? _
 What do you do when the child engages in the behavior? _____

SURVEY OF REINFORCERS

What qualities make this child enjoyable to be around? _____
What does the child like to eat and drink? _____
What things does the child like to do? _____
What kinds of games or toys interest this child? _____
What kind of social reinforcers does this child like? _____
What does your child like to do in his/her spare time? _____
What do you enjoy doing with the child? _____

VI. Other Comments _____

TABLE 9-9 Guidelines for Using a Token Economy

	Before presenting the program to students, make sure you have all the details worked out.
Examples	1. Establish rules that clearly specify requirements, such as how many problems done correctly will earn a point.
	2. Make sure your system is workable and not too complicated. You might discuss it with another teacher to identify possible sources of problems.

	You may want to have different goals for different groups of students.
Examples	1. Focus on cooperative behaviors for students who are disruptive.
	2. For high-achieving students, give tokens for enrichment work, peer tutoring, or special projects.
	3. Match the token to the age of the student—colored chips for younger children, points for older students.

	Offer a variety of rewards at different prices.
Examples	1. Offer rewards that can be purchased for only two ro three tokens, so that all students will be motivated to try.
	2. Offer rewards that make more extensive efforts or saving up tokens worthwhile.

	Gradually increase the requirements for each token.
Examples	1. Begin with one token for each correct answer, then give a token for every three correct answers, and so on.
	2. Offer tokens for five minutes of attention to assignments, then eventually for a whole day of attentive work.

	Gradually change from tangible rewards and privileges to time focused on enjoyable learning experiences.
Examples	1. With young students start with candy or small toys, but move to assisting the teacher and free reading time.
	2. With older students, start with such things as magazines and move toward free time to spend on special projects, the chance to tutor younger children, or the opportunity to work in the computer lab.

Source: Woolfolk, 1990. *Educational psychology,* 4th Ed. Englewood Cliffs, NJ: Prentice-Hall, p. 213. Used with permission.

Contingency Contracting

Some students are well aware of the behaviors they need to change (either decrease or increase). They simply need some form of external reinforcer to facilitate these desired behaviors. One good method of doing this is through the use of contingency contracting. Students enter into a formal contract with the teacher to do certain things in exchange for specific rewards.

Salend (1990) suggests that contingency contracts include the following components.

- A statement of the behavior(s) the student(s) are to increase or decrease in observable terms
- A statement of the environmental conditions during which the strategy will be implemented
- A listing of the type and amount of reinforcers that will be provided and who will provide them
- A schedule of when the delivery of reinforcers will take place
- A listing of the roles teachers and students can perform to increase the success of the system
- A time frame for the length of the contract, including a date for renegotiation
- Signatures of the students and teacher (p. 287).

Figure 9–3 provides a sample of a behavior contract.

FIGURE 9–3 Example of a Behavioral Contract

Official Contract

Parties involved in the contract:

_____ and _____.

Date of Contract: _____

Contract Period: _____

Conditions of the Contract:

I, _____ , representing the _____
school district, will _____

_____

_____

when _____ (student)

does the following: _____

_____

_____

Signed: _____   Date: _____

 _____   Date: _____

There are several things teachers can do to increase the likelihood that contingency contracts are successful. For one thing, the contracts should stress the positive. By phrasing the contract in positive terms, students have something to attain rather than something to avoid. The contract should also reinforce small improvements. If students have too much to accomplish before reinforcement, they may forget their goals and the accompanying reinforcers. The contract must also be simple and easily understood. Students must understand what they are required to accomplish and what the reinforcement will be. Provisions must also be made in the contract for immediate reinforcement of target behaviors. If the student must wait for the reinforcer, the link between the target behavior and reinforcement may be minimized. Finally, provisions should be included that allow the student to withdraw or modify the terms of the contract. Specifying the terms by which students may withdraw or modify the contract prevents students from simply declining to participate (Sulzer-Azaroff & Mayer, 1991).

Good Behavior Games

Good behavior games are fun activities students can play in teams with a focus on appropriate behaviors. Good behavior games take advantage of peer pressure. Teachers may have different groups within the classroom, such as rows of students or boys versus girls, compete for certain privileges (Ellenwood & Felt, 1989). In determining groups for a contest, students with behavior problems should be grouped with those who display appropriate behaviors (Stainback, Stainback, Etscheidt, & Doud, 1986). The contest can target appropriate behaviors by the group, such as not getting out of your seat, not talking, or completing an assignment without disrupting other students.

The number and types of good behavior games are endless. Teachers have used this approach to help manage classroom behaviors for years. Westling and Koorland (1988) suggest the following examples of playing good behavior games.

1. Arrange the class into teams and post the rules for the game. State the reward that the winning team receives (such as free time or first to the lunch room).

2. Students with behavior problems may be placed on the same team to prevent them from penalizing other students, or they may be placed on several teams for dispersion and for peer pressure.

3. A kitchen timer may be used to restrict parts of the game to a specific amount of time.

4. Variations of bingo, monopoly, and other board games may be used to develop good behavior games.

Wood (1987) described a good behavior game called "Clams." The objective of this game, designed for elementary-aged students, is to prevent noise and disruption during periods where this is likely to occur. When noise or disruptions begin to grow, the teacher says "1, 2, 3, CLAMS." Since clams are animals that do not make any sounds, students must immediately stop making any noises. This silence is continued until someone makes a noise. The student making the first sounds loses the game. Since this is viewed as a game by students, it is generally considered a positive activity by students.

Daily Report Cards

Often parents of students with disabilities are eager to collaborate with the teacher to improve specific behaviors. Unfortunately they may not be able to help because of a lack of specific knowledge about what the student does during the school day. Parents are more involved in the intervention process if they are aware, on a daily basis, how the student is doing in the classroom. The daily report card is one means of the teacher informing parents daily about the child's behaviors during the school day (Ellenwood & Felt, 1989). The daily report card is a simplified version of a behavioral contract involving the school, student, and home (Sulzer-Azaroff & Mayer, 1991).

Using this communication device, teachers report on a daily basis how the child is doing in school. The report can be in narrative format; however, for convenience, it is more likely that the report will be in the form of a check list or graded form. For example, the teacher may develop a reporting form with specific behaviors listed that the student should exhibit. The teacher can then indicate on the form, with a specific notation system, how the student is exhibiting each of these behaviors. To ensure that the parents are receiving the report, teachers may require that they sign the card and have it returned daily.

Limit Setting

Limit setting is the formal use of imposed limits on students. All teachers have certain limits of behaviors that they will tolerate without any consequences. Once those limits are exceeded, however, teachers need to consistently apply consequences. Limit setting is when teachers formally acknowledge those limits. This can be accomplished by establishing and posting rules (as noted), using checkmarks on the board to reveal which students are getting close to the imposed limits, or restating rules to students who are getting close to exceeding the limits.

In classrooms without limits, students will frequently "test" the teacher to see how far they can go in bending rules. Objectively stating limits that are reinforced will reduce this "testing." Of course, teachers must implement consequences when the limits are reached or the entire system will lack credibility and will therefore not be effective in managing behaviors.

Group Oriented Strategies

One way to implement behavior management strategies is through the context of a peer group. Salend (1987) calls this group-oriented behavior management strategies. The basic premise underlying this approach is that group members help modify individual behaviors. The following are some advantages of this model over individual management strategies.

1. Group cooperation and collaboration is enhanced.

2. Students learn to be responsible to other group members and how to solicit help from group members.

3. Teachers are able to spend time on more productive activities other than behavior mangement.

4. Group activities help students adapt to multiple settings.

The group system can be used effectively with group behavior games and group activities. Peer pressure could be a negative side effect; however, teachers should encourage positive group interactions to avoid negative peer pressures.

Other Classroom Management Techniques

Regardless of the effectiveness that behavior management techniques frequently have with students, there are times when their use simply does not improve behaviors. There are several reasons why behavior management approaches may be ineffective with some children. These include (Westling & Koorland, 1986):

- *Ineffective Consequences*   Sometimes teachers simply cannot find positive reinforcers, negative reinforcers, or punishments that are effective.

- *Contingencies too Difficult*   For some students, the contingencies set up are too difficult for the student to achieve. If they are not achieved within a reasonable period of time, the student will likely lose interest.

- *Distracting Environment*   Some physical settings present so many competing stimuli that the student cannot focus on the appropriate behaviors.

- *Learning Assignment too Difficult*   The learning activity set up as the requirement may not be achievable by the student.

- *General Inconsistency*   Teachers do not apply consequences, either positive or negative reinforcers, consistently; this causes confusion for students.

- *Inadequate Identification of Target Behavior*   There may be a lack of clarity in the behavior targeted for change.

- *Inadequate Observation and Measurement*   The teacher may have poor ways to observe and measure desired behaviors; small behavior changes may thus go unchanged.

- *Cumbersome System*   The entire behavior management system may be difficult to implement effectively. Teachers need to keep the system as simple as possible.

When other techniques need to be used, teachers and parents have several different approaches they can select. The following describes some of these alternative methods.

INTERSPERSED REQUESTS

Sprague and Horner (1990) describe a method of preventing inappropriate behaviors called interspersed requests. This approach works by first getting students to perform tasks that they can readily accomplish and that they like to do. These tasks should be actions that are capable of being completed successfully, require only a short time to complete, and are likely to be successful. Teachers should have students perform two to five of these kinds of activities, then request that a less desirable task be completed. Studies have revealed that this approach can reduce aggressive behaviors (Sprague & Horner, 1990).

TIME OUT

Time out is when students are physically isolated from other students. They are placed in a separate part of the classroom, time out room, booth, or some other physical setting that results in an isolation from any reinforcement. This type of placement may be necessary if a student is so disruptive that the behaviors are interfering with the remainder of students in the classroom. These procedures have been proven effective in reducing inappropriate behaviors (Rakow & Krutchinsky, 1986; Barton, Brulle, & Repp, 1987; Sherburne, Utley, McConnell, & Gannon, 1988).

There is a wide continuum of activities that can be considered as time out. These include:

- not allowing students to interact with a particular student who remains at his desk,

- having a student put her head down on her desk and not interact with other students,

- having the student sit in a separate section of the classroom,

- physically removing the student from the classroom to another classroom setting, and

- physically removing the student from the classroom to a special time-out room.

This last option is the most restrictive and should be used only as a last resort. The appropriate level of time-out for specific behaviors should be determined by the teacher prior to having to implement time-out options.

School personnel need to be very cautious when using time out. They need to ensure that the child is safe, that the child is monitored routinely, and that time out does not become a habitual placement for some students. Due to the nature of placing students in time-out settings, most states have specific guidelines that must be followed. These could include:

- size and physical characteristics of the time-out area;

- ways to observe students in the time-out area;

- time limits for length of time out (generally not to exceed thirty minutes);

- specific behaviors that can result in time-out placement;

- limitations on the frequency students can be placed in time-out;

- IEP requirements for using time-out placements.

EXCLUSIONARY DISCIPLINE PRACTICES

Suspension and expulsion are two methods of removing students from the classroom and the school when the degree of inappropriate behaviors warrant such extremes. Schools have frequently invoked these two measures for all students who display significantly inappropriate behaviors, not just those who have disabilities. Students who get into fights, are under the influence of alcohol or drugs, or consistently defy teachers may be suspended or expelled.

Suspension is generally a short period of time, usually a few days, when students are not allowed to attend school. Expulsion, on the other hand, is the more extreme of these measures. Expulsion may be keeping students out of school for the remainder of the school year or semester. Expulsion may result in being excluded from the school for several months. While these methods have been used in schools with all children, including those with disabilities, recent court rulings have questioned the practice for students whose disabilities can be shown to be directly related to the inappropriate behaviors.

Rose (1988) surveyed more than 250 principals regarding their use of suspension and expulsion to deal with inappropriate behaviors of students with disabilities. The results indicated that the behaviors most likely to lead to suspensions were disruptive behaviors, such as fighting. Other actions that caused frequent suspensions or expulsions were being tardy or cutting classes, disrespecting rules and people, and being defiant.

In 1988, the United States Supreme Court handed down a ruling in *Honig v. Doe* that dealt with the proposed expulsion of two students with emotional problems and aggressive tendencies. The ruling found for the students and underlined the fact that students cannot be expelled from schools for behaviors that are directly related to their disabilities. As a result, special educators and administrators must take steps to meet the unique needs of students with behavior problems and avoid having to determine the relationship between behaviors and disabilities (Bartlett, 1989). If expulsion is warranted, due process steps must be taken by school personnel.

PUNISHMENT

Punishment can be defined as imposing undersirable consequences following a particular behavior (Slavin, 1988). When at all possible, behavior should be managed or changed using positive means; punishment should be used only when other means are ineffective. Punishment can take several different forms, including time out, which was previously described. Other likely forms of punishment include:

- taking away privileges, such as free time;

- requiring students to do extra work, such as writing exercises;

■ retaining students after school;

■ corporal punishment.

While punishment is a less desirable method of managing behaviors than positive reinforcement, teachers may find it necessary. When using punishment, there are several general suggestions to use. Table 9–10 describes these different ways.

In situations where punishment is used to manage and control students' behaviors, school personnel must consider the legal ramifications (Bartlett, 1989). Moriarity (1986) suggests that school officials consider three principles when using punishment. These include 1. understanding the legal issues involved in the punishment, 2. developing interventions that can be upheld in the courts, and 3. developing interventions that are sensitive to the social and economic status of the community. As a result of litigation, teachers and

TABLE 9–10 Ways to Use Punishment Effectively

■ Maintain administrative permission to use punishment in writing.

■ Do not use punishment for revenge; never use punishment when you are angry.

■ Always be consistent when applying punishment. If rules have been broken, prior-stated consequences must be used.

■ Give a minimum of one warning, but never more than two or three before using punishment.

■ Keep records of punishment used for each student. If the same students are being punished regularly, then the punishment is obviously not being effective.

■ Punishment is more effective if it is brief and more aversive than an on-going punishment.

■ Do not use punishment as the only method of controlling students' behaviors.

■ Once the decision has been made to use punishment, use it immediately following inappropriate behaviors.

■ Students should be placed in time out to "cool off" immediately following punishment.

■ Determine what reinforcers are maintaining the inappropriate behaviors and attempt to remove them.

Source: Westling and Koorland (1988). *The special educator's handbook*. Boston: Allyn & Bacon.

other school personnel must consider their legal position and the rights of students when applying punishment.

MEDICATION

An intervention technique for managing behavior that has become very popular during the past decade is medication. Medication is the most widely used intervention strategy for students classified as having attention-deficit/hyperactivity (Ellenwood & Felt, 1989). A wide variety of medications have been found to be effective with children's behavior problems. These include stimulants, tranquilizers, anticonvulsants, and antidepressants or mood altering drugs (Westling, 1986; Forness & Kavale, 1988).

Although medications are currently used extensively to control behavior problems, there is a significant controversy regarding their use. Probably the most commonly used type of medication for children with behavior disorders is stimulant drugs, such as Ritalin and Dexedrine. These drugs generally result in a very quick increase in attention. Drugs considered tranquilizers include Thorazine, Haldol, and Mellaril. These drugs have a slower effect on students' behaviors, and may result in the reduction of aggressive behaviors (Forness & Kavale, 1988).

Anticonvulsants are primarily used with children who experience seizures. Common drugs in this group include Dilantin, Mysoline, Phenobarbitol, and Tegretol. These drugs, as well as those from the fourth group, antidepressants, have not been studied extensively. In light of the reported fact that many students classified as having emotional problems are likely taking these medications, a lack of research is alarming (Forness & Kavale, 1988).

If medication is used as a means for managing behaviors, several important points need to be considered. First of all, close monitoring of students on medication needs to occur. Teachers need to be aware of the medications students are taking, possible side effects, and specific characteristics to monitor. There needs to be close communication between teachers and parents and teachers and physicians regarding behaviors exhibited by students on medication (Ellenwood & Felt, 1989).

SELF-MANAGING OF BEHAVIORS

A common goal for all students is that they become effective in managing their own behaviors. Being able to control behaviors and follow classroom rules is critical to the success of all students. Teachers quickly develop a dislike for students who consistently cause them discipline problems. Acting out and attention seeking behaviors only disrupt the regular instructional activities and are therefore annoying to the teacher as well as to the other students. Many students without disabilities are capable of achieving this goal; they modify their own behaviors as they deem necessary based on their responding to external cues. Other students who are not disabled, and many students with disabilities, are not capable of self-monitoring their behaviors without interventions (Osborne, Kosiewicz, Crumley, & Lee, 1987). Therefore, teachers need to be aware of ways to teach students to use self-monitoring techniques and to appropriately respond to these techniques to modify behaviors.

There are numerous advantages for students monitoring their own behaviors. These include:

1.   Self-monitoring improves specific behaviors that are in need of modifications. By targeting behavior change for particular actions, students are likely to experience success.

2.   Self-monitoring stresses the role of students in their own behavior management. By participating in their own behavior change program, students are more likely to understand their behaviors and the need to change.

3.   Self-monitoring facilitates the generalization of behavior monitoring and appropriate behaviors to environments outside the school. For students entering the job market, or those simply trying to develop social relationships, this generalization can be invaluable.

4.   Self-monitoring enables teachers to focus their attention on other areas. Without students participating in their own behavior monitoring, teachers may have to focus on this activity.

5.   Self-monitoring helps students learn to take personal responsibility and helps them learn that they can, to some degree, determine their futures (Frith & Armstrong, 1986).

Students with diabilities may be oblivious to their own inappropriate behaviors. Without being cognizant of inappropriate behaviors that are exhibited, students will not likely modify those behaviors. Studies have shown that students with mild disabilities can be trained to self-record and self-monitor their behaviors (Osborne *et al*, 1987). Students can be taught how to monitor their behaviors and then be reinforced for their accomplishments of the target behavior, as well as their effective use of self-monitoring methods (Dunlap, Dunlap, Koegel, & Koegel, 1991). In one study, students with mild mental retardation used self-recording to improve their on-task behaviors and productivity (McCarl, Svobodny, & Beare, 1991).

One method that has been used to help students monitor their own behaviors is the self-monitoring mood chart. This approach enables students to chart their moods and feelings. Safran and Safran (1984) describe a chart that uses five different feelings—sad, withdrawn, bored, frustrated, and mean. Students circle how they fall in each of these areas. The advantage of the mood chart is that it is an easy and inexpensive system for helping students learn how to monitor their own feelings. Figure 9–4 (on page 356) presents an example of a self-monitoring mood chart.

REALITY THERAPY

Reality therapy is a method of teaching behavior self-control to students that was developed by Glasser (1965). Reality therapy is based on six assumptions.

1.   Individuals are responsible for their own behavior; any terms that would tend to excuse the behavior, such as "emotionally disturbed," are avoided.

2.   The past is rejected. Only the present and the future are of value in relating to the person's problem.

FIGURE 9–4 Mood Chart

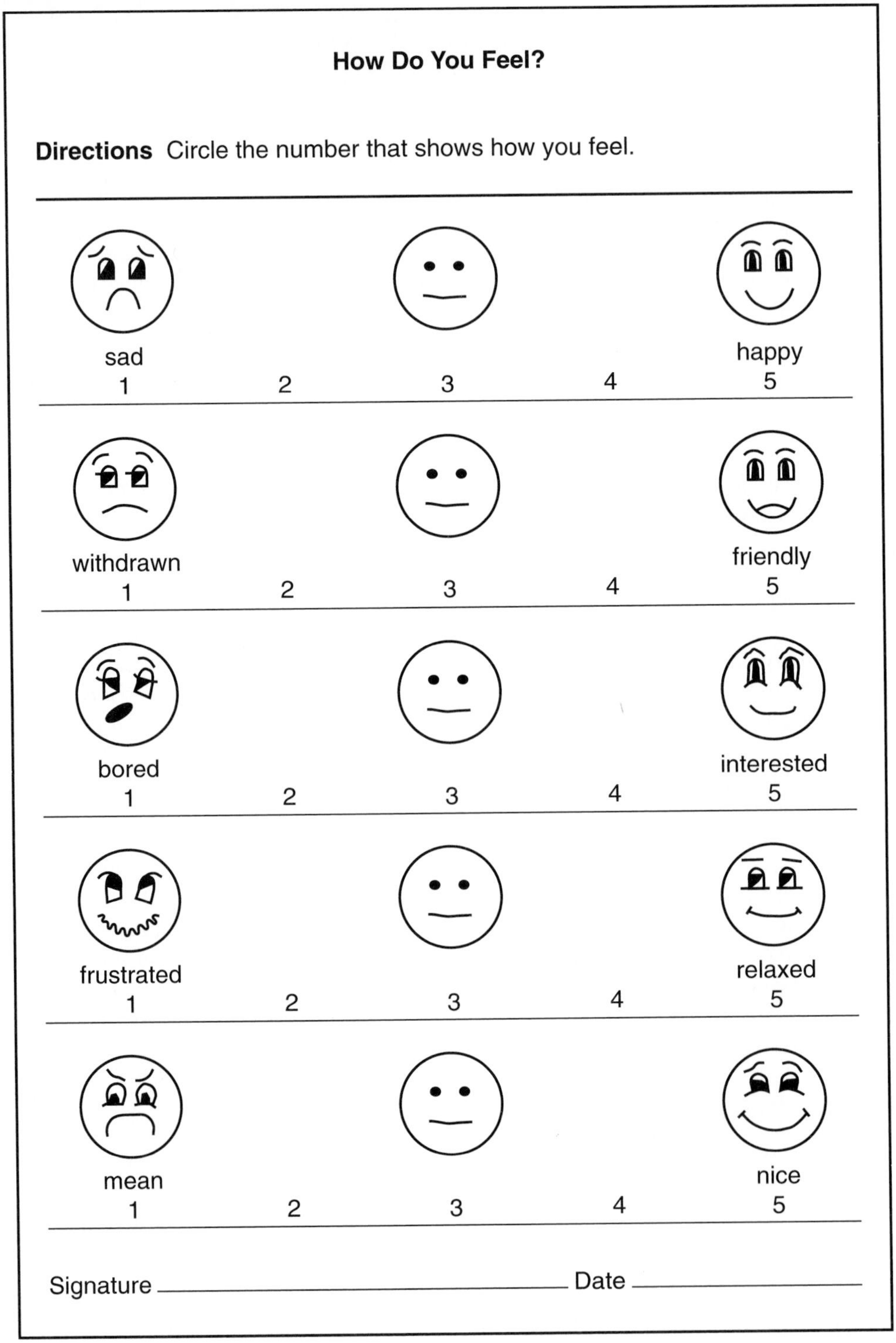

How Do You Feel?

Directions Circle the number that shows how you feel.

sad				happy
1	2	3	4	5

withdrawn				friendly
1	2	3	4	5

bored				interested
1	2	3	4	5

frustrated				relaxed
1	2	3	4	5

mean				nice
1	2	3	4	5

Signature ______________________________ Date ______________

Source: Safran and Safran (1984). The self-monitoring chart: Measuring affect in the classroom. *Teaching Exceptional Children*, *16*, p. 173. Used with permission.

3. The relationship between the teacher and the student is direct. The role of teacher as a transference figure is avoided.

4. Behaviors are never excused because of "unconscious motivation."

5. The morality of behavior is emphasized.

6. Students learn to satisfy needs in a socially acceptable manner. (Masters & Mori, 1986, p. 277)

Glasser believes that inappropriate behaviors are students' attempts to meet their needs, which are not being met in other ways (Wolfgang and Glick, 1986). In reality therapy, teachers constantly remind students of what is acceptable and unacceptable behavior and possible consequences of unacceptable behaviors. In addition, teachers are always in a supportive mode; they are there for the students and provide encouragement for appropriate behaviors (Heuchert, 1989).

When implementing reality therapy, teachers use a three-step format. First, the teacher tries to help the student understand about the inappropriate behaviors. In doing so, the teacher may ask questions such as, "Tell me what happened." and "What do you think will result from those behaviors?" In the second step, the teacher helps the student realize that their rationale for the behavior is faulty. Teachers do not accept irresponsibility of students as an excuse. Finally, the teacher instructs the student in more appropriate behaviors that would have resulted in a more positive outcome (Masters & Mori, 1986).

SUMMARY

This chapter has focused on the management of behaviors in the classroom. It was noted that teachers must manage behaviors in their classrooms if effective instruction is to occur. Students who are disruptive not only interfere with their own learning, but may prevent other students from learning effectively. Classroom management was described as all of the techniques and methods that teachers can use to control their classrooms.

The behavioral characteristics of students with disabilities were described. It was pointed out that students with learning disabilities and mental retardation account for about sixty percent of all students served in special education classes. These students, although their most publicized characteristics deal with academic deficits, experience significant problems with behavior. The third largest group of students served in special education classrooms, those with emotional and behavioral disorders, obviously exhibit behavior problems. Therefore, special education teachers must have sufficient knowledge about classroom management to effectively control their students.

Several different management strategies were discussed. These included general classroom factors, such as grouping, physical arrangement of the classroom and how teachers start and end the learning period. Specific behavior management strategies were also discussed. Different types of reinforcements, reinforcement schedules, and ways to arrange for reinforcements were included. Specific actions that teachers can take to plan and implement effective classroom management techniques were presented.

REFERENCES

Bartlett, L. (1989). Disciplining handicapped students: Legal issues in light of *Honig v. Doe*. *Exceptional Children, 55*, 357–366.

Barton, L.E., Brulle, A.R., & Repp, A.C. (1987). Effects of differential scheduling of timeout to reduce maladaptive responding. *Exceptional Children, 53*, 351–356.

Bender, W.N. (1987). Secondary personality and behavioral problems in adolescents with learning disabilities. *Journal of Learning Disabilities, 20*, 280–285.

Brady, M.P., & Taylor, R.D. (1989). Instructional consequences in mainstreamed middle school classes: Reinforcement and corrections. *Remedial and Special Education, 10*, 31–35.

D'Alonzo, B.J., & Miller, S.R. (1977). A management model for learning disabled adolescents. *Teaching Exceptional Children, 9*, 58–60.

Deaton, A.V. (1987). Behavioral change strategies for children and adolescents with severe brain injury. *Journal of Learning Disabilities, 20*, 581–589.

Deibert, A.N., & Harmon, A.J. (1973). *New tools for changing behavior*. Champaign, IL: Research Press.

DeLuke, S.V., & Knoblock, P. (1987). Teacher behavior as preventive discipline. *Teaching Exceptional Children, 19*, 18–24.

Duke, D.L., & Meckel, A.M. (1984). *Teacher's guide to classroom management*. New York: Random House.

Dunlap, L.K., Dunlap, G., Koegel, L.K., & Koegel, R.L. (1991). Using self-monitoring to increase independence. *Teaching Exceptional Children, 23*, 17–22.

Ellenwood, A.E., & Felt, D. (1989). Attention-deficit/hyperactivity disorder: Management and intervention approaches for the classroom teacher. *LD Forum, 15*, 15–17.

Epstein, M.H., Polloway, E.A., Patton, J.R., & Foley, R. (1989). Mild retardation: Student characteristics and services. *Education and Training in Mental Retardation, 24*, 7–16.

Etscheidt, S. (1991). Reducing aggressive behavior and improving self-control: A cognitive-behavioral training program for behaviorally disordered adolescents. *Behavioral Disorders, 16*, 107–115.

Evans, S.S., Evans, W.H., & Gable, R.A. (1989). An ecological survey of student behavior. *Teaching Exceptional Children, 21*, 12–15.

Feldman, D., Rosenberg, M.S., & Peer, G.G. (1984). Educational therapy: A behavior change strategy for pre-delinquent and delinquent youth. *Journal of Child and Adolescent Psychotherapy, 1*, 34–38.

Forness, S.R., & Kavale, K.A. (1988). Psychopharmacologic treatment: A note on classroom effects. *Journal of Learning Disabilities, 21*, 144–147.

Frith, G.H., & Armstron, S.W. (1986). Self-monitoring for behavior disordered students. *Teaching Exceptional Children, 18*, 144–148.

Gardner, W.I., Cole, C.L., Davidson, D.P., & Karan, O.C. (1986). Reducing aggression in individuals with developmental disabilities: An expanded stimulus control, assessment, and intervention model. *Education and Training in Mental Retardation, 21*, 3–12.

Gearheart, B.R., Weishahn, M.W., & Gearheart, C.J. (1988). *The exceptional student in the regular classroom*, 4th Ed. Columbus, OH: Merrill.

Glasser, W. (1965). *Reality therapy*. New York: Harper & Row.

Gallup, A.M. & Elam, S.M. (1988). The 20th Annual Gallup Poll of the public's attitudes toward the public schools. *Phi Delta Kappan, 70*, 33–46.

Glosser, G., & Koppell, S. (1987). Emotional-behavioral patterns in children with learning diabilities: Lateralized hemispheric differences. *Journal of Learning Disabilities, 20*, 365–368.

Greenwood, C.R. (1991). Longitudinal analysis of time, engagement, and achievement in at-risk versus non-risk students. *Exceptional Children, 57*, 521–535.

Heuchert, C.M. (1989). Enhancing self-directed behavior in the classroom. *Academic Therapy, 24*, 295–303.

Jones, H.Z., & Warren, S.F. (1991). Enhancing engagement in early language teaching. *Teaching Exceptional Children, 23*, 48–50.

Larson, K.A., & Gerber, M.M. (1987). Effects of social metacognitive training for enhancing overt behavior in learning disabled and low achieving delinquents. *Exceptional Children, 54*, 201–211.

Lerner, J. (1988). *Learning disabilities*, 5th Ed. Boston: Houghton Mifflin.

McCarl, J.J., Svobodny, L, & Beare, P.L. (1991). Self-recording in a classroom for students with mild to moderate mental handicaps: Effects on productivity and on-task behavior. *Education and Training in Mental Retardation, 26*, 79–88.

McWilliam, R.A. (1991). Targeting teaching at children's use of time: Perspectives on preschoolers' engagement. *Teaching Exceptional Children, 23, 42–43.*

Maher, C.A. (1987). Involving behaviorally disordered adolescents in instructional planning: Effectiveness of the GOAL procedure. *Journal of Child and Adolescent Psychotherapy, 4*, 204–210.

Maher, G.B. (1989). "Punch out": A behavior management technique. *Teaching Exceptional Children, 21*, 74.

Masters, L.F., & Mori, A.A. (1986). *Teaching secondary students with mild learning and behavior problems*. Rockville, Maryland: Aspen.

Mehring, T.A., & Colson, S.E. (1990). Motivation and mildly handicapped learners. *Focus on Exceptional Children, 22*, 1–14.

Mercer, C.D. (1987). *Students with learning disabilities*. Columbus, OH: Merrill.

Moriarity, J.K. (1986). Discipline and student rights. *Kappa Delta Pi Record, 22*, 91–93.

National Center for Education Statistics, (1988). *The condition of education, 1988 edition*. Washington, D.C.: U.S. Department of Education.

Nelson, C.M., Rutherford, R.B., Center, D.B., & Walker, H.M. (1991). Do public schools have an obligation to serve troubled children and youth? *Exceptional Children, 57*, 406–415.

O'Melia, M.C., & Rosenberg, M.S. (1989). Classroom management: Preventing behavior problems in classrooms for students with learning disabilities. *LD Forum, 15*, 23–26.

Olson, J. (1989). Managing life in the classroom: Dealing with the nitty gritty. *Academic Therapy, 24*, 545–553.

Osborne, S.S., Kosiewicz, M.M., Crumley, E.B., & Lee, C. (1987). Distractible students use self-monitoring. *Teaching Exceptional Children, 19,* 66–69.

Polloway, E.A., Epstein, M.H., & Cullinan, D. (1985). Prevalence of behavior problems among educable mentally retarded students. *Education and Training in Mental Retardation, 20,* 3–13.

Polloway, E.A., Epstein, M.H., Patton, J.R., Cullinan, D., & Luebke, J. (1987). Demographic, social, and behavioral characteristics of students with educable mental retardation. *Education and Training in Mental Retardation, 21,* 27–34.

Ragan, W.B., & Shepherd, G.D. (1977). *Modern elementary curriculum.* New York: Holt, Rinehart & Winston.

Rakow, S.J., & Krustchinsky, R. (1986). Discipline: Some guiding principles. *Kappa Delta Pi Record, 22,* 125–128.

Repp, A.C., Felce, D., & Barton, L.E. (1991). The effects of initial interval size on the efficacy of DRP schedules of reinforcement. *Exceptional Children, 57,* 417–425.

Rose, T.L. (1988). Current disciplinary practices with handicapped students: Suspensions and expulsions. *Exceptional Children, 55,* 230–239.

Safran, S., & Safran, J. (1984). The self-monitoring mood chart: Measuring affect in the classroom. *Teaching Exceptional Children, 16,* 172–175.

Salend, S.J. (1987). Group oriented behavior management strategies. *Teaching Exceptional Children, 20,* 53–55.

Salend, S.J. (1990). *Effective mainstreaming.* New York: MacMillan.

Sherburne, S., Utley, B., McConnell, S., & Gannon, J. (1988). Describing violent or aggressive theme play among preschool children with behavior disorders. *Exceptional Children, 55,* 166–172.

Slavin, R.E. (1988). *Educational psychology: Theory into practice,* 2nd Ed. Englewood Cliffs, New Jersey: Prentice-Hall.

Smith, T.E.C. (1990). *Introduction to education,* 2nd Ed. St. Paul: West Publishing.

Spooner, F., Test, D.W., & Jolly, A.C. (1990). Precision teaching: Using a nonaversive procedure to decrease refusals. *Teaching Exceptional Children, 22,* 55–57.

Sprague, J.R., & Horner, R.H. (1990). Easy does it: Preventing challenging behaviors. *Teaching Exceptional Children, 23,* 13–15.

Stainback, W., Stainback, S., Etscheidt, S., & Doud, J. (1986). A nonintrusive intervention for acting-out behavior. *Teaching Exceptional Children, 19,* 38–41.

Sugai, G. (1986). Recording classroom events: Maintaining a critical incidents log. *Teaching Exceptional Children, 18,* 98–102.

Sulzer-Azaroff, B., & Mayer, G.R. (1991). *Behavior analysis for lasting change.* Fort Worth: Holt, Rinehart and Winston.

Walker, J.E., & Shea, T.M. (1984). *Behavior management: A practical approach for educators,* 3rd Ed. St. Louis: C.V. Mosby.

Westling, D.L. (1986). *Introduction to mental retardation.* Englewood Cliffs, NJ: Prentice-Hall.

Westling, D.L., & Koorland, M.A. (1986). *The special educator's handbook.* Boston: Allyn & Bacon.

Whaley, K.T., & Bennett, T.C. (1991). Promoting engagement in early childhood special education. *Teaching Exceptional Children, 23,* 51–54.

Wiener, J., Harris, P.J., & Shirer, C. (1990). Achievement and social-behavioral correlates of peer status in LD children. *Learning Disability Quarterly, 13*, 114–127.

Wolfgang, C., & Glickman, C. (1986). *Comprehensive classroom management.* Boston: Allyn & Bacon.

Wood, P.C. (1987). A game to prevent disciplinary problems. *Teaching Exceptional Children, 19*, 52–53.

Woolfolk, A.E. (1990). *Educational psychology*, 4th Ed. Englewood Cliffs, NJ: Prentice-Hall.

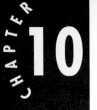

Teaching Social Skills

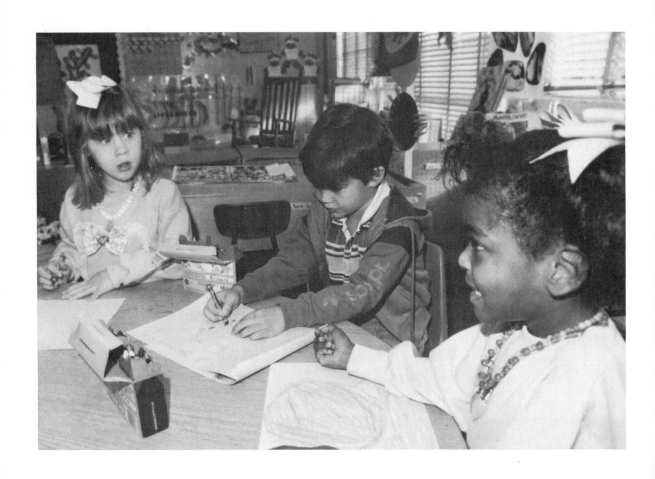

Outline

OBJECTIVES

After reading this chapter, you should be able to:

- define social skills;

- describe the nature of social skills;

- discuss why social skills instruction is important with students with disabilities;

- describe the different ways to assess social skills;

- list the general considerations in teaching social skills;

- describe some of the methods used for teaching social skills;

- describe at least one social skills lesson.

Introduction

Social skills are those skills people perform in everyday life that impact on their acceptance or rejection by others in their environments. People are often liked or disliked, employed or unemployed, and accepted or rejected based on the social skills they exhibit. The ways people look and act go a long way in how they are thought of, and accepted by others. Social skills, therefore, permeate all aspects of our lives from school to work, social to leisure. The criticality of persons possessing appropriate social skills is undeniable (Sargent, 1991).

For many years, educators believed that students with disabilities were best served when instructional time was spent on teaching academic skills, prevocational skills, and vocational skills. Educators thought these skills were the most critical for persons with mental retardation, learning disabilities, and emotional problems to develop to maximize their chances for later success. Social skills training, for the most part, was considered a luxury, something that was taught if there were time available after other topics had been completed.

Recently, educators have begun to realize the importance of social skills instruction because of the essential nature of these skills to successful placement in regular classrooms (Nelson, 1988) and to the future success of adults (Cosden, Iannaccone, & Wienke, 1990). Many students with mild disabilities who have the academic abilities to succeed in regular classrooms experience failure because of deficiencies in social skills (Nelson, 1988).

For most children and adolescents, social skills develop automatically (Sargent, 1991). These skills are frequently learned through modeling, observations, and trial and error. Some parents informally teach social skills to their children by emphasizing the use of courtesy and manners. Social skills can also be learned in Sunday school, scouting, or while participating in athletic events. However, for many students with disabilities, deficits in social skills are common (Nelson, 1988; Cosden *et al.*, 1990).

THE NATURE OF SOCIAL SKILLS

Social skills include a variety of different behaviors and characteristics. Unlike skills in reading, math, and other academic areas, social skills are more difficult to define (Luftig, 1989). In general, they can be described as "those skills necessary to accommodate the demands of society and, at the same time, maintain satisfactory interpersonal relationships" (Masters & Mori, 1986, p. 259).

Swanson and Watson (1989) note that there are three different ways to define social skills. These include definitions that relate to 1. peer acceptance, 2. behavior orientations, and 3. social interpretations. Using the first focus, individuals are considered to have social competence if they are accepted by their peers. The behavioral definition targets behaviors that "maximize the probability of reinforcement being maintained in a social context" (Swanson & Watson, 1989, p. 284).

In definitions that are developed around a social or ecological context, individuals are considered socially competent if they are accepted by their peers, are perceived as socially competent by significant others, and there is some agreement between peer acceptance and the judgment of significant others (Swanson & Watson, 1989). Social competence is facilitated by the presence of social skills. Social skills are therefore a critical set of skills for most people. Individuals with great competencies in social skills can achieve some levels of success strictly based on those skills. Likewise, persons with social skill deficits may be very competent in certain areas but fail simply because of their limited social skills.

Social Skills and Students with Mild Disabilities

As noted, the majority of children and adolescents develop social competence naturally; they do not have to be formally taught social skills. However, for many students with disabilities, social skills competence is significantly lacking (Andersen, Nelson, Fox, & Gruber, 1988; Nelson, 1988; Sargent, 1991). Students with mental retardation (Andrasik & Matson, 1985; Furnham, 1989; Patton, Payne, & Beirne-Smith, 1990; Forness & Kavale, 1991), learning disabilities (Carlson, 1987; Wallace & McLoughlin, 1988; Gresham & Elliott, 1989; Ritter, 1989; Ness & Price, 1990), and emotional problems (Kauffman, 1989) have been shown to exhibit significant deficits in social skills.

In addition to deficits in social skills, research reveals that students with disabilities also have different social goals than their nondisabled peers. Data also suggest that although the majority of students with disabilities display social deficits, some of these students compare equally with their nondisabled peers (Carlson, 1987).

If a lack of social competence resulted in minimal negative consequences, then special education teachers would not need to focus so much of their attention on teaching these skills. However, the reality is that problems in social skills can result in extremely negative consequences for students and adults with disabilities. Many students with disabilities are failing in mainstreamed settings because of poor social skills (Nelson, 1988). Also, studies have found that most adults with disabilities who lose their jobs do so because of poor social skills and inappropriate behaviors, not limited job skills (Sargent, 1988). Sabornie and Beard (1990) reviewed several studies and concluded that deficits in social skills can result in 1. low social status among their nonhandicapped peers, 2. low participation rates in school-related and out-of-school activities, 3. dissatisfaction with their social lives, 4. fewer friendships than their nonhandicapped cohorts, and 5. more loneliness and isolation in school than their nonhandicapped counterparts" (p. 35).

Children and adults with disabilities often have limited skills in many areas, including academic , emotional, and vocational. As a result of their having limitations in these areas, these individuals definitely need to be competent socially. Social competence can go a long way in overcoming the negative consequences of other deficit areas. For example, if a young adult woman has good social skills but limited abilities in written expression, it is likely that she can still get a job that requires meeting and greeting the public; however, if she also has social skill deficits, her chances for success in a job that requires her to deal with people are limited.

One of the major reasons social skills are so important for school-aged children with disabilities is the trend to provide educational services in the least restrictive environment. As a result, the majority of students with mild disabilities receive a significant portion of their educational program in a regular classroom (Smith, Price, & Marsh, 1986). Social competence will greatly facilitate their chances for being accepted by their nondisabled peers and their chances for academic success (Nelson, 1988).

Adults with disabilities also need to have social competence. Getting and maintaining jobs, getting along with neighbors, and general functioning in social settings require a certain level of social competence. Unfortunately, many adults with disabilities have been shown to exhibit major deficits in their social skills (Ness & Price, 1990). These social skill deficits frequently result in interpersonal problems as well as problems on-the-job. Adults with disabilities who exhibit significant social skill deficits have a difficult time leading successful, independent lives.

Assessment of Social Skills

Just as assessment in academic areas is important before developing intervention programs, teachers need to ascertain the social skills competence of individuals prior to implementing training programs. Without an adequate evaluation of a student's social skills, teachers are not able to accurately determine on which skills to focus. Unfortunately, as a result of a lack of agreement on a definition of social competence, assessment is difficult (Herbert, 1986).

Due to disagreements and the nebulous nature of social skills, there are some inherent difficulties in their assessment. Luftig (1989) notes three problems in the assessment of social skills. The first problem deals with the fact that many social behaviors are directly related to a specific situation. Individuals may display certain social behaviors in some settings, and totally different social behaviors in another. Similar to pragmatics in oral expression, individuals often alter their behaviors related to the situation. This makes valid assessment very difficult. If a child is evaluated in a setting where social skill deficits are not obvious, the results may reveal no problems are present, when, in fact, the student exhibits many social skill deficits in other environments or at other times. One way to help deal with this problem is to collect as much information about a student's social skills as possible in a variety of settings and sites.

A second problem in assessing social skills is the different ways people interpret behaviors. For example, what you might think is socially inappropriate might be considered acceptable by another professional. Since people have very different opinions about appropriate dress and actions, it is difficult to evaluate these skills with any degree of standardization. Again, collecting as much information as possible, from a variety of sources, will help deal with this problem.

The final problem with social skills assessment is the reliability of the evaluator. Since a great deal of assessment data in this area is collected using observations and interviews, reliability becomes a major issue (Luftig, 1989). Collecting information from several sources by a variety of different people will help educators validly assess social skills. This means the assessment of social skills has to be a team effort; school personnel cannot limit their analysis of a student's social skills to the evaluation completed by the psychometrist in a two- or three-hour setting.

The problems inherent in assessing social skills have resulted in numerous criticisms of the assessment/intervention process. These include:

- lack of attention to relationships between training procedures and specific subject characteristics,

- nonempirical methods of selecting target behaviors,

- failure to specify situational determinants of selected skills, and

- failure to use socially valid outcome measures (Maag, 1989, p. 6).

Regardless of these problems in assessing social skills, educators must develop an understanding of the social competence of students before they can create and implement appropriate intervention programs. Providing training in specific social skills areas without knowing if students have deficiencies is making inefficient use of time (Maag, 1989). Teachers must identify specific deficits in social skills (Gresham, 1981), in order to implement appropriate instructional programs. Therefore, although difficult, assessment of social skills must be completed.

The assessment of social skills is normally accomplished through formal, standardized instruments, systematic observations, informal assessments, self-reporting systems, and sociometric methods (Luftig, 1989). The following discussion presents examples of each of these areas.

FORMAL ASSESSMENT OF SOCIAL SKILLS

Formal, norm-referenced assessment of social skills is generally accomplished using checklists and behavior rating scales. When using these types of instruments, persons familiar with the student, such as parents, teachers, and other adults in the student's environment, are asked to provide the necessary information. These scales differ significantly. Some are broad based and cover a wide range of social skills, while others may focus on one area, such as how students get along with their peers. Also, some scales require the rater to simply indicate "yes" or "no," while others require a rating based on degree of expression. An advantage of most of these types of instruments is that they are generally easy to complete (Luftig, 1989). An obvious disadvantage in having these forms of assessment is that bias can enter into the ratings.

Despite flaws in collecting assessment data from individuals with biased opinions, information obtained from these assessments can provide very valuable insights into the social skills of students (Masters & Mori, 1986). One reason for this is the closeness between the students being evaluated and those collecting the assessment data. This, in many respects, is much better than a stranger (psychometrist) having a student go to a testing room and asking him questions. Table 10–1 (page 368) describes examples of these kinds of instruments.

TABLE 10-1 Examples of Formal Assessment Instruments to Measure Social Skills

INSTRUMENT	DESCRIPTION
The Behavior Rating Profile (Brown & Hammil 1978)	■ used with students 1st–12th grades ■ completed by parents, peers, teachers, & students ■ helps identify settings where inappropriate behaviors occur
The Devereux Adolescent Behavior Rating Scale (Spivack, Spotts, & Haimes, 1967)	■ used with 13–18 year-olds ■ looks at factors such as poor emotional control & peer dominance ■ looks at behavior toward adults
The Pupil Behavior Inventory (Vinter, Sarri, Vorwaller, & Schaefer, 1966)	■ for 7th–12th grades ■ rates using a 5-point scale ■ rates classroom behavior, academic motivation & performance, social-emotional status, teacher dependence, & personal behavior
The Vineland Social Maturity Scale (Doll, 1965)	■ birth–adulthood ■ includes 8 categories ■ completed by primary caretaker

Source: Masters & Mori (1986).

INFORMAL ASSESSMENT OF SOCIAL SKILLS

Assessment of social skills depends on the informed judgment of various individuals, such as teachers and parents. This assessment can result from formal instruments, like those described in table 10–1, or it can be obtained from teacher developed, informal checklists. Information collected by teachers using these formats can often lead to effective intervention techniques because the information is collected in natural settings and is directly related to what the child normally does. Table 10–2 presents an example of a checklist for social skills.

Checklists and behavior rating forms provide a structured means for collecting, tabulating, and summarizing information. Collecting the information necessary to complete these checklists is generally accomplished in one of several ways, including observations, interviews, peer assessment, self-reports, and sociometric methods.

Observations

One of the most effective means for informally assessing social skills is through observations (Gresham, 1981). Teachers are in ideal situations to observe students in natural

TABLE 10-2 School and Community Social Skills Rating Checklist

Student's Name: _____   Birthdate: _____

Sex: _____ Male _____ Female   Date: _____

School: _____   Rater: _____

Current grade level or class assignment: _____   Special education classification: _____

DIRECTIONS: This social skills rating form is designed to be used with the *Social Skills for School and Community* instructional materials. Rate each of the skills using one of the following ratings:

Rating

3   = The child possesses the skill and performs it adequately and with sufficient frequency.

2   = The child possesses the skill and performs it adequately but not with sufficient frequency.

1   = The student possesses the skill but performs it inadequately (e.g., student leaves out part of the skill or uses wrong language when performing the skill).

0   = The student does not have the skill.

N   = Rater has no knowledge of the child's ability to perform the skill.

NA = The skill is not age appropriate and would only be used by an older student.

Social Skills for School and Community lessons are coded:

P = Primary, **I** = Intermediate, **JH** = Middle School/Junior High, and **SH** = Senior High.

CLASSROOM RELATED BEHAVIORS
SOCIAl SKILLS FOR SCHOOL AND COMMUNITY

Rating	The Student Adequately and Appropriately:	Lesson Prepared at Level
_____ 1.	attends to teacher during instruction.	P-C-1
_____ 2.	maintains correct sitting posture.	P-C-2
_____ 3.	gains the teacher's attention.	P-C-3
_____ 4.	answers questions asked by teachers.	P-C-4
_____ 5.	asks teacher for assistance or information.	P-C-5
_____ 6.	shares materials with classmates.	P-C-6
_____ 7.	keeps own desk in order.	P-C-7
_____ 8.	enters class without disruption.	P-C-8
_____ 9.	follows classroom rules.	I-C-1
_____ 10.	cooperates with work partners.	I-C-2
_____ 11.	ignores distractions.	I-C-3
_____ 12.	stays on task during seatwork.	I-C-4
_____ 13.	completes work on time.	I-C-5
_____ 14.	participates politely in classroom discussion.	I-C-6
_____ 15.	makes relevant remarks during classroom discussion.	I-C-7

continued

CLASSROOM RELATED BEHAVIORS (continued)
SOCIAL SKILLS FOR SCHOOL AND COMMUNITY

Rating	The Student Adequately and Appropriately:	Lesson Prepared at Level
_____	16. follows verbal directions.	I-C-8
_____	17. follows written directions.	I-C-9
_____	18. speaks politely about schoolwork.	I-C-10
_____	19. participates in classroom introductions.	I-C-11
_____	20. completes homework on time.	JH-C-1
_____	21. uses free time in class productively.	SH-C-1
_____ Subtotal	Number of Items Scored _____	

SCHOOL BUILDING RELATED BEHAVIORS
SOCIAL SKILLS FOR SCHOOL AND COMMUNITY

Rating	The Student Adequately and Appropriately:	Lesson Prepared at Level
_____	22. follows procedures for boarding school bus.	P-SB-1
_____	23. follows bus riding rules.	P-SB-2
_____	24. walks through hallways and passes to class.	P-SB-3
_____	25. waits in lines.	P-SB-4
_____	26. uses rest room facilities.	P-SB-5
_____	27. uses drinking fountain.	P-SB-6
_____	28. follows lunchroom rules.	P-SB-7
_____	29. uses table manners.	P-SB-8
_____	30. responds to school authorities.	JH-SB-1
_____	31. deals with accusations at school.	SH-SB-1
_____ Subtotal	Number of Items Scored _____	

PERSONAL SKILLS
SOCIAL SKILLS FOR SCHOOL AND COMMUNITY

Rating	The Student Adequately and Appropriately:	Lesson Prepared at Level
_____	32. says "please" and "thank you."	P-PS-1
_____	33. speaks in tone of voice for the situation.	P-PS-2
_____	34. takes turns in games and activities.	P-PS-3
_____	35. tells the truth.	P-PS-4
_____	36. accepts consequences for wrong doing.	P-PS-5
_____	37. maintains grooming.	I-PS-1

PERSONAL SKILLS (continued)
SOCIAL SKILLS FOR SCHOOL AND COMMUNITY

Rating	The Student Adequately and Appropriately:	Lesson Prepared at Level
_____	38. avoids inappropriate physical contact.	I-PS-2
_____	39. exhibits hygienic behavior.	I-PS-3
_____	40. expresses enthusiasm.	I-PS-4
_____	41. makes positive statements about self.	I-PS-5
_____	42. expresses anger in nonaggressive ways.	I-PS-6
_____	43. accepts praise.	JH-PS-1
_____	44. stays out of fights.	JH-PS-2
_____	45. deals with embarrassment.	JH-PS-3
_____	46. chooses clothing for social events.	JH-PS-4
_____	47. deals with failure.	SH-PS-1
_____	48. deals with being left out.	SH-PS-2

_____ Subtotal   Number of Items Scored _____

INTERACTION INITIATIVE SKILLS
SOCIAL SKILLS FOR SCHOOL AND COMMUNITY

Rating	The Student Adequately and Appropriately:	Lesson Prepared at Level
_____	49. greets peers.	P-II-1
_____	50. borrows from peers.	P-II-2
_____	51. asks other children to play.	P-II-3
_____	52. expresses sympathy.	I-II-1
_____	53. asks peers for help.	I-II-2
_____	54. makes invitations.	I-II-3
_____	55. introduces self.	JH-II-1
_____	56. makes introductions.	JH-II-2
_____	57. initiates conversations.	JH-II-3
_____	58. joins activities with peers.	JH-II-4
_____	59. congratulates peers and adults.	JH-II-5
_____	60. makes apologies.	JH-II-6
_____	61. excuses self from groups and conversations.	JH-II-7
_____	62. expresses feelings.	SH-II-1
_____	63. expresses affection.	SH-II-2
_____	64. stands up for a friend.	SH-II-3
_____	65. asks for dates.	SH-II-4
_____	66. gives compliments.	SH-II-5
_____	67. makes complaints.	SH-II-6

_____ Subtotal   Number of Items Scored _____

continued

INTERACTION RESPONSE SKILLS
SOCIAL SKILLS FOR SCHOOL AND COMMUNITY

Rating	The Student Adequately and Appropriately:	Lesson Prepared at Level
_____	68. smiles when encountering acquaintances.	P-IR-1
_____	69. listens when another child speaks.	I-IR-1
_____	70. participates in group activities.	I-IR-2
_____	71. helps peers when asked.	I-IR-3
_____	72. accepts ideas different from own.	I-IR-4
_____	73. meets with adults.	I-IR-5
_____	74. maintains conversations.	JH-IR-1
_____	75. responds to teasing and name calling.	JH-IR-2
_____	76. responds to constructive criticism.	SH-IR-1
_____	77. recognizes feelings of others.	SH-IR-2
_____	78. respects the space of others.	SH-IR-3
_____	79. responds to peer pressure.	SH-IR-4
_____	80. deals with an angry person.	SH-IR-5
_____	81. makes refusals.	SH-IR-6
_____	82. answers complaints.	SH-IR-7

_____ Subtotal   Number of Items Scored _____

COMMUNITY RELATED SKILLS
SOCIAL SKILLS FOR SCHOOL AND COMMUNITY

Rating	The Student Adequately and Appropriately:	Lesson Prepared at Level
_____	83. asks for direction in public.	JH-CR-1
_____	84. gives directions.	JH-CR-2
_____	85. exhibits sportsmanship as a game participant.	JH-CR-3
_____	86. exhibits polite behavior and sportsmanship as a spectator.	JH-CR-4
_____	87. disposes of wastepaper and debris in public.	JH-CR-5
_____	88. respects the rights of others in public.	JH-CR-6
_____	89. respects private property.	JH-CR-7
_____	90. exhibits good audience behaviors.	JH-CR-8
_____	91. responds to public authority.	JH-CR-9
_____	92. asserts self to gain service.	JH-CR-10
_____	93. deals with public officials over the phone.	SH-CR-1

_____ Subtotal   Number of Items Scored _____

WORK RELATED SOCIAL SKILLS
SOCIAL SKILLS FOR SCHOOL AND COMMUNITY

Rating	The Student Adequately and Appropriately:	Lesson Prepared at Level
_____	94. sets goals for work.	SH-W-1
_____	95. negotiates on the job.	SH-W-2
_____	96. responds to unwarranted criticism.	SH-W-3
_____	97. asks for feedback on the job.	SH-W-4
_____	98. minds own business on the job.	SH-W-5
_____	99. chooses a time for small talk.	SH-W-6
_____	100. refrains from excessive complaining.	SH-W-7

_____ Subtotal   Number of Items Scored _____

SCORING
SOCIAL SKILLS FOR SCHOOL AND COMMUNITY

Strength Index	Subtotals	Items Scored
Step #1: Add		
Classroom Related Behaviors	_____	_____
School Building Related Behaviors	_____	_____
Personal Skills	_____	_____
Interaction Initiative Skills	_____	_____
Interaction Response	_____	_____
Community Related Skills	_____	_____
Work Related Skills	_____	_____
TOTALS	_____	_____

Step #2:   Divide the total score by the items scored.

Total score _____ ÷ Items scored _____

Step #3:   Multiply the quotient by 100.

$$\underset{\substack{\text{Total} \\ \text{Score}}}{\_\_\_\_} \div \underset{\substack{\text{Items} \\ \text{Scored}}}{\_\_\_\_} = \underset{\text{Quotient}}{\_\_\_\_} \times 100 = \underset{\substack{\text{Composite} \\ \text{Strength} \\ \text{Score}}}{\_\_\_\_}.$$

Growth Index
Post intervention rating.

     Total score of second rating: _____

     Minus (–) total score of first rating: _____

     Growth Score: _____

Source: Sargent, L. R. (1991). *Social skills for school and community*, 269–273. Reston, VA: Council for Exceptional Children, Division on Mental Retardation. Used with permission.

settings and interactions to obtain valuable assessment information. They are in a position to observe students over several time periods, which will enable them to obtain more useful information than a single observation.

There are basically three types of observations that can be used when assessing social skills.

1. *Event Recording*   This is the recording of specific behaviors with respect to duration and frequency.

2. *Time Sampling*   Using this method, behaviors are recorded during a specific time. This could answer the question "Does this behavior occur during the first five minutes of the class period?"

3. *Running Record*   A running record is used when the observer attempts to record all of the behaviors observed. Usually a coding system must be used with this approach (Gearheart & Gearheart, 1989).

Using event recording, teachers focus on one or two specific social skills. For example, a teacher might want to know how often a student displays "rude" behaviors to other students. The teacher would keep a frequency count of the number of times the student was rude to other students, as well as the duration of the episodes. The teacher might also keep a frequency count of interpersonal behaviors by the student that are considered appropriate. Time sampling of rude behaviors would target a specific time frame. For example, if the teacher thought that the rude behaviors were occurring during the first period of the school day, frequencies would be recorded only during the first few minutes of the period.

Teachers using a running record approach would have to be prepared for a much more extensive system for data recording. Teachers might choose this type of observation in situations where students are experiencing significant, generalized, social deficits. By recording all behaviors of a student during the day, or during several class periods, the teacher would be in a position to better understand the kinds of behaviors, frequencies, and duration of the behaviors throughout the day. This could result in the teacher realizing that certain inappropriate social behaviors occurred during certain periods of the day. This type of conclusion could lead to better intervention programs.

Regardless of which recording system is used, observations can occur in natural settings, such as the classroom, or contrived settings specifically established for the observation. Being able to observe the social skills of students in a variety of settings will make the information collected more valid. Whereas students may not "be themselves" in a contrived setting where information about social skills may be collected, they will more likely reflect their true social skills if observed over time and in several natural settings.

Observations in Natural Settings   By observing students in natural settings, teachers are able to understand the relationships between environmental antecedents and their consequences. This approach lends itself to operationally defining social skills and observing them in an environment where they normally occur (Maag, 1989). An advantage of this type of observation is that repeated measurements can be made without interruptions (Gresham, 1981). The most important advantage, however, is that the behaviors are observed in natural settings and are therefore likely to reflect a true picture of the student's social skills. The validity of the assessment should be high.

Examples of natural settings where social skills can be observed include classrooms, cafeterias, gym, auditorium, playground, home, and neighborhood. To obtain as accurate and comprehensive a picture as possible about a child's social competence, several observations should be made in more than one setting. This will enable information to be collected in a variety of social situations.

When observing students in natural settings, the teacher needs to do so in an unobtrusive manner. If the students realize that their behaviors are being observed for a specific purpose, they may actually alter those behaviors. Therefore, observations and the recording of the observations should be done as inconspicuously as possible. To do so, teachers should consider the following actions.

1. Observe students in settings where the presence of the teacher is routine.

2. Do not make obvious notes about students' behaviors.

3. Keep records incidentally, as if recording notes related to other activities.

4. Do not make obvious notes after an incident has occurred that would clue the students about the purpose of the note-taking.

5. Have the data sheet arranged in such a way that only frequencies have to be recorded rather than long, written notes.

6. Use some sort of code to reflect notes rather than specific descriptors, such as "talking back," "rude," or "unfriendly."

Observations in Contrived Settings   Often, teachers and evaluators set up situations in order to observe social skills. These "unnatural," or contrived situations are created when students are role playing various behaviors to produce specific social skills for assessment purposes.

There have been a lot of criticisms directed at role playing social situations for assessment purposes. The major criticism appears to be the lack of correspondence between the role-play situation and natural settings. However, even though this criticism has some validity, by setting up role-play situations to assess social skills, teachers are able to observe certain behaviors that are difficult to elicit in natural settings (Maag, 1989). Consumers of assessment information collected in contrived settings must keep in mind that these behaviors may or may not reflect actual behaviors in more natural situations.

Peer and Self-Report Assessment of Social Skills

Another informal means of social skills assessment is through peers and self-reports. For both of these sources of information, teachers and evaluators must take into consideration personal bias. Peers and individuals are likely to interpret social skills in a prejudicial context. While this fact should be taken into consideration during analysis of the assessment information, it should not preclude collecting information from these sources.

Peer Assessments   Asking peers about the social skills exhibited by individual students can be an excellent source of assessment data. Information collected from peers is often very valid because there is daily interaction between the person and peers (Luftig, 1989). Also, information can be collected from several peers and analyzed together. Peer

TABLE 10–3 Peer Evaluation Checklist

Characteristic/Behavior	Yes/No
1. Generally likes to be alone.	
2. Has many friends.	
3. Gets along well with other students.	
4. Likes school.	
5. Gets along well with teachers.	
6. Is usually in a good mood.	
7. Feels good about him or herself.	
8. Gets along well with parents.	
9. Rarely gets sick; generally healthy.	
10. Rarely gets angry.	
11. Generally ignores things he or she does not like.	
12. Worries about bad things a lot.	
13. Has trouble sleeping.	
14. Enjoys being around people.	
15. Gives up easily when cannot do something.	

Source: Adapted from Masters & Mori (1986).

evaluations are normally informal checklists. Table 10–3 presents an example of a peer checklist.

Teachers should never single out individual students when collecting information from peers. Rather than asking the class or some students to rate other, specific students, make the activity a group exercise. For example, have students complete a questionnaire or survey form that answers questions such as:

1. Which student in class is the friendliest?

2. Which student in class is the most unfriendly?

3. With which student in class do you enjoy working on class projects?

4. Which student(s) in class are difficult to get along with?

5. Which students in class have the best manners?

Group activities with these kinds of questions can help teachers gain a great deal of insight into the social skills of all students in the class without calling undue attention to specific students.

Self-Evaluations Students can be interviewed to determine their self-perceptions of social skills, or they can simply complete a questionnaire. Collecting information from students themselves is probably the most direct and efficient method for obtaining information concerning the social skills of a particular student (Maag, 1989). Of course, the obvious drawback is that students may not be honest. They may want themselves to look like they are better adjusted and exhibit more appropriate social skills than they actually do.

Teachers obviously have to take personal bias into consideration when analyzing the results of students' self-evaluations. Ways teachers can add validity to the process include 1. comparing the student's self-evaluation with data collected from other sources, 2. comparing the student's self-evaluation on social skills with other self-evaluations, such as academic self-evaluations and sports self-evaluations, and 3. having students complete self-evaluations more than one time to determine any differences from one rating to another.

Another way students can use self-evaluations in determining social skills is through self-monitoring. Students can keep open-ended diaries as well as rating their behaviors in specific social situations (Maag, 1989). Self-monitoring helps keep students aware of their behaviors at the time of occurrence and may therefore act as a cue for certain, appropriate actions. Figure 10–1 provides an example of a self-monitoring form.

FIGURE 10-1 Checklist for Self-Monitoring

Accepting Praise

Name: _____ Date: _____

School: _____

Directions: Fill in this form when someone praises you.

1. Who praised you? _____

                                            Circle

2. Did you listen to the person? yes no
3. Did you smile? yes no
4. Did you say thank you? yes no
5. Did you tell yourself not to brag? yes no
6. Did you say something bad about yourself? yes no
7. How did you do? ____good ____ok ____not so good

Source: Sargent, L.R. (1991). *Social skills for school and community*, p. 281. Reston, VA: Division on Mental Retardation, Council for Exceptional Children. Used with permission.

Sociometric Measures One additional method often used to assess social skills is through sociometric measurement. Sociometric assessment techniques determine how individual students are accepted in a group (Gresham, 1981). In the most popular form of sociometric assessment, students are asked to nominate one or more of their peers who they would like to work with on some activity (Wallace & McLoughlin, 1988). Examples of topics that could be used to collect information include:

- lunch partner,
- math partner,
- roommate,
- project leader,
- team member,
- "buddy" on a school trip (Guerin & Maier, 1983).

After the information is collected, a sociogram can be developed, which is a graphic illustration of the students different students choose. Figure 10–2 presents an example of such a sociogram.

Teachers wishing to collect information and develop a sociogram could use the following steps.

1. Determine which students should be included in the potential pool of students. This is usally the specific class the student has to interact.

2. Tell the students you are going to play a group game and you want them to help choose the teams. Make sure that you explain that the game is not related to academic skills (this should eliminate students being selected simply because of their academic competence).

3. Tell the students that each team has three players and that they should choose any two students in the class they want on their team.

4. Tell the students that in order to make the teams as fair as possible, they need to indicate which two students they definitely do not want on their team.

5. Collect the information and chart how often students get selected and by which students. Also determine which students are designated as those not wishing to be on a particular team.

6. After the information is collected, it is important for the teacher to follow through with some sort of group activity so the students will think that the exercise was actually related to the stated purpose.

Another form of sociometric measurement is called the Q-sort. Using this method, students are asked to sort a deck of printed cards that have various descriptors, such as

FIGURE 10-2   Example of a Sociogram

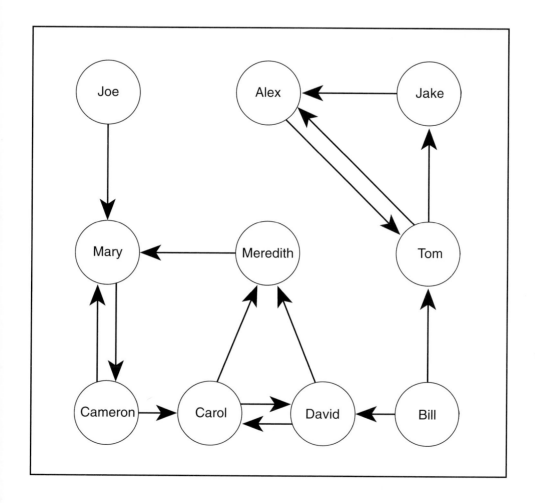

"disrupts class," "enjoys school," and "has many friends," based on "most like me" to "least like me." The student sorts the cards based on an ideal person and then on himself. A comparison is therefore provided between the student's evaluation of an "ideal" person and himself (Masters & Mori, 1986).

Q-sort cards can also be categorized onto a formboard with a Likert-like system. Figure 10–3 (on page 380) shows an example. By using the Q-sort method, teachers can not only find out how students feel about themselves, but they can also determine which social skills need attention first (Minner & Beane, 1985).

Still another method of using sociometric measures is the "guess who" technique. Using this model, teachers have students match various descriptors, which may include positive and negative, with names of students in the classroom (Hopkins, Stanley, & Hopkins,

FIGURE 10-3 Sample Formboard for Q-Sort.

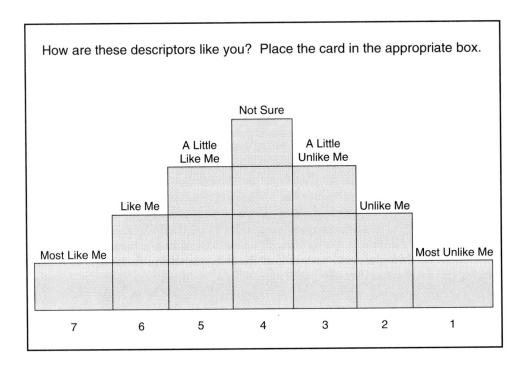

Source: Adapted from Minner, S., & Beane, A. (1985). Q-Sort for special education teachers. *Teaching Exceptional Children, 17*, 279–281.

1990). This, as well as other sociometric results, must be maintained with the strictest of confidentiality. It would only do harm to students to find out that their classmates assign negative descriptors to them or that they were "chosen" on only one team.

Teaching Social Skills

If students with disabilities are to have a chance to develop and enhance social skills, they must be provided with opportunities to learn these skills. However, just as the need for academic intervention programs differs among students with disabilities, so do the needs of these students for social skills training. Some students with mild disabilities may not need training in this area. For those students who require the training, it should be considered just as important, programmatically, as academic remediation (Sabornie & Beard, 1990).

Social skills training can occur in a variety of settings, including natural interactions in the classroom. However, since many students with mild disabilities have failed to develop social competence in natural settings and within natural interactions, specific social skills training may be necessary (Sargent, 1991). If students have not learned social skills incidentally by the time the problems become apparent, then special steps probably need to be taken to provide training opportunities.

These could include:

- implementing commercial programs to teach social skills;

- developing and implementing teacher-made activities to teach social skills;

- using direct instruction to teach specific social skills;

- including social skills training on the IEPs of some students who are experiencing significant skill deficits.

Special educators are beginning to realize the importance of social skills training. In fact, social skills programs are becoming more apparent in the special education curriculum for most students with disabilities (Nelson, 1988; Elksnin, 1989). The growth of social skills training has been so widespread that it is safe to say that social skills training is currently one of the most popular approaches for working with disabled students (L'Abate & Milan, 1985). Although additional reasearch needs to be completed regarding the efficacy of social skills instruction, the majority of research to this point suggests that such training efforts can result in positive gains for students with disabilities (Gresham, 1981; Anderson *et al.*, 1988; Blackbourn, 1989; Elksnin, 1989; Herbert, 1989).

GENERAL CONSIDERATIONS IN TEACHING SOCIAL SKILLS

Just as there are some general considerations when teaching reading, math, social studies, and other content areas, there are some general programming considerations for teaching social skills. Just saying you are going to teach social skills without planning specific social skills programs will probably be as unsuccessful as trying to teach students how to read without any thought to the reading curriculum, reading materials, or specific reading approach. Successfully teaching social skills does not simply happen. Teachers should consider several areas before implementing a social skills teaching program.

Group Instruction

By the very nature of social skills focusing on "social" activities, it should be taught in groups. A recommended group size is three to six students (Carter & Sugai, 1989). By teaching social skills in small groups, students are able to learn and practice specific behaviors with other group members. Other reasons for small group instruction include 1. peers usually provide better role models than adults and feedback is more meaningful and reinforcing in groups (Michelson & Mannarino, 1986) and 2. it is much more natural to teach students how to intereact with peers if peers are present during the training.

When teaching social skills to students using group instruction, the composition of the group is very important. Teachers should mix the groups with socially competent students and students who are experiencing deficits in social skills. This gives students the opportunity to model appropriate social skills and receive reinforcement for their actions. Teachers should also consider a continuous monitoring of the groups for possible regrouping when teaching different social skills. Again, having good role models for students who are experiencing difficulties is important. Since all students do not exhibit all social skills equally well, a restructuring of the composition of groups to ensure a balance in skill levels might be necessary.

Individualize the Curriculum

The social skills instructional activities should be individualized. As noted by Maag (1989), providing instruction in an area where a student is not experiencing a deficit is not efficient use of instructional time. Therefore, teachers should determine where social skill deficits exist and target these deficiencies with programming activities (Carter & Sugai, 1989).

The best way to individualize social skills training is through the individual education program. If teachers are going to develop goals and objectives related to social skills, and spend instructional time to help students achieve those goals and objectives, the activities should be documented in the student's IEP.

Cost-Effectiveness of the Curriculum

There are many commercially developed training programs for social skills currently on the market. Teachers need to be aware of the different types of programs and make sound judgments concerning which ones to purchase. If possible, materials should be reviewed before they are purchased. A discussion later in this chapter deals with selecting commercial training programs.

Some publishers will allow materials to be previewed. In these situations, school personnel should make every effort to find out about the materials before they are purchased. Asking other teachers and personnel from other districts, as well as trying to find reviews of materials in professional journals, are all excellent ways to find out information about specific materials prior to their purchase.

Another possible source of social skills training materials that will help school personnel determine cost effectiveness is the regional resource center or regional service center. Many states have regional centers that loan instructional materials and provide other services to local public schools. These facilities are likely to maintain supplies of social skills curricula.

Field Test the Curriculum

Even though materials may appear to be good or be recommended by other teachers, they may not meet the specific needs of some students. In order to develop an understanding of which programs work with different types of students, teachers should, if at all possible, field test the program. If the company does not allow for field testing prior to purchase, there are other sources where field test results may be found. Often, field test information is available in the technical manuals that accompany curriculum packages, or they may be reported in the literature. Such field test information can tell school personnel:

- the types of students the materials have been used for;

- the conditions under which the materials have been used;

- how the reliability or consistency of the materials has been; and

- the range of coverage of the materials (Carter & Sugai, 1989).

Teachers can field test social skills curricula using several different approaches. One method is to actually try a social skills lesson on a particular set of students. In order to field test materials using this approach teachers should:

- identify the social skill that will be taught;

- determine if the materials include that particular social skill;

- select a group of students for training;

- devise and implement some means of pre- and posttesting students' competence in the social skill;

- implement the social skill training lesson;

- conduct a posttest to determine effectiveness of the training.

When field testing materials, teachers need to determine not only the effectiveness of the materials with students, but the cost of the materials, ease in using the materials, and training and time commitment of the teacher.

Use Assessment Data

Without adequate assessment information, it is impossible to know what skill deficits students are experiencing and, therefore, what kinds of interventions are needed. Assessment data should also be used to determine the effectiveness of programming with particular students. Teachers should use on-going monitoring to asses the day-to-day efficacy of the program. This enables teachers to alter ineffective programming.

Maintenance and Generalization

A major goal in social skills instruction is to enable students to generalize their newly acquired social skills in different settings (Wood, 1982; Blackbourn, 1989). If this is not achieved, then the training is of limited value (Sargent, 1991). Knowing how to use a particular social skill in a classroom situation, but not understanding how to implement the skill in the "real world," does not help the student achieve social success. Likewise, if students learn social skills and these are not maintained over time, then the efforts have been minimized. Early research into the generalizability of social skills training revealed that, although students learned these skills and could apply them in the setting where they were learned, generalization to other settings often did not occur (Wood, 1982). Therefore, teachers need to implement specific strategies to facilitate generalization of learned social skills.

There are several ways to improve the likelihood that students will maintain and generalize social skills. These include:

- using multiple trainers;

- training in multiple settings;

- teaching a variety of response variations that will be maintained by the natural environment;

- selecting a representative range of instructional examples, nonexamples, reinforcers, and materials that are likely to be encountered outside the training setting,

- reinforcing social skills when they occur in new settings and under different conditions. (Carter & Sugai, 1989, p. 37)

In addition to these general considerations, Fiedler and Chiang (1989) suggest that teachers remember that social skills only occur in a particular way in a specific setting. Therefore, the assessment of social skills may not be sufficiently comprehensive to accurately determine a student's social functioning. As a result, teachers need to monitor closely students' social skills to ensure that programs being used are effective, learned skills are being maintained, and that newly detected deficit areas are addressed. Teachers can provide social skills training in a number of different ways, including commercial training programs and teacher-developed activities. There is no one method that works best with all students; therefore, teachers may choose one approach or a combination of approaches for their social skills training program.

COMMERCIAL SOCIAL SKILLS PROGRAM

There are numerous commercially prepared programs for social skills instruction. Most are designed to improve peer acceptance of students (Vaughn & Lancelotta, 1990). Since the recent rapid expansion in social skills training programs, materials companies have developed many different social skills training programs. For the most part, these programs are more comprehensive and sophisticated than earlier versions of programs.

Evaluation of Commercial Programs

Although programs appear to be getting better, teachers and other school district personnel who are responsible for purchasing social skills programs should consider the following factors before purchasing and using commercial programs.

- *Efficacy of Approach*   Has there been any research that validates the training program?

- *Cost*   Prices generally range from about $22.00 to $1,400.

- *Target Group*   Does the age range suggested for the program fit your school's needs?

- *Target Setting*   Can the program be used in both special education and regular education settings?

- *User Friendliness*   How easy is the program to implement?

- *Style of Approach*   Is the program strictly instructional, cognitive, or problem-solving?

- *Number of Skills Taught*   Most programs teach from 8 to 136 skills.

- *Concern for Generalization*   Is there evidence that the skills learned are generalizable? (Sabornie & Beard, 1990, p. 37)

Figure 10–4 (on page 386) presents a checklist that can be used to evaluate social skills programs.

Most schools have a mechanism for reviewing materials prior to their purchase. Certainly this is true for textbook adoptions, and it may be true for major materials or curricular purchases. If not, then teachers should develop and implement a mechanism for previewing materials. This would include 1. developing a review panel consisting of teachers, students, parents, and representative from the administration; 2. adopting a checklist or format for formal review of the materials; 3. establishing a mechanism for actual field testing of the materials, as previously outlined.

Specific Commercial Programs

The following section describes examples of social skills commercial programs available (Gearheart & Gearheart, 1989).

Skill Streaming the Adolescent and *Skill Streaming the Elementary School Child* (Goldstein, Sprafkin, Gershaw, & Klein, 1980; McGinnis, Goldstein, Sprafkin, & Gershaw, 1984) provide step-by-step programs for implementing a social skills curriculum. The elementary program includes classroom survival skills, friendship-making skills, dealing with feelings, alternatives to aggression, and dealing with stress. Adolescent program includes beginning social skills, advanced social skills, dealing with feelings. alternatives to aggression, dealing with stress, and planning skills.

The program consists of five distinct steps.

1. Specific steps that are learned to a mastery level, with actual examples to illustrate these steps (modeling).

2. Practice with the steps in simulated problem situations (role playing).

3. Information as to how the student has performed the steps (feedback).

4. Practice in real-life situations (transfer of training).

5. Approval for successful use of the skill (reinforcement). (McGinnis, Sauerbry, & Nichols, 1985, pp. 160–161).

The first phase of the skill-streaming program is modeling various skills by the teacher. This shows students exactly what they should do rather than simply telling them. Modeling is most effective when the skills used are some that the students actually need. The next phase is when students practice the newly developed skill in a role-play situation. This helps students understand how to perform the skill. As the behaviors exhibited by the student during role play become more and more like the model's behavior, student and teacher approval is given. The final phase of skill-streaming is transfer of the training to real-life situations (McGinnis *et al.*, 1985).

FIGURE 10-4 Checklist for Commercial Training Programs in Social Skills

Name of Curriculum: _____

Purpose of the Program
___ 1. Are instructional objectives clearly stated in the manual?
___ 2. Was the program designed for mildly handicapped students?
___ 3. Was the program designed for nonhandicapped students?
___ 4. If the program was designed for nonhandicapped students, can it be adapted for use with handicapped populations?

Validation of the Program
___ 1. Has the program been field-tested?
___ 2. Do the results of the field testing document the program's effectiveness?
___ 3. If the program is recommended for use with specific target populations (for example, learning disabled students, behaviorally disordered students), was it used with these groups during field testing?

Content and Structure of the Program
___ 1. Is the material appropriate for stated objectives?
___ 2. Is the content relevant to the experiences and environment of the target population?
___ 3. Are directions for teaching presentations included?
___ 4. Does the teacher need special training to use the materials?
___ 5. Are the same instructional steps followed for teaching each new skill?
___ 6. Are *all* materials needed to teach individual lessons included in the training program?
___ 7. Does the program allow for sufficient practice of newly learned skills?
___ 8. Are provisions made to motivate students to use skills?
___ 9. Are suggestions included for adapting the material to individual needs?
___ 10. Are provisions made to ensure maintenance and generalization?

Evaluation Procedures
___ 1. Are procedures included for identifying students who would benefit from this training program?
___ 2. Are on-going evaluation procedures included?
___ 3. What procedures are used to assess mastery of each skill?

Source: Used with permission, Elksnin, L.K. (1989). Teaching mildly handicapped students social skills in secondary settings. *Academic Therapy, 25*, pp. 165–166.

The *ACCEPTS Program* (Walker, McConnell, Holmes, Todis, Walker, & Golden, 1983) is designed for elementary students and is one of the most popular social skills programs for this age group. Social skills training is provided by the teacher using direct instruction. The steps included in the program are 1. skill to be learned is defined; 2. examples and nonexamples of the behavior are given; 3. students practice the skill through role playing; 4. feedback is provided students; and 5. learned skills are generalized with the aid of contracts (Sabornie & Beard, 1990).

Developing Understanding of Self and Others (DUSO) (Dinkmeyer & Dinkmeyer, 1982) is a program for kindergarten through fourth grade students. It includes lessons on self awareness, awareness of others, making choices and decisions, and communication skills.

Metacognitive Approach to Social Skills Training (MASST) (Sheinker, Sheinker, Peterson, & Craft, 1988) is designed for students in the fourth through twelfth grades, and teaches students how to monitor their behaviors and develop alternatives. Examples of topics include "How I see myself," "How my peers see me," and "Who controls my feelings?"

Teaching Social Skills to Children (Cartledge & Milburn, 1986) differs from the others in that it is not a structured program. Rather, teachers are given the tools necessary to develop their own social skills intervention programs. Topics include 1. the cognitive-affective approach, 2. coaching techniques, 3. activities to teach skills, and 4. the adolescent.

ASSET (Hazel, Schumaker, Sherman, & Sheldon-Wildgen, 1982) focuses on improving social skills in eight different areas: 1. giving positive feedback; 2. giving negative feedback; 3. accepting negative feedback; 4. resisting peer pressure; 5. solving problems; 6. negotiating; 7. following instructions; and 8. conversing. Homework assignments and the required involvement of parents are two unique components of the program (Sabornie & Beard, 1990).

TEACHER-DEVELOPED ACTIVITIES

Often teachers choose to develop their own intervention programs to help students learn social skills rather than using commercial programs. These programs, if well conceived and implemented, can significantly improve the social skills of students with disabilities (Kerr, Nelson, & Lambert, 1987). Generally, teacher-developed social skills instruction revolves around daily occurrences in the classroom. Teaching students how to interact among themselves, how to use good manners and be courteous, and how to exhibit teacher pleasing behaviors are common in teacher-developed activities. This is an advantage over commercial programs that may have to be implemented using contrived situations specifically designed to teach a certain social skill.

While many teachers may say they work on social skills in their classroom, they frequently do not approach social skills instruction in a systematic manner. This is likely to result in social skills not being taught effectively. For this reason, teachers who rely on their own programs need to include social skills goals and objectives in students' IEPs as a way of ensuring that social skills training occurs.

There are several different activities that teachers should consider when teaching social skills. While these suggestions can apply to commercially prepared materials, they are also very germane for teacher-developed training.

1. *Whole Skill Prompts*   A typical prompt to an elementary school pupil would be something like "Show me how you are supposed to pay attention," and "Tell me

how to ask someone to play and then you can go ask someone to play." The nature of the prompts must be changed to fit the particular child.

2. *Coaching* Coaching simply means telling the student what to do and then providing feedback.

3. *Skill Challenges* A skill challenge occurs when a contrived social or classroom situation is created where a pupil must demonstrate use of a particular skill.

4. *Homework* Social skills lessons generally call for formal homework at the junior and senior high levels and informal homework for elementary-aged children.

5. *Skill Review Session* These sessions consist of a review of reasons for using the particular skills, the skill components, and modeling by one or two proficient class members.

6. *Daily Role Playing* Through feedback given during and after the role play practice sessions, skills will be shaped to correct performance.

7. *Skill of the Week* When a new skill is introduced, it may be emphasized by posting the skill components.

8. *Reteaching the Lesson* The same lesson may be retaught (usually in an abbreviated form) at a later date.

9. *Reteaching at Different Levels* Several of the social skills will need to be retaught as students become older (Sargent, 1989, p. 280).

INSTRUCTIONAL METHODS FOR SOCIAL SKILLS

Whether teachers use commercially prepared materials, teacher-developed activities, or a combination of both, they generally rely on similar instructional methods. These include modeling, prompting, coaching, practice, and several others. The following describes several of these techniques. Table 10–4 summarizes these methods and give advantages and disadvantages of each.

Modeling

Modeling is a teaching technique that can be used to teach a wide variety of knowledge and skills. When using this approach, students observe and imitate appropriate social skills exhibited by others in an exemplary form (Andersen *et al.*, 1988). Observing the "model" exhibiting appropriate social skills and being rewarded for it makes it likely that the student will imitate these behaviors (Masters & Mori, 1986). Modeling is easy to implement (Carter & Sugai, 1988; Carter & Sugai, 1989) and has been shown to be most successful when the model is similar in age, sex, and social status to the students and when the model is highly skilled and helpful (McGinnis, 1985). In general, modeling has been determined to be an effective way to teach a variety of new behaviors (Carter & Sugai, 1989; Woolfolk, 1990).

Appropriate social skills can be modeled using live demonstrations or symbolic models, such as film or videotape, audiotape, mental imagery, puppets, and books. Live demonstrations are generally performed by teachers or socially competent peers. As a result of many students with disabilities having poor discriminatory skills, the actual social skills that are

TABLE 10-4 Summary Descriptions of Tactics to Teach Social Skills

INSTRUCTIONAL STRATEGY	DESCRIPTION	ADVANTAGES	DISADVANTAGES
Modeling	Exposing target student to display of prosocial behavior.	Easy to implement.	Not sufficient if used alone.
Strategic Placement	Placing target student in situations with other students who display prosocial behaviors.	Employs peers as change agents. Facilitates generalization. Is cost effective.	Research data inconclusive when used alone.
Instruction	Telling students how and why they should behave a certain way, and/or giving rules for behavior.	Overemphasizes norms/expectations.	Not sufficient if used alone.
Correspondence Training	Students are positively reinforced for accurate reports regarding their behavior.	Facilitates maintenance and generalization of training. Is cost effective.	Very little documentation of effectiveness.
Rehearsal and Practice	Structured practice of specific prosocial behavior.	Enhances skill acquisition.	Not sufficient to change behavior if used alone.
Positive Reinforcement or Shaping	Prosocial behaviors or approximations are followed by a reward or favorable event.	Strong research support for effectiveness.	Maintenance after treatment termination is not predictable.
Prompting and Coaching	Providing students with additional stimuli/prompts that elicit the prosocial behavior.	Particularly effective after acquisition to enhance transfer to natural settings.	Maintenance after treatment termination is not predictable.
Positive Practice	A consequence strategy in which student repeatedly practices correct behavior.	May produce immediate increases in prosocial behavior.	Long-term effectiveness not documented. Less restrictive approaches should be used first.
Multimethod Training Packages	Multicomponent instructional package that incorporates several behavioral techniques.	Greater treatment strength and durability. Applicable to a wide range of children and settings.	

Source: Carter, J., & Sugai, G. (1989). Social skills curriculum analysis. *Teaching Exceptional Children, 22,* p. 38. Used with permission.

being demonstrated need to be identified during the modeling. When using symbolic models, such as a videotape, the tape can be stopped and appropriate skills discussed (Sargent, 1991).

   Sargent (1988) gives an example of teaching the skill of paying attention to the teacher using modeling:

1. Explain to the pupils that it is important to pay attention to the teacher in all their classes.

2. Appoint a pupil to act as a teacher. The pupil's job will be to act as the teacher at the front of the classroom while the actual teacher takes a seat in the classroom.

3. As the "teacher" begins a simulated lesson, the teacher narrates how she is attending to the "teacher" by maintaining eye contact, moving her head to follow the "teacher" and listening to what the "teacher" is saying.

4. Different students can then take turns narrating how they are attending to the teacher. During a later lesson, the teacher can actually call on a student and ask how he is attending to the main activity in the classroom.

Role Playing

"Role playing is a technique in which students act out their problems in a less threatening atmosphere while seriously attempting to understand the conflict in their lives." (Masters & Mori, 1986, p. 278). Students are able to practice various social skills during role-playing activities; this turns out to be a rehearsal for real-life implementation (Andersen *et al.*, 1988). Role plays should occur only after students have observed a skilled model perform the particular skill. The teacher observes the role-playing situation and provides immediate feedback to the participants (Fiedler & Chiang, 1989).

An example of using role playing to teach the social skill of politely greeting visitors to the classroom follows.

1. Tell the students in your class the importance of being polite to visitors.

2. Explain the importance of a polite greeting in response to a visitor's greeting.

3. Have a student pretend to be a visiting school board member and enter the classroom and say, "Good morning class."

4. Instruct the class to respond, "Good morning," after the visitor's initial greeting.

5. Rotate which students get to role play the visitor.

Strategic Placement

Placing students who need to develop certain social skills in settings where they can readily observe and model these skills is called strategic placement (Carter & Sugai, 1988; Carter & Sugai, 1989). There will likely be some students in every classroom who display appropriate social skills in an exemplary manner. Teachers should take advantage of this on-site training opportunity and place students who need to learn skills in close proximity with those that exhibit good skills. This enables direct observations, modeling, and practice opportunities.

An important element in using strategic placement is that students are learning social skills in natural settings. The classroom, lunchroom, auditorium, playground, bus, or other locations provide students with an opportunity to observe appropriate social skills in "real" situations.

Teachers can implement this strategy by requiring certain students who need social skills training to sit next to students who typically display appropriate social skills. The teacher should be near by to positively reinforce the model student's appropriate social skills and then the modeled social skills exhibited by the student who is learning.

Direct Instruction

For some students, directly teaching social skills is an important component of a social skills curriculum. Some students simply need to be taught specific social skills and how to use them in certain situations. Research has demonstrated that direct instruction methods work effectively in teaching social skills to students with disabilities (Wood, 1982; Sargent, 1988; Sargent, 1991).

There are six specific components in a direct instruction approach, regardless of the skills being taught. These are 1. specifying the objectives, 2. devising strategies, 3. developing teaching procedures, 4. selecting examples, 5. sequencing skills, and 6. providing practice and review (Carnine, Silbert, & Kameenui, 1990). When using this approach with social skills instruction, the same steps should be included.

For example, if a teacher wants to teach students how to make positive statements about himself, the following procedures could be used. These three steps include each of the six components noted above (Sargent, 1991).

1. Specify that the objective of the lesson will be for students to make positive statements about themselves without bragging.

2. Develop direct teaching activities that will help students learn this appropriate behavior. This could include role playing, modeling, and giving examples in a story about how two different students used this skill, one appropriately and one inappropriately.

3. Provide students the opportunity to practice saying appropriate things about themselves that are positive but not bragging. Other students could evaluate these statements and determine which ones are good (and why) and which ones are bad (and why).

Direct instructional approaches for social skills instruction differ in some areas, however, they nearly all use certain strategies, including modeling, role playing, practice, and feedback (Sargent, 1991). The key element in any direct instruction approach is to directly teach specific skills in "the most effective and efficient manner possible" (Carnine *et al.*, 1990).

Correspondence Training

Correspondence training is simply instructing students to accurately report their social behaviors (Carter & Sugai, 1988; Carter & Sugai, 1989). Since it is critical that students understand their strengths and weaknesses in all areas, including social skills, they are encouraged to be aware of these behaviors and report them accurately. After reporting on behaviors, teachers and students can discuss the effectiveness of certain behaviors and the consequences, both positive and negative, that result.

One method of doing this is to ask students whether or not an observed behavior reflects a positive or negative social skill. Students may need help in focusing their attention on their own actions. By directly asking them about specific behaviors and discussing with them the positive and negative components of those behaviors, students will learn to "tune in" to their own actions. This discussion could be a group discussion in front of the entire class or a one-on-one discussion between the student and teacher. The teacher should determine which is appropriate. If the episode could result in a learning experience for the entire class, without embarrassment to the student involved, then it might be appropriate for the class to discuss it. Teachers must, however, keep in mind any potential embarrassment that might result in a group discussion.

Rehearsal and Practice

After learning appropriate social skills, students need the opportunity to practice their use. Just as students with disabilities must practice newly acquired academic skills in order to maintain them, they must also practice social skills (Sargent, 1988; 1989). Teachers should set up situations where this practice can occur. This can be in natural settings, or through the use of role-play situations.

Several of the previous examples included rehearsal and practice. Having students rehearse how to use appropriate social skills and then practice the use of that social skill will help them to assimilate the skill into their natural behaviors.

Positive Reinforcement or Shaping

These are simple behavior management techniques of positively reinforcing and shaping work effectively when teaching students social skills (Gresham, 1981). Exhibiting appropriate social skills needs to be reinforced to increase the likelihood that they will reoccur. Appropriate social skills that go unnoticed and unreinforced, especially newly acquired social skills, may disappear.

Positive Reinforcement   When appropriate social behaviors are exhibited by students, positive reinforcement should be provided. Positive reinforcement is when something positive happens to a student who exhibits a desirable behavior (Woolfolk, 1990). The use of positive reinforcement is used in teaching all kinds of skills, from self-help skills to higher level skills, such as social skills. The premise is that if something pleasant occurs following a particular behavior then that behavior is likely to be repeated.

The use of positive reinforcement in social skills training is simply the application of behaviorism to teaching students social skills. When students exhibit appropriate behaviors, some positive reinforcement results. This could include verbal praise, a pat on the back, or a more concrete reinforcer. A key in positive reinforcement when teaching social skills, as with any skill, is that the reinforcer must be viewed as something positive by the student. Providing stickers to a teen-age student as positive reinforcement for appropriate social skills may not be considered as something positive. Therefore, teachers must ensure that the positive reinforcers are indeed considered positive by the students. When determining an appropriate positive reinforcer, teachers should not overlook verbal praise. Many students rarely receive verbal praise and therefore will respond very favorably to the teacher telling them how well they are doing. It is generally a good idea to have students participate in the selection of positive reinforcements.

Chapter 9 describes specific ways to implement positive reinforcement strategies. When using this approach to teach social skills, the following steps should be taken.

1. Identify the social skill that will be taught.

2. Determine the frequency of the targeted skill (or frequency of the skill used inappropriately).

3. Identify appropriate, positive reinforcers.

4. Develop a reinforcement schedule.

5. Reinforce the appropriate social skill with the designated positive reinforcer, using the identified reinforcement schedule.

6. Determine the frequency of the desired social skill.

Shaping   Shaping can be defined as "the systematic, immediate reinforcement of successive approximations of the target behavior until the behavior is established" (Walker & Shea, 1984, p. 71). Shaping social skills would require the following steps.

1. Select an appropriate target social skill.

2. Obtain reliable baseline data regarding how the particular social skill is exhibited.

3. Select appropriate reinforcers that are effective with the particular student.

4. Reinforce successive approximations as the social skill is exhibited.

5. Reinforce the social skill each time it is demonstrated.

6. Reinforce the behavior using a variable reinforcement schedule to maximize its likelihood of continuation (Walker & Shea, 1984).

Shaping enables teachers to reinforce progress rather than waiting for the complete accomplishment of the social skill (Woolfolk, 1990). Through shaping, students should get closer and closer to exhibiting, totally, the desired social behaviors.

Prompting and Coaching

Prompting and coaching are methods to provide students with additional stimuli that results in the display of appropriate social skills (Carter & Sugai, 1988; 1989). Prompts for social skills could include a variety of things, including 1. directly telling students what to do, 2. physical cues, such as a hand motion, or 3. the physical arrangement of the environment.

Prompting is an excellent method for helping students develop appropriate social skills, however, anytime prompts are used to facilitate the development of skills, they eventually have to be eliminated, that is, faded (Walker & Shea, 1984). Without the fading, students may never be able to exhibit appropriate social skills without the presence of prompts. Therefore, although prompts may help students initially develop social skills, they must be eliminated if the social skills are to truly be assimilated into the student's natural behavior repertoire.

An example of a verbal prompt could apply to the previous example about teaching appropriate greeting behaviors to a class. The teacher could teach the use of appropriate group greetings with the verbal prompt of "class." Students would then know that when someone walks in the room and the teacher says "class" that a group greeting is in order. This would be paired with a facial gesture which would eventually replace the verbal prompt. Finally, the teacher would be able to eliminate all prompts and the students would express the greeting voluntarily.

Coaching is simply telling students what to do, when to do it, and providing appropriate feedback (Sargent, 1989). It also is used a great deal in direct instruction. When parents tell their children to say "thank you" they are coaching a particular social skill. Likewise, teachers who tell their students to smile in their English class are coaching them in a social skill. Coaching is a very effective method of getting immediate results; the primary drawback is the necessity for students to eventually display the behaviors without coaching.

Class Dialogues

Gearheart and Gearheart (1989) discuss the approach of teaching social skills through class dialogues. This method focuses on planned discussions around a particular topic, such as mutual concerns and problems, changing behaviors, and importance of appropriate social behaviors.

Class dialogues can help students feel more comfortable about themselves as a result of open discussions with their peers. The model, similar to approaches that focus on self-help groups, enables students to understand that their problems may be shared by many of their peers and that they are "OK" even though they experience certain difficulties.

Videotape Feedback

Another approach to helping students develop social skills is through videotape feedback (Gearheart & Gearheart, 1989). Students are able to watch themselves and their peers interact in various settings and are able to discuss and analyze their social skills. Strengths and weaknesses that are observed are discussed, and students are able to suggest ways to improve various social skill deficits.

Bibliotherapy

Bibliotherapy has been used extensively to help students develop a better understanding of themselves and others. This approach can be used to help teach social skills by having students read books and articles related to social skills and discussing the content. In order for bibliotherapy to be most effective, teachers must prepare for leading a structured discussion. Without structure, the discussions can quickly lose focus and result in a waste of time.

The structured discussion should focus on the following.

1. Recalling the main story line or character with an emphasis on feelings, values, or attitudes.

2. Discussing the manner in which the story character coped with the problem.

3. Exploring similar problems in students' lives and the ways in which they attempted to deal with them.

4. Evaluating the consequences of students' solutions to the problem.

5. If necessary, suggesting alternative solutions to the problem. (Masters & Mori, 1986, p. 271)

Magic Circle

This approach to teaching social skills uses group discussion as the primary instructional tool. Students sit in a circle (magic circle) and discuss their feelings, acceptance of other students and adults, and other topics that could relate to social skills. The role of the teacher is to serve as the group leader and keep the discussion on track. Although these discussions may range from very short to long, the average length of time is about twenty minutes. Magic circle is primarily designed for students in grades kindergarten through sixth (Gearheart & Gearheart, 1989).

STATUS OF SOCIAL SKILLS INSTRUCTION

The importance of social skills instruction, especially for students with mild disabilities, should be apparent. Without specific training activities, many of these students will not develop competence in social skills sufficient to enable them to be successful in school situations or post-secondary environments. Therefore, public schools must continue to assume a greater role in social skills instruction.

A recent study (Cosden, Iannaccone, & Wienke, 1990) investigated the status of social skills instruction. Using a sample of twenty-eight teachers in secondary schools, the study revealed the following.

■ The majority of teachers believe that social skills instruction for students with disabilities should be a shared responsibility between regular and special education teachers.

■ The majority of teachers indicated that they wanted to be more involved in proactive social skills training than they were.

■ The majority of teachers indicated that they had no or limited resources to use in social skills training.

■ Most teachers agreed that they needed more competencies in the area of social skills instruction than they possessed.

■ Related to the importance of social skills training, the majority of teachers believed that it helped students in a number of areas, including student-teacher relationships.

It appears from this study that teachers understand the importance of social skills training and are interested in implementing such training. However, the data also suggest that these teachers feel as if they are ill prepared to provide the needed training and that there are limited resources in the schools to help them do so (Cosden *et al.*, 1990). This information, along with the finding by Smith and Dowdy (1989) that teachers are including social skills goals and objectives in IEPs, is encouraging.

EXAMPLES OF SOCIAL SKILLS LESSONS

A recent publication (Sargent, 1991) presents 100 proactive lessons for teaching social skills to students primary through high school. Following are five examples of lessons from this source.

EXAMPLES OF SOCIAL SKILLS LESSONS

Social Skills Lesson—Primary
Attending to Teacher during Instruction

Objective: Students will attend to the teacher during instruction.

Performance Criteria: This skill will be performed adequately when the student:

1. Maintains upright sitting posture.

2. Sits facing the direction of the teacher.

3. Directs eyes at teacher during instruction (i.e., when teacher is giving directions, or demonstrating).

4. Responds immediately to directions.

5. Moves head to follow teacher with eyes as she/he moves.

6. Directs eyes in the direction where the teacher points.

7. Maintains eyes on teacher during the entire course of instruction.

8. Gives occasional nonverbal gestures to indicate understanding (e.g., head nod, facial changes).

Materials: Prizes (e.g., small pieces of candy, small amounts of popcorn, or tokens), pictures posted in the front of the classroom.

Procedures:

Step #1. Establishing the Need

a. Tell the students that you are going to play a looking game and that there are prizes for those who play the game carefully. The game is played by watching the teacher as she talks. Sometimes the teacher will tell where the prizes are and sometimes the teacher will point in the direction of the prize. A student can win a prize if they are the first to raise their hand and tell the class where the prize is. The rules include a stipulation that a student cannot win more than once and may not retrieve his or her prize until the game is over.

b. After playing the game, ask students to tell what is necessary to win a prize in the game. Elicit that they must listen and watch the teacher.

c. Ask students to identify consequences of attending to the teacher. Elicit that students will learn more, teachers will be happy, and parents will be happy.

continued

Step #2. Identify the Skill Components

    a.   Elicit through discussion or provide students with the following:

        1)   Sit up straight.

        2)   Listen carefully.

        3)   Look where the teacher points and where the teacher moves.

        4)   Follow teacher's directions.

        5)   Nod or smile to show understanding.

    b.   Write steps on chalkboard or overhead.

    c.   Rehearse the steps with the students. Repeat the sequence in unison at least twice.

    d.   Have students restate or paraphrase the steps.

Step #3. Model the Skill

    a.   Explain to the students that it is important to pay attention to the teacher in all their classes.

    b.   Appoint a student to act as the teacher. The student's job will be to tell the class what he or she is wearing and to tell where three of his or her classmates sit in the classroom.

    c.   Before the student begins to speak, the role playing teacher uses the think aloud procedures to point out that he/she is sitting straight, facing the speaker, and looking at him/her. The teacher narrates how he/she is attending to the speaker by moving her head to follow the speaker and looking where the speaker points.

Step #4. Role Play

    a.   Tell students that you will be talking to them about the picture that is posted in the front of the room. Their job will be to pay attention and follow the attending procedures. Encourage all class members to sit up straight, face in the direction of the teacher, and look at the teacher.

    b.   Talk about the picture and move and point.

    c.   Ask students how they did. Did they sit straight, look where the teacher pointed, etc.?

    d.   Using another picture, repeat the role playing and have each student monitored and given feedback by another student.

continued

Step #5. Practice

    a.   For four or five days subsequent to the lesson, begin class with the unison repetition of the steps for paying attention.

    b.   During instruction provide feedback and reinforcement to students for their attending behavior.

    c.   Give students an assignment to pay attention when enrolled in a regular class. Have them report on how they did.

    d.   Continue to intermittently provide feedback and reinforcement on attending behavior.

Step #6. Generalization

    a.   If students are not attending to instruction while integrated into regular classrooms, ask co-operating teachers to remind and reinforce students to attend to instruction.

NOTE: Consideration must also be given to the fact that lack of attention may mean that the subject matter is beyond the student's comprehension.

    b.   Ask regular education teachers to report on good attending behavior. After receiving good reports, reinforce the students and take the opportunity to restate the attending procedures.

    c.   Ask students to report on how well they attended in regular classes.

Social Skills Lesson—Intermediate
Following Classroom Rules

Objective: Students will follow classroom rules when the teacher is present and when the teacher is out of the room.

Performance Criteria: This skill will be performed adequately when the student:

1. Restates rules when asked.

2. Follows specific rules without prompting.

3. Can identify consequences for not following rules.

4. Follows rules when the teacher is out of the room.

Materials: Poster board.

Procedures:

Step #1. Establishing Need

    a. This lesson should be taught at the beginning of the school year.

continued

`b. Read optional story to introduce the lesson.

Rules to Follow

    Mr. Craig's fifth grade class at Barton Elementary was scheduled to go on a field trip to a space museum, but they never went. Here is why.

    Mr. Craig's class was more fun than almost any others in the school. The lessons were interesting, Mr. Craig told good jokes, and everyone learned a lot. To make sure everyone in class could learn and enjoy school, Mr. Craig had some rules that the children had to follow. Most of the time all the children followed the rules. Unfortunately, the week before the field trip, several of the children forgot to follow the rules. The trouble began when Bobby walked into class and pushed all of Mary's papers onto the floor. The next day, Mary and Audrey stole all of Bobby's pencils and sharpened them down to the nubs. Later that same day, Bill and Jim were out of their seats throwing erasers across the room and Ann and Leslie just seemed to talk the whole afternoon. Mr. Craig kept them all after school that night.

    On the third day of the week things were just as bad. This time Sarah and Jennifer wouldn't stop talking, John and Lenny were throwing erasers, and Greg and Donald got into a pushing match. Things were so bad that Mr. Craig warned the class that any more rule breaking and the class wouldn't be able to go on the field trip.

    On Thursday, things went pretty well until about 10 o'clock. When everyone came in after recess, they took their seats just like they were supposed to. After a minute or so, Greg blurted out "Oh no, I've got gum all over the seat of my pants." Someone had put freshly chewed gum on Greg's chair. That was not only a mean trick, but it was against the rules in Mr. Craig's class to chew gum. Mr. Craig asked who put the gum on Greg's chair and when nobody admitted doing it, he simply called the principal and cancelled the field trip.

    Everyone in the class was disappointed and angry.

continued

   c.   Ask students what would have happened if the children in the story had followed the classroom rules.

   d.   Ask students if they had classroom rules to follow in previous years. Elicit that they did.

   e.   Ask what happened to them when they broke the rules. Elicit whatever consequences are realistic.

   f.   Ask class members if they would prefer to avoid the consequences for breaking rules.

Step #2. Identify the Skill Components

   a.   Put a list of classroom rules on poster board and leave posted.

   b.   Have the class rehearse the rules orally.

   c.   Point out to class that rules should be followed without being reminded.

   d.   Point out to the class that the rules must be followed even when the teacher is gone from the room.

   e.   Tell class members that they will have to repeat rules when asked.

Step #3. Model the Skill

   a.   Pretend to be a student entering the classroom and beginning seatwork.

   b.   Narrate how the rules are being followed using the think aloud procedure.

   c.   Ask students to recall all the rules that were followed.

Step #4. Role Play

   a.   Direct each student to spend one minute role playing the skill and thinking aloud to show which rules he or she was following.

   b.   Give each student feedback on his or her performance.

Step #5. Practice

   a.   For the week following introduction of the classroom rules, rehearse the list of the rules daily. Occasionally review the rules throughout the school year.

   b.   Remind students to follow the class rules and then provide intermittent reinforcement for correctly performing the behaviors.

continued

Step #6. Generalization

a. Consult with regular class teachers from whom the students with disabilities receive instruction. Ask them to prompt and reinforce the students with disabilities for following classroom rules.

b. Make up a list of general classroom rules applied in your building. Give a list to each student and have them mark down which rules they followed during instruction in the regular classroom.

c. Ask students to report on themselves. Praise students for self-reporting.

Social Skills Lesson—Intermediate
Asking Peers for Help

Objective: Students will be able to ask peers for help.

Performance Criteria: This skill will be performed adequately when the student:

1. Tries to accomplish task by self.

2. Decides that help is needed.

3. Considers the most appropriate source for help (peer, teacher, parent, other).

4. Rules out going to an adult for help.

5. Checks to see if peer is busy.

6. Goes to peer.

7. Tells peer that he/she is having trouble or needs assistance.

8. Politely asks peer for help.

9. Says "thank you" after help is provided.

Materials: Skill monitoring cards, chalkboard, feedback cards.

Procedures:

Step #1. Establishing the Need

a. Read the following brief story to the children:

Jim's Problem

Mr. Reese's fifth grade class was in the middle of their math lesson when Jim, a member of the class, started banging on his desk and yelling, "I can't do it, I can't do it." Of course, that made every-one take notice. Then all of the kids in class started talking and one boy started to tease Jim.

Well, as you can imagine, Mr. Reese was becoming angry with all of the noise and Jim was not only frustrated, he was angry for being teased. Jim pounded his desk one more time, yelled at Bobby for teasing him, and slammed his math book shut.

Mr. Reese had almost no choice but to punish Jim for making all that noise. Jim was told he would have to stay after school for 30 minutes. Since Mr. Reese was angry with the class, everyone had to stay in for recess that day.

b. Ask students what Jim might have done instead of pounding his desk and yelling, "I can't do it." Elicit that he could ask someone for help. Further, elicit that he could have asked a peer for help.

continued

c. Ask students to identify examples of when they might need to ask someone for help. Elicit examples for times in special and regular classes.

Step #2. Identify the Skill Components

a. Tell students that there are some good ways to ask for help and that you will put them on the board. List and discuss the following steps:

1) Try to solve the problem yourself. (Discuss the fact that people don't like to help unless the student tries first.)

2) Decide if you need help and who can help.

3) Check to see if the person is busy.

4) Go to the person and tell the person that you are having trouble.

5) Ask for help politely.

6) Say thank you when the help is given.

b. As the skill steps are introduced, it may be helpful to chain them through an oral read-along procedure. This means read steps 1 and 2, then 1, 2, and 3, then 1, 2, 3, and 4, etc.

Step #3. Model the Skill

a. Create a classroom type of example and model the skill of asking a peer for help. Use the think aloud procedure to narrate each of the skill components.

b. Have students recall the skill components they observed. Then model the skill without narrating the steps. Again, ask students to identify the skill components they observed.

Step #4. Role Play

a. Have each student role play a situation of his or her own choosing where they would need to ask for some help. Encourage students to use both in-class and out-of-class examples.

b. Provide feedback to the students and ask other students to provide feedback. To elicit feedback from some students, it may be helpful to develop feedback cards where the student holding that card is responsible for providing feedback.

Step #5. Practice

a. This is a skill which can be practiced during the course of the week following introduction of the lesson. Remind students that they may need to ask someone for help and review the steps with the students each day.

continued

b. Set up challenge situations where students are given tasks where the help from another individual would be necessary. This might be a simple task such as moving a desk or carrying books to another classroom. Be sure to praise students for following correct procedures. Some students will need prompting with statements such as, "you might want to find a helper."

c. At a review session, have the skill modeled by one or two students.

Step #6. Generalization

a. Inform other staff members that the class is working on how to ask for help. Request that they prompt this behavior when needed.

b. Send notes home to parents describing the social skill of asking for help. Request parents to ask their children how the skill is performed.

c. Ask students to report on their use of the skill outside the classroom. Some students may benefit from use of skill monitoring cards.

Social Skills Lesson—Middle School/Junior High
Staying out of Fights

Objective: Students will use alternatives to aggression to stay out of fights.

Performance Criteria: This skill will be adequately performed when the student:

1. Stops and considers why they want to fight.

2. Considers the potential short-range outcomes (i.e., risks vs. gains).

3. Decides what the long-range outcomes would be.

4. Consider other ways to handle the situation besides fighting (e.g., negotiating, standing up for his or her rights, asking for help, or pacifying the individual).

5. Chooses the best alternative to fighting.

Materials: Chalkboard, homework form.

Procedures:

Step #1. Establishing the Need

a. Begin with a discussion on how junior high students tend to get into fights. Ask students to tell whether or not they have ever witnessed any fights between agemates. Elicit from students the consequences of fighting. List some of the consequences on the chalkboard.

b. Point out to students that one of the severest consequences of fighting is arrest for assault and battery.

c. Through discussion, make it clear to students that avoiding fighting often means avoiding punishment from school authorities or parents.

Step #2. Identify the Skill Components

Describe the steps for keeping out of fights. Write each of the following on the chalkboard and discuss them with the students:

1. Stop and think why you want to fight.

2. Think about whether or not it will do you any good.

3. Think about what might happen if you get caught.

4. Think about what can be done besides fighting, e.g.:

    a) ask for help.

    b) talk it over.

continued

    c)   stand up to the person.

    d)   do something to make the person happy.

    e)   walk away.

5.   Choose what to do.

Step #3. Model the Skill

a.   Describe a situation where a person is treated unfairly or injured. For example, a student sets his lunch tray down at a cafeteria table and leaves to go back to the lunch line to get a napkin. While picking up the napkin, a second student comes along, takes the chair, and moves the first student's lunch tray to another table.

b.   Model four different ways to respond to the rude fellow student. Narrate the thinking steps through the think aloud procedure.

c.   Ask students to comment on whether or not the skill steps on the board are followed.

Step #4. Role Play

a.   Ask students to think up situations where they might consider fighting and role play for the class.

b.   For students who cannot think of a situation, suggest an argument with a sibling, being teased by a peer, or being pushed by an aggressive student.

c.   Provide feedback to students on how well they role play. For students who do not perform well, prompt them through the skill to ensure correct performance.

d.   Ask students to provide feedback to their classmates. To elicit feedback from some students, provide feedback cards and make them responsible for providing feedback on a single skill component.

Step #5. Practice

a.   Provide students with homework assignments and ask students to practice the skill at home or with a friend.

b.   Hold a skill review session and have students repeat skill steps. Have one or two students model the skill.

c.   Warn students in advance that they will be challenged to demonstrate the skill. Have students challenge one another for contrived situations.

continued

Step #6. Generalization

    a.   Ask students to report on whether or not they had avoided fights. Provide praise to students who have.

    b.   Ask other school officials to praise the students with disabilities for being good at avoiding fights.

Social Skills Lesson—Senior High
Minding One's Own Business on the Job

Objective: Students will mind their own business in a job setting.

Performance Criteria: This skill will be performed adequately when the student:

1. Identifies the tasks related to his or her own job.

2. Refrains from physically interfering with the tasks of co-workers.

3. Refrains from commenting on the job performance of co-workers.

4. Refrains from publicly complaining about work performance of a co-worker.

5. Refrains from asking personal questions of co-workers during work hours.

6. Stays on task during designated work hours.

Materials: Chalkboard, general homework forms.

Procedures:

Step #1. Establishing the Need

a. Ask students to identify some things that they don't like about other people. Elicit or suggest that they may not appreciate people who do not mind their own business. Have the students provide some examples of people not minding their own business.

b. Have students identify some consequences for not minding one's own business on the job. Elicit that they can (1) slow other workers down, (2) make co-workers angry, (3) start arguments, (4) take time away from their own work, and (5) possibly get fired. Write the possible consequences on the board.

Step #2. Identify the Skill Components

a. Elicit from the students the following rules and write them on the chalkboard:

1) Stick to your own job.

2) Stay out of the way of someone doing their job.

3) If someone is doing their job wrong, let the boss take care of it.

4) Don't ask personal questions on the job.

b. Discuss each of the rules and give examples and elicit consequences for not following the rules. Have students imagine as many situations as possible where the skill will be used.

continued

Step #3. Model the Skill

a. Create a typical work situation and model the skill. Use the "think aloud" procedure to demonstrate following the rules.

b. Some situations which may be modeled are as follows:

1) Two individuals working as bus boys and one of them is not cleaning the tables in his area correctly.

2) Workers on an assembly line and one is slowing down the work.

3) Two workers in a store and one has a skin problem. Model avoiding asking personal questions about the problem.

Step #4. Role Play

a. Have students suggest a work situation that they might find themselves in and then role play the skill. They should think aloud to demonstrate the cognitive components.

b. Have class members provide feedback.

c. Prompt all students through correct performance and provide praise.

d. Have students evaluate their own performance.

Step #5. Practice

a. Each day during the week following introduction of the skill, remind students that minding their own business is the skill of the week. Tell students to practice the skill during the course of other instruction. Take a few minutes at the end of each class period to have students evaluate their own performance as you lead them through the skill components. Have students provide feedback on each other's behavior.

b. Using the general homework form, give students a homework assignment to practice the skill on their work training job or while they are in attendance in another class.

c. Have the skill modeled by a student at a periodic skill review session.

Step #6. Generalization

a. Ask student's work supervisor or regular class teacher to prompt students to use the skill.

b. Make "minding one's own business" an evaluation item for part of the student's work training. Insure that employers and work supervisors give students feedback on this behavior.

c. Systematically ask students to self-report on skill usage. Praise students for self-reporting.

Source: Sargent, L.R. *Social Skills for School and Community*, pp. 29, 30, 93, 94, 132, 133, 157, 158, 255, 256. Reston, VA: Council for Exceptional Children, Division on Mental Retardation. Used with permission.

SUMMARY

This chapter has focused on teaching students with disabilities social skills. It was pointed out in the beginning section that social skills training has not always been a priority among special educators. Just a few years ago, teachers assumed that their primary, and often only role was to provide academic instruction to students with disabilities. However, as a result of these students having difficulties in mainstreamed classes, and follow-up studies revealing that adults with disabilities often failed in jobs due to limited social skills, the instructional importance of social skills training has developed.

The second section of the chapter discussed assessing social skills. It was noted that due to disagreements about what social skills are, it is difficult to assess this area. However, regardless of the difficulties and criticisms leveled against attempts to evaluate social skills, it is still a critical step that must be accomplished before appropriate social skills training can be implemented.

Several different types of social skills assessments were discussed, including formal checklists and behavior rating scales. Teacher developed checklists and observational records were also presented. Finally, a brief discussion concerning peer and self evaluations was included. Sociometric techniques were also discussed.

Following the assessment section, the chapter focus shifted to ways to teach social skills. Both commercially prepared materials and teacher developed activities were presented. Among the primary techniques used to instruct students in social skills, modeling, role playing, practice, direct instruction, and bibliotherapy were discussed.

Social skills are obviously critical for students with disabilities in regular classrooms, as well as adults in post-secondary environments. Better programs for social skills instruction and research validating specific techniques are being developed. These advances should result in increased and improved training efforts in the future.

REFERENCES

Andersen, M., Nelson, L.R., Fox, R.G., & Gruber, S.E. (1988). Integrating cooperative learning and structured learning: Effective approaches to teaching social skills. *Focus on Exceptional Children, 20,* 1–8.

Blackbourn, J.M. (1989). Acquisition and generalization of social skills in elementary-aged children with learning disabilities. *Journal of Learning Disabilities, 22,* 28–33.

Carlson, C.I. (1987). Social interaction goals and strategies of children with learning disabilities. *Journal of Learning Disabilities, 20,* 306—311.

Carnine, D., Silbert, J., & Kameenui, E.J. (1990). *Direct instruction reading,* 2nd Ed. Columbus, OH: Merrill Publishing.

Carter, J., & Sugai, G. (1988). Teaching social skills. *Teaching Exceptional Children, 20,* 68–71.

Carter, J., & Sugai, G. (1989). Social skills curriculum analysis. *Teaching Exceptional Children, 22,* 36–39.

Cartledge, G. & Milburn, J.F. (Eds.) (1986). *Teaching social skills to children*: Innovation approaches (2nd ed). New York: Pergamon Press.

Cosden, M.A., Iannaccone, C.J., & Wienke, W.D. (1990). Social skills instruction in secondary education: Are we prepared for integration of difficult-to-teach students? *Teacher Education and Special Education, 13,* 154–159.

Dinkmeyer, D., & Dinkmeyer, D., Jr. (1982). *Developing understanding of self and others* (rev. ed.), Circle Pines, MN: American Guidance Service.

Elksnin, L.K. (1989). Teaching mildly handicapped students social skills in secondary settings. *Academic Therapy, 25*, 153–167.

Fielder, C.R., & Chiang, B. (1989). Teaching social skills to students with learning disabilities. *LD Forum, 15*, 19–21.

Forness, S.R., & Kavale, K.A. (1991). Social skills deficits as primary learning disabilities: A note on problems with the ICLD diagnostic criteria. *Learning Disabilities Research & Practice, 6*, 44–49.

Furnham, A. (1989). Social skills training with adolescents and young adults. In Hollin, C.R., & Trower, P. (Eds.). *Handbook of social skills training*. Oxford: Pergamon Press.

Gearheart, B.R., & Gearheart, C.J. (1989). *Learning Disabilities*, 5th Ed. Columbus, OH: Merrill.

Goldstein, A.P., Sprafkin, R.P., Gershaw, N.J., & Klein, P. (1980). *Skillstreaming the adolescent*, Champaign, IL: Research Press.

Gresham, F.M. (1981). Social skills training with handicapped children: A review. *Review of Educational Reasearch, 51*, 139–176.

Gresham, F.M., & Elliott, S.N. (1989). Social skill deficits as a primary learning disability. *Journal of Learning Disabilities, 22*, 120–123.

Guerin, G.R., & Maier, A.S. (1983). *Informal assessment in education*. Palo Alto, CA: Mayfield Publishing.

Herbert, M. (1989). Social skills training with children. In Hollin, C.R., & Trower, P. (Eds). *Handbook of social skills training*. Oxford: Pergamon Press.

Hopkins, K.D., Stanley, J.C., & Hopkins, B.R. (1990). *Educational and psychological measurement and evaluation*, 7th Ed. Englewood Cliffs, NJ: Prentice-Hall.

Kerr, M.M., Nelson, C.M., & Lambert, D.L. (1987). *Helping adolescents with learning and behavior problems*. Columbus, OH: Merrill.

L'Abate, L. & Milan, M.A. (1985). *Handbook of social skills training and research*. New York: John Wiley & Sons.

Luftig, R.L. (1989). *Assessment of learners with special needs*. Boston: Allyn & Bacon.

Maag, J.W. (1989). Assessment in social skills training: Methodological and conceptual issues for research and practice. *Remedial and Special Education, 10*, 6–14.

Masters, L.F., & Mori, A.A. (1986). *Teaching secondary students with mild learning and behavior problems*. Rockville, Maryland: Aspen.

McGinnis, E., Goldstein, A.P., Sprafkin, R.P., & Gershaw, N.J. (1984). *Skillstreaming the elementary school child*. Champaign, IL: Research Press.

Minner, S., & Beane, A. (1985). Q-Sort for special education teachers. *Teaching Exceptional Children, 17*, 279–281.

Nelson, C.M. (1988). Social skills training for handicapped students. *Teaching Exceptional Children, 20*, 19–23.

Ness, J., & Price, L.A. (1990). Meeting the psychosocial needs of adolescents and adults with LD. *Intervention in School and Clinic, 26*, 16–21.

Ritter, D.R. (1989). Social competence and problem behavior of adolescent girls with learning disabilities. *Journal of Learning Disabilities, 22*, 460—461.

Sabornie, E.J., & Beard, G.H. (1990). Teaching social skills to students with mild handicaps. *Teaching Exceptional Children, 23*, 35–37.

Sargent, L.R. (1988). *Systematic instruction of social skills (Project SISS)*, 2nd Ed. Des Moines, IA: Iowa Department of Education.

Sargent, L.R. (1989). Instructional interventions to improve social competence. In Robinson, G.A., Patton, J.R., Polloway, E.A., & Sargent, L.R. (Eds.). *Best practices in mild mental disabilities*. Reston, VA: Division on Mental Retardation, Council for Exceptional Children.

Sargent, L.R. (1991). *Social Skills for school and community*. Reston, VA: Council for Exceptional Children.

Schinke, S.P., & Gilchrist, L.D. (1984). *Life skills counseling with adolescents*. Austin, TX: PRO-ED.

Smith, T.E.C., Price, B.J., & Marsh, G.E. *Mildly handicapped children and adults*. St. Paul: West Publishing.

Vaughn, S., & Lancelotta, G.X. (1990). Teaching interpersonal social skills to poorly accepted students: Peer-pairing versus non-peer-pairing. *Journal of School Psychology, 28*, 181–188.

Walker, H.M., McConnell, S., Holmes, D., Todis, B., Walker, J., & Golden, N. (1983). *The Walker social skills curriculum: The ACCEPTS program*. Austin, TX: Pro-Ed.

Walker, J.E., & Shea, T.M. (1984). *Behavior management*. St. Louis: C.V. Mosby.

Wallace, G., & McLoughlin, J.A. (1988). *Learning disabilities: Concepts and characteristics*, 3rd Ed. Columbus, OH: Merrill.

Wood, F.H. (1982). Affective education and social skills training: A consumer's guide. *Teaching Exceptional Children, 14*, 212–216.

Woolfolk, A.E. (1990). *Educational psychology*, 4th Ed. Englewood Cliffs, NJ: Prentice-Hall.

Transition Planning for Adolescents with Mild Disabilities

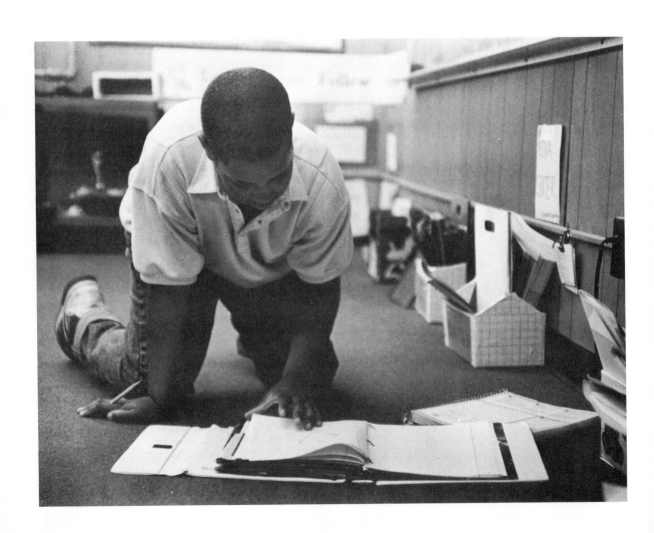

Outline

OBJECTIVES

After reading this chapter, you will be able to:

- describe the developmental changes associated with adolescence;

- discuss the additional challenges that a disability imposes on the adolescent period;

- identify the influence of societal changes on adolescents;

- specify the components of a high school special education curriculum;

- discuss the various roles of the high school special education teacher;

- summarize important legislation related to education and employment;

- describe the components of an employment curriculum;

- discuss model transition programs.

Introduction

Each year thousands of students with disabilities exit high school facing new demands in post-secondary education programs, independent living settings, and, ultimately, employment. Too often their high school education has not focused on the skills needed to make a successful transition into these new environments. Studies have shown that many of these students are likely be unemployed, underemployed, or employed part time to a greater degree than nondisabled individuals (Wehman, Kregel, & Barcus, 1985; Mithaug, Martin, & Agran, 1987; Rusch & Phelps, 1987; Neel, R.S., Meadows, N., Levine, P., & Edgar, E.B., 1988; Edgar, 1988). These negative findings in follow-up studies have served to stimulate ongoing interest in developing more effective high school programs for students with disabilities; however, to date these programs do not appear to be preparing students adequately for post-secondary programs, employment, or independent living (Polloway, Patton, Payne, & Payne, 1989; Smith & Dowdy, 1989).

Data from the students also suggest that they realize their lack of preparedness. Dowdy, Carter, and Smith (1990) surveyed students with learning disabilities and non-learning disabled students in high schools concerning their transition needs. While both groups expressed an interest in having more assistance with career decisions, significant differences were found between the students. Students with learning disabilities had a greater desire for more information about how to find a job, how to keep a job, and how to live independently than their nondisabled peers. Parents were credited by both groups as providing the majority of support in preparing them for life after high school. Friends were actually credited with providing more support in these efforts than teachers or counselors.

Another indication of the ineffectiveness of schools in meeting the needs of students is the high drop-out rate among adolescents with disabilities. Zigmond (1988) reported that the school drop-out rates for this group were highest after the ninth grade. The adolescent age group has been identified as the group most in need of services (U.S. Department of Education, 1988). The 12th Annual Report to Congress on the Implementation of the Education of the Handicapped Act (U.S. Department of Education, Office of Special Education and Rehabilitation Services, 1990) revealed that in 1987–1988 only 42 percent of students with disabilities graduated with a diploma; 11 percent graduated with a certificate. The report also indicated that the drop-out rate for students with disabilities was 27.4 percent. The highest drop-out rate was 40 percent for students with emotional conflict; 26 percent of the students with learning disabilities and mental retardation dropped out. Edgar (1987) reported that a study of students with learning disabilities and behavior disorders revealed a 42 percent drop-out rate for these populations. The high proportion of adolescents with mild disabilities dropping out of school in comparison to the normal population suggests that these students are a high risk for dropping out. Measures should be taken to make school more appealing and meaningful for students with disabilities.

Much improvement is needed in our educational approach for adolescents with disabilities to change the prognosis for these young adults. Teachers must address the effects of the natural maturation process of adolescence as well as the special complications that evolve as students with disabilities face these changes. At the same time, they must deal with significant changes in the school environment as they move from the more supportive, nurturing elementary and middle school settings into high school. This chapter will address the period of adolescence including the physical, cognitive, personality, and societal changes. Various models of transition and the roles of high school teachers will be explored to identify the most effective procedures for preparing each young person for the demands of the future.

Adolescence

The adolescent phase of development is a transitional period of great change that presents unique challenges and adjustment for children, parents, and others who interact with the adolescent. The child's challenge is to develop independence and maturity as he or she leaves the restrictiveness of childhood. Parents face the need for a change in the long-standing dependent relationship with their child, as they must offer new freedom and greater responsibility. Their primary challenge is to cope effectively during this tumultuous period, providing support during the many crises and conflicts which are inevitable. Because so many parents work outside the home, teachers have more responsibility than ever to prepare these young people for the many adult roles which they will assume. Understanding the increasing task demands of the adolescent period and the complicated physical, psychological and personality, and cognitive changes that affect each adolescent regardless of disability are essential for a successful transition to adulthood.

The period of adolescent development has been described in many ways. It can be defined as "1. the transitional period between childhood and adulthood, 2. the period during which an emotionally mature person reaches the final stages of physical and mental development, and 3. the period of attainment of maturity" (Smith, Price, & Marsh, 1986, p. 212). It is well documented as a period of difficult adjustment, great turmoil, and conflict. The physical, psychological and personality, and cognitive changes characteristic of this period will be addressed separately.

PHYSICAL CHANGES

The physical changes generally begin during the onset of adolescence described by Mercer (1987) as early adolescence, between the ages of twelve and fifteen. During this time puberty begins as the body changes, becoming sexually active and capable of reproduction. The ovaries of the female and the prostate gland and seminal vesicles of the male gradually become enlarged. An accelerated period of growth usually begins that generally lasts about two years. Although males typically begin their growth spurt later than females, males generally grow more and faster with more musculature developing. Males and females can become excessively concerned when they feel that their development is unusually slow. Males may express their concern about their limited masculinity. During this period, males also frequently develop enlarged breasts and fattiness around their middle. This is very normal, and both disappear within a year or two, leaving a more "normal," socially acceptable masculine appearance (Cruickshank, 1978). The increase in height, strength, and stamina is significant in both sexes, with females developing wider hips and males developing wider shoulders (Scarr, Weinberg, & Levine, 1986).

Similar to the way in which females have their growth spurt before males, their sexual development also occurs before males. The onset of menarche formally signifies the beginning of sexual maturity for females; the age of onset varies from approximately 9.5 years to 14.5 years. The average beginning of the monthly menstrual cycle is 12.8 years (Kerr, Nelson, & Lambert, 1987). The average age for males to reach sexual maturity is 13.5 years, approximately three years after females. Male sexual maturity is characterized by their ability to develop and ejaculate sperm. Other examples of physical maturity include the lowering of the male voice and the development of breasts in females. Mercer (1987) notes that as sexual maturity is evolving, the adolescent must develop a new identity and learn a new set of rules. Expressing this new sexuality appropriately is often a difficult task.

Adolescents frequently spend a great amount of time and energy worrying about the normalcy of their physical development and their own sexual behavior. They are in a struggle to establish a sense of self. This focus on self, which is typically not present in childhood, results in a preoccupation with appearance, clothes, and adherence to peer-group norms (Mercer, 1987). If the adolescent does not approve of his or her own looks, the result can be feelings of inferiority, self-consciousness, and withdrawal (Evra, 1983). Many adolescents go through a period where they simply do not like themselves.

PSYCHOLOGICAL AND PERSONALITY CHANGES

Adolescents also go through a difficult period of emotional changes. The importance of peer acceptance, doubts about their new self image, acceptance of their changing bodies and new sexuality, and growing tension with their parents create unpredictable emotional states. Adolescents frequently describe their feelings as being mixed up. They may snap at their parents, cry easily, and behave in ways that they cannot explain (Polloway & Smith, 1992).

The late development experienced by many young people, can be even more devastating to adolescents. Cruickshank (1978) cites a study in which boys who matured late were found to exhibit less behavior control, appear less attractive, be less poised, and interact with others with greater tension. They were also described as bossy, less attentive, talkative, and more restless. Conversely boys who matured earlier showed more self-control, self-confidence, and a greater ability to laugh at themselves. They also engaged in more socially appropriate behavior. The personality traits of both early and late maturers tended to persist into adulthood. Cruickshank proposed that these antisocial, rebellious characteristics may not be inherent personality traits but more a result of the young person's lack of understanding and subsequent response to the way they are treated.

Although females were less affected by late maturation than males, a few differences were found (Cruickshank, 1978). Early maturing girls tended to be better adjusted and have fewer feelings of inadequacy than the later developing girls, who were found to have higher levels of anxiety. Interestingly, the early developing females were considered more of an abnormal person among their peers. Overall, females seem better able to cope with changes in development than males.

The physical growth of adolescents soon results in the appearance and stature of adults. This mature appearance frequently causes adults to expect more adult-like behavior from adolescents than they are emotionally capable of handling (Mercer, 1987). This is a difficult period of adjustment in which adolescents are faced with the need to become more independent and separate from their families, yet they need familial ties and support. These personality and psychological changes can result in greater conflict and stress than the physical changes as teenagers attempt to find their niche in the adult world. They tend to rebel for more independence and self-responsibility before they are ready to handle the consequences of their behavior (McDowell, 1981).

Opportunities are available for the adolescent to be mobile and functionally independent. Unlike the life of a child, which focuses on school and family, the adolescent moves about the community and beyond independently, generally unsupervised. Parental control and thus societal control is weakened. The increase in the importance of peers occurs as the influence of the family declines (Larson, Kubey, & Colletti, 1989). At this time more than any other in one's life, the peer group exerts the single most important influence, particularly in behavior and dress. Rogers (1977) points out that adolescent peers help broaden perspectives, develop independence from families, and offer encouragement and support for rebellion. Confrontation and conflict can result when the values held by peers differ significantly from those of the families (Evra, 1983). In trying to establish a personal identity and also conform to peer expectations, adolescents sometimes engage in undesirable behaviors that result in trouble in school and at home (Mercer, 1987). It is particularly important to maintain open lines of communication during this time period. If parents and teachers have maintained a secure and well-structured relationship, it will be helpful in allowing adoles-cents to draw on the adult "ego bank" for the needed security and supports (Cruickshank, 1978).

McDowell (1981) summarizes these changes that occur as the adolescent struggles with autonomy as the evolution of maturation around seven major issues: identity, status, independence, sex and sexuality, relationships and intimacy, decision making, and values. As teens strive to be accepted for their own merit, their self-perception or identity can be a source of great stress. Nicknames and labels are frequently used during this period, with status in the group connoted by your individual label. Obtaining membership in the most prestigious teen clubs can be an obsession for teenagers who have not developed a sense of self-identity. Participation in gangs is the extreme extension of this need for group acceptance and status. The search is for belonging, often without regard for the societal acceptance of the group that has accepted them. During the struggle for independence, the adolescent frequently breaks rules and challenges limits established by authority. Often the values established in the family are at least temporarily challenged. All significant relationships are redefined during adolescence. Constant stability, love, caring, and support from significant adults is critical for adolescents to move successfully through this period of conflict and to eventually develop intimate relationships with others (McDowell, 1981).

COGNITIVE CHANGES

During the period of adolescence, individuals evolve from being concrete thinkers to having the capability for higher levels of abstract thinking and problem solving. While IQ basically remains stable, mental abilities develop to allow the generation of a variety of hypotheses and exploring solutions using deductive reasoning (Mercer, 1987). However, the adolescent's lack of experience can often interfere with good judgment.

During adolescence, young people begin to see the hypocrisy in society and express disgust when they see adults behaving in a manner different from the way they have been expected to behave. This is often the first period of rebellion when parental or societal values are first questioned (Cruickshank, 1978). Adolescents are observed brainstorming about world issues, often offering oversimplified solutions to world problems.

Another cognitive development is the emergence of language skills necessary to meet the increased expressive and receptive demands of high school content classes and to understand the more complex social interactions (Polloway & Smith, 1992). Even understanding and participating in humorous conversations and jokes becomes a difficult challenge as adolescents begin using double entendres, puns, and expressive body language. Many teachers are not understanding about disabilities and feel that accommodations should not be made at the high school level. Students unable to meet class standards simply receive failing grades.

In addition to the changes in characteristics, every adolescent goes through a series of developmental tasks. These task demands that face adolescents have remained fairly consistent since they were proposed by Havighurst in 1953. Following is a modified list proposed by Smith, Price, and Marsh (1986).

1. The creation of a sense of sexual identity.

2. The development of self-confidence in social situations.

3. The integration of social values into the individual's code of conduct.

4. The acceptance of physical changes.

5. The attainment of emotional independence.

6. The exploration of career interests.

7. The identification of individual interests and talents.

8. The awareness of individual strengths and limitations.

9. The development of sexual interests outside the family unit.

10. The development of relationships with peers.

11. The completion of formal educational activities.

12. The preparation for marriage, parenting, and adult relationships (p. 212).

The presence of a handicap can make the fulfillment of these tasks much more difficult. It is important for parents and professionals to understand the normal characteristics and tasks of adolescence as well as the problems that can occur as a function of the presence of a disability. Table 11–1 provides a summary of these difficulties.

TABLE 11-1 Developmental Tasks and Resultant Questions

DEVELOPMENTAL TASKS	QUESTIONS TO CONSIDER
Creation of a Sense of Sexuality as Part of a Personal Identity	■ How is this affected by the presence of a physical handicap? ■ Does poor school performance and low social status impact this?
Development of Confidence in Social Interactions	■ Do negative classroom experiences play a role? ■ Is social inadequacy assumed by others to be an automatic result of being handicapped?
Infusion of Social Values into a Personal Code of Behavior	■ Are handicapped students often protected by adults to such a degree that they do not have experiences which allow them to develop a sense of what social values exist? ■ Does the handicap and/or other's reaction to it prevent experimentation with social behavior?
Acceptance of Biological Changes	■ Are handicapped students denied accurate information about their own bodies and sexual maturity? ■ Is it sometimes difficult for handicapped students with lower intellectual performance to glean information by osmosis or to comprehend the information?
Attainment of a Sense of Emotional Independence	■ Are handicapped students given the same opportunity as other adolescents to make their own decisions? ■ Is it more difficult for a handicapped adolescent to deal effectively with emotion?
Contemplation of Vocational Interests	■ Are handicapped students limited in vocational choices because of preconceived notions of their ability? ■ Are vocational training options too tightly tied to labels and not to true individual ability?
Identification of Personal Talents and Interests	■ Is it more difficult for handicapped students to identify positive trails within themselves as a result of negative events experienced?
Awareness of Personal Weaknesses and Strengths	■ Do students focus more on their limitations than strengths? ■ Do handicapped students have an inaccurate self-concept?
Development of Sexual Interests with Nonfamily Members	■ Is it more difficult to develop heterosexual contacts if the adolescent is handicapped?

continued

TABLE 11–1 Developmental Tasks and Resultant Questions (cont'd.)

DEVELOPMENTAL TASKS	QUESTIONS TO CONSIDER
Development of Sexual Interests with Nonfamily Members	■ Do public prejudices serve as barriers to the development of sexual interests?
Development of Peer Relationships	■ Are there fewer opportunities for handicapped adolescents to develop peer relationships? ■ Are some students isolated socially by the limitations of their label more than by the actual effects of the condition?
Completion of Formal Educational Activities	■ Has Public Law 94–142 increased the likelihood of this? ■ Should handicapped students receive special diplomas which identify them as handicapped?
Preparation for Marriage, Parenting, and Adult Relationships	■ Do handicapped students receive information concerning family responsibilities? ■ Do some community attitudes operate against adolescents so that adult relationships are difficult to achieve?

Source: Smith, T.E.C., Price, B.J., & Marsh, G.E. (1986). *Mildly handicapped children and adults.* St. Paul, MN: West., p. 214. Reprinted with permission.

Adolescents with Disabilitites

The characteristics specific to adolescents with mild disabilities exacerbate the normal difficulties of adolescence (Dossetor & Nicol, 1989). Although these characteristics manifest themselves to varying degrees across categories and more importantly, between individual children, the deficits in cognitive, academic, and social and behavioral functioning described in Chapter 2 create tremendous hurdles for students with disabilities. The cognitive and social and behavioral differences generally have an even greater impact than the academic difficulties. Collectively, they can seriously limit interactions with peers, success in school settings, and relationships within families.

THE IMPACT OF COGNITIVE DIFFERENCES

Generally the cognitive deficits used to describe children with mild disabilities persist into adolescence. These include below-average general intellectual functioning, field-dependent cognitive styles, attention and memory problems, poor problem-solving skills, and deficits in planning and organizing.

Because of the more serious cognitive limitations of adolescents with mental retardation, the impact is intensified. While they generally have the same physical development of nondisabled adolescents, they do not have the cognitive ability to cope with the new differences within themselves or the new demands of their environment (Drew, Logan, & Hardman, 1988). They are faced with the responsibility of preparation for employment and developing the competency in social skills that will allow them to be accepted in society. These adolescents need very concrete experiences to learn academics and to become competent in social skills and independent living skills. Their limited cognitive ability frequently creates problems in identifying appropriate career goals. It is a great challenge for parents and educators to help the adolescent with mental retardation realize limitations without damaging their fragile self-concept (Drew *et al.*, 1988).

To some degree, cognitive deficits affect all adolescents with disabilities. Because of limited problem-solving and language skills they are often not able to effectively participate in the type of "intellectual exercise" commonly observed with adolescents. It is necessary for teachers and parents to discuss this new level and type of interaction and advanced language abilities observed among their peers without disabilities. Without an understanding of the changes in their peers, adolescents with disabilities may try to compensate by engaging in distracting behaviors, such as teasing, using foul language, or being sexually inappropriate (Cruickshank, 1978). The result may be removal from the group and the feeling of being left out and having no friends.

Social acceptance is extremely important to students with disabilities; it is probably more important than acceptance from parents and other adults. Limited language and cognitive abilities can impact on this approval, resulting in peer rejection and low self-esteem, which could have long lasting effects (Polloway & Smith, 1992). Some students will benefit from being taught strategies for problem solving and how to use more complex kinds of humor such as puns or the double entendre. At the very least students should be taught how to respond in socially appropriate ways during these sophisticated group exchanges.

THE IMPACT OF SOCIAL AND BEHAVIORAL CHARACTERISTICS

A review of Chapter 2 suggests that adolescents with disabilities are often characterized by a low self-concept, ineffective levels of motivation, behavior problems, hyperactivity, and poor social skills. Ness & Price (1990) also report psychological problems including feelings of anger, incompetence, inadequacy, and frustration. Characteristic behaviors included boldness, impulsivity, excessive dependency, and shyness. These characteristics can have a serious impact on a student's success in academic classrooms and the ability to establish important social networks. Job success is also compromised many times by an individual's inability to function socially regardless of an ability to perform the job. Teachers of students with disabilities must carefully observe the social and behavioral characteristics of their students, determine the impact of the behaviors, and identify strategies to remediate or make effective accommodations.

Low motivation and self-concept are frequently found among teens without disabilities, so these characteristics do not always set the students with disabilities apart. However, if high levels of motivation can be sustained and adolescence can be reached with a positive self-concept, the prognosis for success in high school and beyond is significantly greater (Epstein, Polloway, Patton, & Foley, 1989). The manifestation of inappropriate behavior, hyperactivity, and poor social skills are especially apparent and considered inappropriate in high school settings. Without successful treatment or intervention, these characteristics often persist through adolescence and may be manifested in adulthood (Mercer, 1987; Kauffman, 1989; Polloway *et al.*, 1989).

The normal adolescent years are characterized by increased opportunities for independence, longer periods without supervision and feedback, and greater responsibilities for personal problem solving. Certainly the lower intellectual levels of many students with disabilities limit their judgment capabilities. While they may have a normal desire for self-direction, the cognitive limitations interfere with good judgment and, therefore, limit the probability for success. In trying to emulate the normal behavior of their peers, they may overstep the limits and get in serious trouble with parents, school authorities, and sometimes the law. Even the students with learning disabilities and behavior disorders whose intellectual functioning fall in the normal range, may have other cognitive difficulties that interfere with functioning.

A common characteristic of children with learning and behavior disorders is their inability to predict the consequences of their behavior. For example, they may reason that if they act like one of the popular students, all of the students will like them too. Often they don't have the physical ability or mental capacity to pull off the simulation successfully or they overdo the performance. As a result, they may be successful in making fools of themselves or getting into trouble for the overzealous behavior. The damage to the student's reputation from episodes like these is often long lasting; rarely do second and third chances get offered (Cruickshank, 1978). A study by Polloway, Epstein, Patton, Cullinan, and Luebke (1986) reported that teachers' ratings indicated that more than twenty percent of the older students with mild mental retardation were rejected by their peers. This lack of success socially, the adolescents' typical disapproval of their own looks, and the common failures and frustrations with academic demands can result in serious damage to self-esteem and coping abilities.

THE IMPACT OF ACADEMIC DEFICITS

A primary characteristic of adolescents with learning disabilities and mental retardation and often of those with behavior disorders is the presence of academic disabilities (Mercer, 1987; Polloway, Patton, Payne, & Payne, 1989; Kauffman, 1989). To qualify for special education placement, the disability must interfere with successful functioning in the regular program to such a degree that special services are required. This typically means the humiliation of lower grades and negative attention from teachers in mainstream classes. With emphasis placed on excellence in education in the nineties, students with disabilities have more pressure to succeed and less tolerance for their limitations than ever before.

Academic ability is obviously needed for success in mainstream content classes; however, it is also important in planning for most future endeavors. A high school diploma is obtained in most states only through successful completion of the required Carnegie units, not successful completion of the IEP. This diploma and an acceptable grade point average are required for many competitive jobs and admission to most post secondary institutions. Aside from the embarrassment of poor academic achievement, this characteristic may have a serious impact on success in other environments after high school.

Many of the typical demands of daily living also require a degree of academic ability. Particularly as our society becomes more infused with technology, higher levels of cognitive and academic skills will be required. Operating a bank account, filling out forms for basic needs, such as a car registration or marriage license, and applying for a job can be impossibilities and sources of great humiliation.

Although academic difficulties are not as automatic among adolescents with behavior disorders, the inappropriate behaviors often interfere with success in the mainstream classes and ultimately result in below average academic achievement (Kauffman, 1989). Thus the disability of these young people creates all of the barriers of achievement deficits and success is further complicated by their behavior differences. Students with mental retardation are described as having deficits in all academic areas, poor memory and problem-solving skills, language deficits, and deficient thinking skills (Polloway *et al.*, 1989). The definition and placement criteria for learning disabilities, is a deficit in one or more academic areas. One difficulty for them is the variability across academic subjects. Regular class teachers often do not understand how a student can be accomplished in one subject and do poorly in another. These differences are frequently mislabeled as poor motivation and a lack of effort.

Societal Influences on Adolescents

Many of the unique challenges facing adolescents are a reflection of the interaction of the significant change, turmoil, and insecurity inherent in the adolescent developmental period and the changes and problems occurring in society. These include sexual role identity, adolescent pregnancy, alcohol and drug abuse, and suicide. While all adolescents will not face all of these challenges to the same degree, the problems are widespread enough to warrant discussion. Additional problems exist for adolescents with disabilities because of the altered perception and patterns of interactions of others in response to the disability.

CHANGING ROLES

The rapidly changing roles for males and females are a significant source of confusion for adolescents. In contemporary society there is no set difference between the sexes, yet, there are some unspoken expectations that still prevale in some households and school environments. These subtle expectations and societal nuances are particularly difficult for young persons with disabilities to interpret. Adolescents must be encouraged to express their confusion and be given opportunities to role play some of the difficult social interactions they face.

PREGNANCY AND AIDS

One of the difficulties associated with poor self-esteem and the need for peer approval is the pressure for teenagers to become sexually active, which may result in an unplanned pregnancy. Unplanned pregnancy among teens is an increasing problem. Despite the widespread media coverage about AIDS, significant numbers of adolescents are apparently practicing unsafe sex. Adolescents with disabilities may not understand if only abstract information is provided on contraceptives or may not understand the consequences of the sexual behavior. Ongoing sex education and counseling must be an important component of the educational plans or parental guidance for adolescents with disabilities.

ALCOHOL AND DRUG ABUSE

Drug and alcohol abuse is also a serious problem among adolescents. Anderson and Magnusson (1990) reported that forty-eight percent of the boys sampled admitted having been drunk by the age of fourteen years five months. Eleven percent reported having been drunk ten times or more by that age. The self-esteem problems, the obsession with peer approval, and the need for any form of recognition are the basis for many adolescents turning to alcohol or drugs for escape. Hammer and Vaglum (1990) found that the years of transition between adolescence and adulthood were the highest in the consumption of alcohol for males and females.

The characteristics of adolescents with disabilities make them particularly at risk for drug and alcohol abuse. In 1988 Johnson studied drug and alcohol abusers and noted the following characteristics.

1. Low self-esteem
2. Stress
3. Problems with social interactions
4. Problems with values and character development
5. Depression

Each of these characteristics has been used throughout the literature to describe persons with disabilities. Their lack of achievement and acceptance in society create low self-esteem and stress. Cognitive and language deficits create problems with social interactions and difficulty in consistently making moral choices. All of these contribute to the feelings of depression.

SUICIDE

Suicide is now the second leading cause of death among adolescents. Ritter reports that, "suicide and self-harm have reached epidemic proportions among adolescents" (1990, p. 83). Suicide is a higher risk for adolescents with disabilities than their nondisabled peers.

Students with learning disabilities and behavior disorders experience frustration and depression that can lead to suicide. Poor social skills, characteristic of students with disabilities, have also been linked to depression (Spirito, Hart, Overholser, & Halverson, 1990). Guetzloe (1988) cites stress, low self-esteem, and depression as related to suicide. She also points out the high-risk factor for students with disabilities, since these are frequent descriptors for this population. Signs of depression and threats of suicide must be given serious consideration when manifested by all adolescents. However, it is particularly important for persons with disabilities who may not realize the finality of suicide. Some students have threatened suicide by saying that they will do it to punish their parents or another person who has hurt them. They describe wanting to see their reaction. Limited cognitive levels or perceptual deficits may interfere with their understanding of the consequences of their behavior.

PERSONAL INTERACTIONS

One of the biggest problems that adolescents with disabilities face is adult domination, which is often much greater for them than for their normal peers. Children with disabilities begin to think that adulthood has arrived for them as physical changes become apparent and as they observe other adolescents having more freedom. As with other adolescents, they often express these new feelings of maturity in rather immature ways. Adults recognize the behavior as immaturity and respond by offering more restrictions during a period when the controls should be loosened. This begins a vicious cycle of mistrust that often results in rebelliousness, tension, and turmoil (Cruickshank, 1978). These differences can be very difficult to resolve to the satisfaction of both parties. They can cause serious and lasting interpersonal barriers with the adult figures who are needed for support and guidance during these confusing years.

The perceptions and interactions of other individuals with adolescents with disabilities can also create barriers. Often teachers, family members, and friends treat these young people differently because they know of the disability; they project those differences in abilities through their language or actions whether they are real or not. For example, these individuals may offer fewer invitations for advanced social activities, ask questions that require yes or no responses instead of abstract reasoning, and may not include the young people with disabilities in planning and organizing activities. This can cause serious self-esteem problems. In a study by Young, Rathge, Mullis, and Mullis (1990), it was noted that the number of negative events and stress in a person's life was correlated with self-esteem. Negative parental interaction has also been correlated to low self-esteem (Scarr *et al.*, 1986).

To combat the negative effects of reduced expectations and negative interactions, adolescents with disabilities should be treated as adolescents first. The normalcy of their development and behavior should be given first consideration. After that the differences can be isolated and dealt with directly (Cruickshank, 1978). As noted in Chapter 10, the area of social skills affects all areas of a person's life including home, school, leisure, and employment. A high school curriculum must address these issues and others facing adolescents on a daily basis and encompass the skills and abilities needed for a successful future.

High School Special Education Curriculum

A comprehensive high school curriculum must address both current and future needs of individual students. Polloway, Patton, Payne, and Payne (1989) describe such a program as:

- responsive to the current needs of individual students;

- capable of encouraging maximum interaction wtih nondisabled peers;

- related to the service delivery options such as resource or self-contained classes;

- developed from a comprehensive assessment of adult potential;
- focused on the needs for transition across a life span;
- sensitive to diploma requirements and goals for graduation.

The literature often overviews various curricular approaches to high school students with disabilities as if teachers, administrators, or parents can evaluate the pros and cons of each and make a selection. Indeed, teachers often make choices on the basis of what they are comfortable teaching. Since many special education teacher training programs in the past have focused on elementary methods, it is understandable that teachers might choose a curriculum which would primarily address the needs of elementary children.

The basic skills remediation approach is an example of a curriculum that is basically an upward extension of an elementary model. In this approach, students are provided individualized remedial instruction for basic academic skill deficits. Instead of seeing the need for a new approach to teach adolescents, teachers adopting this model seem to have the philosophy that their methods for teaching phonics and other basic academic skills surpass those used by their students' previous teachers. They give remediation one more try. Some are still trying when students graduate or, worse, drop out of school. Alley and Desher (1979) cited this approach and four others commonly used in high schools.

Also cited was the tutorial approach in which students with disabilities take most content subjects in regular classes, with the efforts of the special education teacher spent preparing the students for the next test or assignment. An improvement over this approach is the learning strategies approach in which students with disabilities are prepared for the challenges in regular classes by instruction in how-to-learn strategies rather than the specific content addressed in the mainstream classes (Deshler & Schumaker, 1986).

A third model, the functional curriculum, focuses more on the skills students need to live successfully in society. This model teaches academics through content related to careers and independent living demands. Finally, the work study model provides instruction in specific job related skills. Each of these curricular approaches has strengths and limitations in addressing the wide variety of needs and the heterogeneous nature of students with mild disabilities. Most are specifically addressing only one of the current or future needs of the students. The role of the special education teacher as depicted in Figure 11–1 must be much more comprehensive.

The Role of the Special Education Teacher

The efforts of the special education teacher must address the current demands placed on the students they teach as well as the future challenges they will face. As shown in Figure 11–1, the role of the high school special education teacher includes preparing students for content classes, the high school graduation exam, post-secondary training programs, independent living, employment, and counseling for today's crises.

FIGURE 11-1 Role of the Special Education High School Teacher

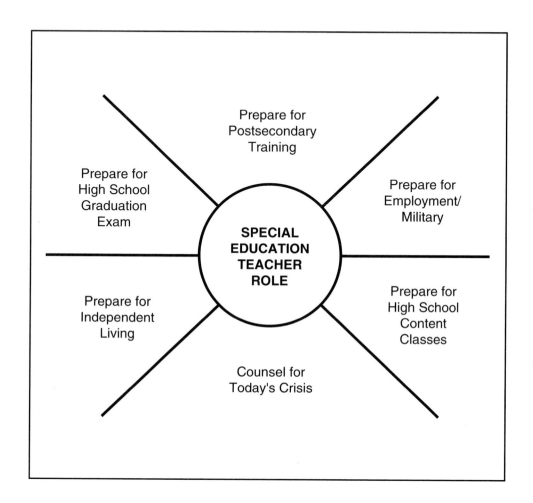

COUNSELING FOR TODAY'S CRISES

The emotional crises faced by a group of adolescents could tie up a teacher's instructional time each day. Earlier sections have addressed the tremendous peer pressure exerted on these students, the difficulty with new identities, relationships, and sexual roles, the prevalence of alcohol and drug problems, as well as the increasing number of teenage pregnancies and the problems of suicide. While these situations can be critical, and are certainly of major concern to the adolescent, teachers must find ways to provide support and counsel for each day's crises and do much, much more. The goal of high school should be to prepare students for their adult lives; however, some teachers work as if their only goal is to get their students through high school!

PREPARING FOR CONTENT CLASSES

The demands on adolescents change dramatically between elementary and high school. Many of these changes can lead to problems for students with disabilities. Mercer (1987) identifies the following high school classroom expectations.

1. Develop complex skills in written expression.

2. Attend to lectures and take elaborate notes.

3. Complete a broad array of courses in the content areas.

4. Read for different purposes with a high level of comprehension.

Buttrill, Niizawa, Biemer, Takahashi, & Hearn (1989) report other demands, including;

1. working independently;

2. reading textbooks on high reading levels; and

3. participating in oral activities in the classroom.

Students without disabilities do not receive a course on how to be successful in meeting the new challenges of the content classes in high schools. Memory strategies, test-taking skills, the ability to listen and take notes simultaneously, time management, and organization skills seem to come naturally for them. However, it is generally accepted that whatever the students with mild handicaps need to learn, they need to be taught (Deshler & Schumaker, 1986). Because of the importance of success in the regular education classrooms, Chapter 8 of the text was developed to provide a comprehensive review of methods that can be implemented to augment the efforts of the regular classroom teacher. The focus on study skills, strategies for learning, and accommodations is very applicable to the demands of the high school environment. The social skills strategies addressed in Chapter 10 are also critical to the students' success in mainstream classes and the future employment, post-secondary, and independent living challenges as well.

PREPARING FOR THE HIGH SCHOOL GRADUATION EXAM

The high school graduation exam or high school exit exam is a fairly recent phenomenon brought about during the push for excellence and the literacy campaigns of the 1980s. Students with disabilities are not required to take the exam in many states, but it is usually a requirement for the regular high school diploma. If a transitional goal includes post-secondary training, the exam is almost a necessity.

The intervention approach that focuses on developing the basic academic skills necessary for passing the graduation exam is the academic remediation approach. When academic abilities are significantly deficient and the desire for passing the basic competency exam is great, academic remediation is an appropriate choice (Mercer, 1987). However, this approach has been criticized by many as seriously limiting (Deshler, Schumaker, Lenz, & Ellis, 1984). In fact Deshler *et al.* (1984) note that remediating basic skills is simply an extension of the elementary program and not effective in impacting the complexities of the demands of high school. Mercer (1987) proposes that academic remediation seems most appropriate for students in the ninth and tenth grades who are functioning below fourth grade level. Unfortunately, to make significant strides in academics with students who are this far behind, teachers tend to totally focus on skill training. Little time is devoted to other areas that are needed for success in future demands, such as independent living and employment. Even if academic skill development is a primary goal, the materials and activities used should be interwoven with career and independent living instruction (Mercer, 1987).

PREPARING FOR INDEPENDENT LIVING

Although daily living skills are generally thought to be more important for the more cognitively limited students with mental retardation, it is a mistake to assume that students with learning disabilities and behavior disorders will need no instruction in these areas. The follow-up studies of adult-adjustment for adults with disabilities suggest that problems exist in the areas of daily living skills, personal and social adjustment, and occupational development. Cullinan, Epstein, and Lloyd (1983) report that the environmental conflicts, personal disturbances, and learning disorders characteristic of persons with behavior disorders suggest the need for intervention in the areas of vocational, career, sexuality, and drug abuse education. In a study by Halpern, Close, and Nelson (1986) the independent living skills cited as problematic for adults with mental retardation included:

- managing money,
- developing social networks,
- maintaining a home,
- managing food,
- conflicts over asking for help versus doing what they are told,
- employment,
- transportation, and
- handling and avoiding problems.

In a survey sponsored by the National Association for Children and Adults with Learning Disorders, now called the Learning Disabilities Association of America (Chesler, 1982), adults with learning disabilities reported having difficulties in:

- social skills and relationships,
- career counseling,
- self-confidence and self-esteem,
- dependency,
- vocational training,
- obtaining and maintaining a job,
- reading,

- spelling,

- managing personal finances, and

- organizing skills.

Independent living is most likely an attainable goal for individuals with mild disabilities. However, living in today's more complex world may require direct instruction for success. Each adolescent should be assessed in terms of potential for independent living and to determine areas of potential difficulty. Several excellent resources are available that offer a functional living curriculum. Knowles (1984) identified the life demands of adults at various stages of life. This comprehensive overview of the demands on young adults could be used as goals for the transitional component of the IEP. This outline is included in table 11–2.

TABLE 11–2 Life Problems of American Adults

Vocation and Career	*Home and Family Living*
Exploring career options	Courting
Choosing a career line	Selecting a mate
Getting a job	Preparing for marriage
Being interviewed	Family planning
Learning job skills	Preparing for children
Getting along at work	Raising children
Getting ahead at work	Understanding children
Getting job protection or military service	Preparing children for school
Getting vocational counseling	Helping children in school
Changing jobs	Solving marital problems
	Using family counseling
Personal Development	Managing a home
	Financial planning
Improving your reading ability	Managing money
Improving your writing ability	Buying goods and services
Improving your speaking ability	Making home repairs
Improving your listening ability	Gardening
Continuing your general education	
Developing your religious faith	*Enjoyment of Leisure*
Improving problem-solving skills	
Making better decisions	Choosing hobbies
Getting along with people	Finding new friends
Understanding yourself	Joining organizations
Finding your self-identify	Planning your time
Discovering your aptitudes	Buying equipment
Clarifying your values	Planning family recreation
Understanding other people	Leading recreational activities
Learning to be self-directing	
Improving personal appearance	
Establishing intimate relations	
Dealing with conflict	
Making use of personal counseling	

continued

TABLE 11–2 Life Problems of American Adults (cont'd.)

Health	Community Living
Keeping fit	Relating to school and teachers
Planning diets	Learning about community resources
Finding and using health services	Learning how to get help
Preventing accidents	Learning how to exert influence
Using first aid	Preparing to vote
Understanding children's diseases	Developing leadership skills
Understanding how the human body functions	Keeping up with the world
Buying and using drugs and medicines	Taking action in the community
Developing a healthy life style	Organizing community activities for children and
Recognizing the symptoms of physical and mental illness	youth

Source: Knowles, M (1986). *The adult learner: A neglected species.* Houston: Gulf Publishers, pp. 146–148. Reprinted with permission.

Kokaska and Brolin (1985) also offer a functional living curriculum that addresses nine major areas. Table 11–3 (on page 434) contains a listing of these areas, which may be used to structure an intervention program in independent living.

These materials are excellent guides; however, a creative teacher should also anticipate the future challenges specific to the local community and incorporate them into the instructional process. The curriculum and activities should be constantly assessed in terms of currency of the demands. For example, as automated bank machines and other technology are introduced into society, the new advances should be incorporated into the life skills curriculum (Patton, Cronin, Polloway, Hutchison, & Robinson, 1989).

Real materials can be collected from the local offices in the community. The bank can supply materials to teach skills for opening and managing a savings and checking account. Field trips to grocery, drug, and retail stores can provide situations for problem solving and training. The daily newspaper should be thoroughly used for keeping up with the national and local news and for finding and using various sections, such as want ads, grocery and store advertisements, and identifying important information for leisure activities. A trip through the offices of the local court house will provide important forms, such as applications for driver's license, car tag, marriage license, voter registration, and so on.

Other areas that should be addressed in a life-skills curriculum are budgeting, transportation, and use of the telephone. When teachers find ways of incorporating these realistic teaching tools, students will become more motivated because of the practical application they can see for their adult lives. Some excellent commercial materials are also available, such as the *Essential Life Skills Series* published by National Textbook Company; this may be ordered from Communication Skills Builders, 3830 Bellevue E., Tuscon, AZ, 85733.

In addition to using real life experiences and materials, an effective method for presenting the independent living skills curriculum is through infusing the presentation of the materials into the content areas of a high school curriculum. The Adult Performance Level Curriculum (APL, 1975), developed at the University of Texas, provides another functional description of adult literacy through forty-two identified life skills. To begin training for

TABLE 11–3 Life-Centered Career Education: Curriculum Area and Competencies

Daily Living Skills

1. managing personal finances
2. selecting and managing a household
3. caring for personal needs
4. raising children and meeting marriage responsibilities
5. buying, preparing, and consuming foods
6. buying and caring for clothing
7. exhibiting responsible citizenship
8. utilizing recreational facilities and engaging in leisure
9. getting around the community

Personal-Social Skills

10. achieving self-awareness
11. acquiring self-confidence
12. achieving socially responsible behavior
13. maintaining good interpersonal skills
14. achieving independence
15. making adequate decisions
16. communicating with others

Occupational Guidance and Preparation

17. knowing and exploring occupational possibilities
18. selecting and planning occupational choices
19. exhibiting appropriate work habits and behaviors
20. seeking, securing, and maintaining employment
21. exhibiting sufficient physical and manual skills
22. obtaining specific occupational skills

Source: Loyd, R. J. & Brolin, D. E. (1989). *Life centered career education: Trainer's manual.* Reston, Virginia: Council for Exceptional Children, p. 77. Reprinted with permission.

these adult skills during the high school years, LaQuey (1981) led a project to modify these skills for the secondary curriculum. The major skill domains included in APL (1975) include reading, writing, listening and speaking, computation, problem solving, and interpersonal relations. These skills are taught within five content curricular areas: Consumer Economics, Health, Occupational Knowledge, Community Resources, and Government and Law. Table 11–4 provides an example of how functional skills can be integrated into the curriculum through the five content areas.

Using this table as a guide, creative special education teachers in collaboration with their partners in regular education can find ways to legitimately introduce the functional academic and life skills needed by individual students with mild disabilities through the content areas required in the high school.

PREPARING FOR POST-SECONDARY TRAINING PROGRAMS

The alternatives available for post-secondary training for persons with mild disabilities include colleges and universities, community colleges, vocational and technical schools, adult education programs, military training, and on-the-job training. Each setting will vary along

TABLE 11–4   Examples of tasks in APL Model of Functional Competency

	CONSUMER ECONOMICS	OCCUPA- TIONAL KNOWLEDGE	HEALTH	COMMUNITY RESOURCES	GOVERN- MENT AND LAW
Reading	read an ad for a sale	read a job description	read first aid directions	read a movie schedule	read about rights after arrest
Writing	fill in income tax form	complete a job application	write a menu	complete an application for community service	write your congressman
Speaking, Listening, Viewing	ask question to IRS	listen to an employer talk about a job	listen to a doctor's directions	use the telephone	describe an accident
Problem Solving	decide which house to rent	decide which job suits you	decide when to call a doctor	use stamp machines in the post office	decide which candidate to vote for
Interpersonal Relations	relate to a sales clerk	be successful in a job interview	interact with hospital personnel	ask directions	interact with police successfully
Computation	compute sales tax	calculate paycheck deductions	decide how many times a day to take a pill	calculate the time it takes to travel a distance	calculate the cost of a speeding ticket

Source: From *APL Model of Functional Competency,* 1981, Austin: University of Texas. Reprinted by permission.

a continuum of services including admissions requirements, eligibility for support services, the advisement system, support services, faculty/staff awareness, instructional modifications, administrative modifications, and the coordination and communication network (Vogel, 1990).

Because of the heterogeneity of persons with disabilities, it is important to analyze each setting in terms of the specific needs and abilities of the prospective student. Vogel (1990) provided a system for assisting rehabilitation counselors in determining the match or mismatch between persons with learning disabilities and post-secondary institutions. The same process would be effective for teachers as they assist their students with other mild disabilities. Vogel's system, presented in table 11–5 (on page 436), suggests an analysis of the individual in terms of their goals, interests, characteristics, and disability. This information is compared to the results of the analysis of the mission, institutional strengths, support services, and other characteristics of the post-secondary setting under consideration.

TABLE 11–5 Criteria for Matching Individuals with Appropriate Post-secondary Training Sites

THE CLIENT	THE SETTING
Goals	*Institutional Mission*
certificate	degree options
degree	vocational options
	major options
Interests	
academic	*Strengths*
extra-curricular	academic programs
career/occupational interests	extra-curricular programs
	curriculum
Client Characteristics	internships
age	
maturity	*Institutional Characteristics*
background	size
social-interpersonal skills	location
dependence/independence	student body characteristics
organizational abilities	core/general requirements
motivation	exit competencies
stamina	counseling center services
	dean of student services
Learning Disability	
type	*Support Services*
severity	diagnostic testing
self-knowledge	special advising
strengths	special courses
processing abilities	remediation
attentional abilities	support groups
basic skills	counseling
study habits	notetakers
self-esteem	accommodations
coping strategies	modifications
compensatory strategies	institutional policies

Source: Vogel, S A. (1990). Postsecondary counseling for adults with learning disabilities in Dowdy, C. A., & Perrry, B. D. (Eds.). *Bridge to success for adults with learning disabilities: A training series.* Birmingham, AL: University of Alabama at Birmingham, p. 14. Reprinted with permission.

In the first step of the analysis, the goals and interests of the individual are compared to the mission of the institution and the strengths of the various programs. The client's characteristics, such as social-interpersonal skills and degree of independence, are assessed and compared to the characteristics of the institution (for example, the size and the counseling services available). Finally, the disability is evaluated in terms of strengths and limitations and the support services provided in the training program are reviewed to determine whether the needs and strengths can be accommodated.

Vogel has also developed an excellent checklist that can be used to collect data on the various options being considered. The checklist is included in table 11–6 (on pages 438–439).

Teachers should participate in the analysis of local training options and maintain a file for review by other students and families. If a training option is selected that does not provide adequate support for the disability, the mismatch between the training program and the student may be addressed as part of the high school program. For example, if the student has limited self-knowledge and the setting does not have special advising or advocates on site, extra effort should be made to develop self-advocacy skills before entering the new environment.

Although not a panacea, Section 504 of the Rehabilitation Act of 1973 and the American with Disabilities Act of 1990 provide mandates that can also make post-secondary training institutions a reality for more persons with disabilities. Section 504 states that:

> No otherwise qualified handicapped individual in the United States shall, solely by reason of his handicap, be excluded from the participation, be denied the benefits of, or be subjected to discrimination under any program or activity receiving federal financial assistance.

Vogel (1990) reviews the following important interpretations for the legislation. The term "qualified" refers to a person who meets the standard academic and technical standards required for the educational program. Questions may not be asked about the disability during the admission process unless it is voluntary or the information is needed for insurance purposes. Accommodations are legally mandated in order to assure access to programs. Programs do not have to alter their requirements. The modifications generally alter the method of input or the methods of evaluating the student's learning.

Common accommodations for input proposed by Vogel include allowing students to tape classes, providing textbooks several weeks before classes begin to allow tape recording, and providing a detailed syllabus and list of readings and assignments in oral and written form in advance of the deadline. Accommodations commonly used to assess students learning include testing in distraction-free environments with extended time and giving oral exams instead of written exams or altering the test format between essay and objective. Clark and Kolstoe (1990) cite other services that are not legally mandated but are more commonly found, including transportation, notetakers, tutors, personal and academic counseling, and faculty consultation. Special student-assistance centers also frequently offer workshops in problem areas, such as time management, studying for exams, taking exams, listening and notetaking, reading for different purposes, outlining, and writing term papers.

Modifications in the academic requirements, curriculum, or institutional policies are not legally mandated in Section 504; however, they are sometimes made on an individual basis (Vogel, 1990). Fairly common modifications include substituting courses or allowing extended time to complete a course. These changes would not be allowed if they compromised the integrity of the program (Vogel, 1990).

Although not all students with mild disabilities desire to pursue a post-secondary education, this will be a realistic goal for many. Often students look forward to freedom from the rigors of getting a high school education and simply do not have the motivation to face more academic challenges. Other students do not have the cognitive abilities and academic

TABLE 11–6   Support Services Checklist

LD SUPPORT SERVICES CHECKLIST

Postsecondary institution: _____

Information source: _____

Are the following available, who provides these services, and where?

1. Special academic advisement_____

    Person responsible_____   Office_____(specify)

2. Early registration_____ Person responsible or office_____

3. Advocacy_____ Person responsible _____

4. Course-related tutoring_____ Person responsible_____

    a. Hours per week_____

5. Basic skills tutoring (remediation)

    a. Reading   _____

    b. Writing   _____

    c. Math   _____

6. Skill-building courses/workshops

    a. Test taking   _____

    b. Writing   _____

    c. Time management _____

    d. Other   _____

7. Counseling

    a. Individual   _____

    b. Group   _____

    c. Career/vocational _____

    d. Transition   _____

    e. Job placement   _____

8. Support groups_____ Person responsible_____

9. Readers_____

continued

TABLE 11-6 Support Services Checklist (cont'd.)

LD SUPPORT SERVICES CHECKLIST, PAGE 2

10. Scribes/notetakers_____

11. 4-Track players_____ Location_____

12. Assistance in ordering books on tape_____ Person responsible_____

    Assistance in tape recording reprints/handouts_____ Person responsible_____

    Kurzweil equipment available _____ Location_____

13. Listening and studying facilities_____ Location_____

    Person responsible_____

14. Word processors_____ Location_____

15. Modified examination procedures_____ Person or office_____

16. Written policies and procedures regarding modified college regulations and requirements (academic and administrative, e.g., English, math, or foreign language competency)_____

Source: Vogel, S. A. (1990). Postsecondary counseling for adults with learning disabilities in Dowdy, C. A., & Perry, B. D. (Eds.). *Bridge to success for adults with learning disabilities: A training series.* Birmingham, AL: University of Alabama at Birmingham, pp. 7–8. Reprinted with permission.

skills to qualify as candidates for these programs. New studies have suggested, however, that for those with the prerequisites, post-secondary training may be critical to optimal employment.

Brown (1989) provided an analysis of the implications of the report from the Hudson Institute (1987) entitled *Workforce 2000 Work and Workers for the 21st Century* for persons with disabilities. The three major trends reported were:

1. Higher levels of academic achievement will be required with very few jobs available for people deficient in reading, writing, and math.

2. There will be a decrease in manufacturing jobs and an increase in jobs in the service industry.

3. There will be an increase in minorities, women, and immigrants in the workforce, with an increase in older workers and a decrease in younger workers.

More than half of the new jobs created between now and the year 2000 will require some education beyond high school, almost a third will be filled by college graduates (Hudson Institute, 1987). Brown (1989) also reported that the jobs with the highest expected growth rate will require post-secondary training. Following is a list of jobs expected to experience the highest percentage growth: lawyers and judges (seventy-one percent); natural, computer, and mathematical sciences (sixty-eight percent); health diagnosing and treating occupations (fifty-three percent); technicians (forty-four percent); engineers, architects, and surveyors (forty-one percent); social scientists (forty percent); marketing and sales (thirty-nine percent); managerial and management-related (thirty-nine percent); service occupations (thirty-seven percent); teachers, librarians, and counselors (thirty-one percent); social, recreational, and religious workers (thirty-one percent); mechanics, installers, and repairers (twenty-three percent) (Hudson, 1987).

These data suggest that there will be opportunities for workers with disabilities, particularly, if those workers have obtained additional training beyond high school. Therefore, the role of the special education teacher is more crucial than ever in preparing students to meet the challenges of post-secondary training. Teachers must be able to assess the demands of the training sites and develop individualized programs to give them the skills to succeed. Following are several excellent sources available to assist in programming in these areas.

1. AHSSPPE (1987). *Unlocking the doors: Making the transition to postsecondary education.* Columbus: Author.

2. American Association of Community and Junior Colleges (1988). *Community colleges and students with disabilities.* Alexandria, VA: AACJC Publications. (Available from AACJC, 80 South Early Street, Alexandria, VA 22304, 1-800-336-4776.)

3. HEATH Resource Center (Spring, 1987). *Learning disabled adults in postsecondary education.* Washington, DC: Author. (Available free from HEATH, One Dupont Circle, NW, Suite 800, Washington, DC 20036, 1-800-544-3284.)

4. Human Resources Center (1988). *Assisting students with learning disabilities in transition from high school to community college.* Albertson, NY: Author.

5. Scheiber, B. & Talpers, J. (1987). *Unlocking potential: College and other choices for learning disabled people—A step-by-step guide.* Bethesda, MD: Adler & Adler. (Address: Adler and Adler, 4550 Montgomery, Avenue, Bethesda, MD 20814.)

6. National Association of Trade and Technical Schools. *How to choose a career . . . and a career school for the student with a disability.* (Address: NATTS, 2251 Wisconsin Ave., NW, Washington, DC 20007.)

7. Vogel S. A. (1985). *The college student with a learning disability: A handbook for college LD students, admissions officers, faculty, and administrators.* Lake Forest, IL: Author. (To write: LDA Bookstore, 4156 Library Road, Pittsburgh, PA 15234.)

8. *125 ways to be a better student.* Linquis System, P.O. Box 747 E. Moline, E. Moline IL 61244, 1-800-7764332.

9. *Becoming a master student.* College Survival, Inc., 2650 Jackson Blvd., Rapid City, SD 57702.

10. *Getting smarter.* David S. Lake, 19 Davis Drive, Belmont, CA 94002.

PREPARING FOR EMPLOYMENT

One of the biggest issues in the area of employment for persons with disabilities is the identification of a realistic vocational goal at the individual's maximum vocational potential. It is very important to consider the interests of the student and the concerns of the parents as these goals are being identified. Some young people will be very determined to pursue a career goal which may or may not be appropriate. More often students will not be able to identify a career or job for which they would like to prepare. Vocational evaluations are available that can evaluate strengths and limitations and offer recommendations for specific jobs or job fields. Vocational evaluators are important team members in the transition process. Clark and Kolstoe (1990) delineate their seven major roles.

1. Assess aptitudes, interests, intellectual capacity, and personal-social adjustment.

2. Assess work skills, work attitudes, work history, and work habits.

3. Assess independent living skills of mobility, hygiene, communication, personal and social skills, consumer skills, and home living skills.

4. Assess physical capacity.

5. Assess job-seeking skills.

6. Write reports that are useful for developing IEPs.

7. Interpret the results of the vocational evaluation to the students, families, and school personnel.

Frequently the results of the vocational evaluation will suggest that the original vocational goal of the student and possibly the family is totally unrealistic. Most vocational assessment batteries will then recommend jobs that are considered realistic based on the results of the aptitude and physical capacity measures. The danger of depending solely on these results is that the recommended jobs are often totally unrelated to the student's personal career goals; their dreams are ignored or squelched.

A more sensitive approach may be to begin with the career goal and begin to test against that goal, staying in that job field if the original preference is not realistic. For example, if a young person with a 78 IQ expresses an interest in becoming a surgeon, it would be obvious that the vocational goal is inappropriate. However, the persons trying to assist the student in identifying a realistic goal should first try to determine what attracts the student to that job. In the case of a surgeon, the student might express a desire to help people, might like the excitement and activity of a hospital, or might want to make a lot of money. He might simply have a relative or know a neighbor whom he respects who has that job. The professional's task is to explore other realistic possibilities within that job field or one which meets several of the job features.

The *Dictionary of Occupational Titles* (1977) provides a listing of jobs in various job fields and an analysis of the related jobs. One job that falls under surgeon is surgeon's assistant. Unfortunately, this job requires an extensive training program and is probably out of reach for a person with a mild mental retardation or a severe learning disability. A more realistic job might be a patient escort within the hospital. This job would allow the student to work in a hospital, help people, and procure hospital benefits and a decent salary. Training might include teaching the student the vocabulary specific to the hospital setting and the social skills appropriate for greeting and relaxing the patients.

This kind of career guidance, job development, and job preparation requires creativity and flexibility on the part of the teacher, parents, vocational evaluator, and high school and vocational counselors. Vocational preparation and successful job placement have long been problems for persons with mental retardation. Payne and Patton (1981) explain that vocational programs for the mildly handicapped have been narrowly focused, teaching skills for a narrow selection of jobs. Sometimes vocational programs focus on jobs that are outdated and do not exist when the individual seeks employment. On some occasions young people have received no vocational training. Recent legislation has provided the mandate to make vocational training and employment settings accessible to all individuals with disabilities.

Federal Legislation Related to Employment

Brolin (1989) pointed out that few individuals with disabilities received services related to employment until the 1960s. The first effective impetus for these services was brought about by the passage of the Vocational Rehabilitation Act of 1973 (Public Law 93–112). This act made rehabilitation services available to all qualified persons with disabilities and vocational training was established as a service. Section 504 of the act is called the basic civil rights legislation for the handicapped, making it illegal to discriminate against individuals with disabilities in providing vocational training and employment (Drew *et al.*, 1988). The interpretation of the law (Federal Register, May 4, 1977) clarified the areas discrimination as:

1. advertising, recruitment, and processing job applications;

2. hiring, making alterations in job status, and rehiring;

3. compensation, including pay rate;

4. classification of jobs and lines of progression;

5. sick leave and leaves of absence;

6. fringe benefits;

7. participation in and funding for training and other job related activities;

8. all social and recreational programs that are approved by the employer.

Even this strong piece of legislation did not open all the doors to employment for persons with disabilities.

To strengthen the intent of the law, Congress passed the Rehabilitation Act Amendments of 1986 (Public Law 95–506) mandating services on a priority basis for the severely handicapped. In some cases this has been a deterrent for persons with learning disabilities, mild mental retardation, and behavior problems because counselors must justify that individuals eligible for Rehabilitation Services have severe disabilities that require multiple services over an extended period of time. Some states are under an order-of-selection mandate that limits services to the severely handicapped when funding is limited. It is important for teachers and other persons advocating for Rehabilitation

Services to understand the legal mandates imposed on the personnel working for this agency. For a more thorough discussion of the concept of eligibility and severe handicap refer to Dowdy, Smith, & Nowell (1992).

On July 27, 1990, President Bush signed into law the Americans with Disabilities Act (ADA). Because of the impact, the day has been called "another independence day" for persons with disabilities. The main focus of ADA is on the areas of employment, transportation, public accommodations, and telecommunications. While all parts of the new legislation are important, the area of employment has particular importance for the area of transition. The law states that employers with fifteen or more employees cannot discriminate against persons with disabilities when hiring, or in pay or promotion decisions. In addition, employers are required to make "reasonable accommodations" to assist persons with disabilities in performing the job. This is by far the strongest piece of legislation designed to lessen discrimination in the workplace. Important legislation in the field of education has also been passed to mandate the preparation of students with disabilities for transition.

Federal Legislation Related to Education

The Education of the Handicapped Act (EHA) (Public Law 94–142) (1975) provided a free appropriate education for all individuals with disabilities between ages three and twenty-two. The educational plans could include vocational training, additional preparation for employment, independent living skills, and training for success in post-secondary education settings; however, transition goals were not required. The magnitude of the transition component was dependent on the creativity and agreement of the IEP Committee.

The Carl Perkins Vocational Education Act of 1984 (Public Law 98–524) was a major piece of legislation affecting vocational programming for students with disabilities. This law required that fifty-seven percent of the federal funds allotted to states for vocational education was to be used for special programs for special groups, including ten percent of the money to be spent on students with disabilities. The law also stipulated that state and local funding was to be used to match equally the federal appropriations to states for the disabled and disadvantaged. Prior to the ninth grade, parents were to be informed of the vocational options available to their children. These services included vocational assessment, special instructional services, career development, career guidance, and counseling services.

Under the enactment of the Education of the Handicapped Act Amendments of 1990 (Public Law 101–476) transition services and plans for students with disabilities are now mandated by the time the student is sixteen. This act renamed EHA to the Individuals with Disabilities Act (IDEA). Section 602(a) (19) of IDEA defines transition services as:

> A coordinated set of activities for a student, designed within an outcome-oriented process, which promotes movement from school to postschool activities including postsecondary, vocational training, integrated employment (including supported employment), continuing and adult education, acquisition of daily living skills, and functional vocational evaluation.
>
> The coordinated set of activities shall be based upon the individual student's needs, taking into account the student's preferences and interests, and shall include instruction, community experiences, the development of employment and other postschool adult living objectives, and, when appropriate, acquisition of daily living skills and functional vocational evaluation.

Section 602 (a) (20) of the new law specifies that an IEP must now include:

A statement of the needed transition services for students beginning no later than age sixteen and annually thereafter (and when determined appropriate for the individual, beginning at age fourteen or younger), including, when appropriate, a statement of the interagency responsibilities or linkages (or both) before the student leaves the school setting. In the case where a participating agency, other than the educational agency, fails to provide agreed upon services, the educational agency shall reconvene the IEP team to identify alternative strategies to meet the transition objectives.

Employment Curriculum

A comprehensive curriculum that leads to successful, satisfying employment should be available as an integral component of every students' IEP. Mercer and Mercer (1985) suggest a comprehensive career development model that begins in kindergarten with exposure to various careers and continues with new activities introduced at various grade levels in the additional areas of career orientation, career exploration, career preparation, and job entry and skill refinement. While it is ideal to think that career education would be an ongoing process in kindergarten through twelfth grades it is more realistic to anticipate that students enter ninth grade with very little knowledge on careers.

Dowdy, Carter, and Smith (1990) found that a majority of students with learning disabilities in high school grades nine through twelve want more help with career decisions and more information on how to get a job, how to keep a job, and how to live independently. The focus on employment should be particularly addressed in educational programs for students with disabilities during the high school program. Even students who will participate in post-secondary training programs will eventually find themselves seeking employment. This process is unique and complicated. Therefore, training in this area should be thorough and comprehensive. At the minimum, students should be provided opportunities for career exploration and instruction in how to get a job and how to keep a job.

Career Exploration   Although it is generally accepted that career awareness and exploration should begin during the early years of school, it must not be assumed to have begun then. Students with disabilities frequently enter high school without a vocational goal and with little knowledge of the world of work. Through a variety of activities including field trips, films, books, and discussion, students should be given opportunities to explore a broad spectrum of occupational categories. As noted earlier, the *Dictionary of Occupational Titles* (1979) can be a valuable tool for this type of exploration. Job categories included in this reference include:

1. professional, technical, and managerial occupations;

2. clerical and sales occupations;

3. service occupations;

4. agriculture, fishery, forestry, and related occupations;

5. processing occupations;

6. machine trades occupations;

7. benchwork occupations;

8. structural work occupations;

9. miscellaneous occupations (transportation, utility, mining, stocking, and so forth).

After reviewing the occupational categories, the student should identify specific job clusters to explore further. These include:

1. agricultural,
2. business and office,
3. communications and media,
4. construction,
5. consumer and homemaking education,
6. environment,
7. fine arts and humanities,
8. health,
9. hospitality and recreation,
10. manufacturing,
11. marine sciences,
12. personal services,
13 public services,
14. transportation.

When students have narrowed their interests to a few job clusters, each job cluster should be researched to address the following job parameters.

1. Work activities
2. Physical demands
3. Working conditions
4. Job qualifications required
5. Schedule of working hours
6. Pay scale

When the results of the exploration of the job clusters are reviewed by the student, further focusing can take place. At this point it is very helpful for students to interview individuals on their preferred jobs and actually spend time job shadowing or observing and assisting for days or weeks with the individual employed on the job.

Job Seeking Skills One of the most important skills in which students need to feel competent is the ability to find a job. This begins with teaching the language commonly found in job applications and newspaper employment ads. Students must also be able to identify job sources and telephone or visit job sources successfully. Interview skills are critical to this process and can be easily role played in the classroom. It is particularly effective to have community volunteers from various businesses come in to participate in the interviews. The employers, the individual interviewing for the job, and classmates can participate in the evaluation of the interview. Table 11–7 (on pages 446–451) provides a task analysis of job seeking skills that were developed and used in the Sparks Center Transition

TABLE 11-7 Task Delineation for Job Seeking Skills

SKILL: *JOB SEEKING*

This scope and sequence of skills was developed for _____. Any skills previously acquired by _____ will be documented by the corresponding objective with a check (✓). A blank has been placed to the left of each objective for the insertion of the date as each new skill is mastered. For specific annual and short-term goals refer to the IEP Implementation Sheet. (To meet individual needs of students, the written information may be presented on tape and the responses required from the student may be given orally.)

Date of Skill Acquistion	Behavioral Objective
	COMPILING PERSONAL INFORMATION
	1. Given a list of words used for completing a job application, _____ will read the words and write or tell the meaning of each word. (Criterion: 80%)

Job Application Language
A Survival Vocabulary

Personal Information Words:

_____	Name	_____	Last	_____	Height	_____	Own Home
_____	Date	_____	First	_____	Weight	_____	Married
_____	Age	_____	Rent	_____	Zip Code	_____	Divorced
_____	City	_____	Middle	_____	Phone No.	_____	Date of Birth
_____	State	_____	Single	_____	Children	_____	Dependents
_____	No. & Street			_____	Citizen	_____	Present Address
_____	Previous Address			_____	Social Security No.		

Education and Training:

_____	School	_____	Circle	_____	Grade
_____	Year	_____	Attended	_____	Skills
_____	High School	_____	Completed	_____	Other
_____	Special Training				

Work History:

_____	One	_____	List	_____	Starting
_____	Position	_____	With	_____	Below

continued

TABLE 11-7   Task Delineation for Job Seeking Skills (cont'd.)

Date of Skill Acquistion	Behavioral Objective

Work History (cont'd.):

_____ Apply	_____ Salary	_____ From
_____ Ever	_____ Explain	_____ Employers
_____ Four	_____ Month	_____ Convicted
_____ Experience	_____ Before	_____ Please
_____ Discharged	_____ Reason for Leaving	

Health Record:

_____ Have	_____ Any	_____ Details
_____ You	_____ Speech	_____ Injured
_____ Were	_____ Defects	_____ Notify
_____ Give	_____ Hearing	_____ Physical
_____ Case	_____ Vision	_____ Emergency

References:

_____ Three	_____ Former	_____ Least
_____ Business	_____ Whom	_____ Relatives
_____ Known	_____ Excluding	_____ Persons
_____ Acquainted		

2. Given a job application, _____
    will write responses for each item. (Criterion: 100%)

3. Given a classified ad describing a job position, _____
    _____ will write a letter-of-application containing
    the information requested. (Criterion: 100%)

4. Given a model of a resume, _____
    will write a resume using his/her own personal information. (Criterion: 100%)

IDENTIFYING JOB SOURCES

5. Given class discussion and activities identifying job sources (example: news-
    paper, community resources, bulletin board, friends, etc.), _____
    will identify five sources for obtaining a job. (Criterion: 100%)

TELEPHONING OR VISITING JOB SOURCES

   (The following objective requires prerequisite skills in the use of the telephone and
   transportation which are detailed in the Community Living Task Delineation.)

continued

TABLE 11-7 Task Delineation for Job Seeking Skills (cont'd.)

Date of Skill Acquistion	Behavioral Objective
	6. Given the names of the job sources listed below, _____ will locate the telephone number and call (or locate the address and visit) the job source, obtaining information regarding services. The information obtained will be presented. (Criterion: 100%) _____ State Employment Agency _____ State Vocational Rehabilitation _____ _____ _____ _____ _____ _____ **INTERVIEWING SKILLS** 7. Given class discussion and activities introducing the job interview, _____ _____ will list _____ of the following points*: _____ 1. Decide what you will need and be sure to bring it. _____ 2. Look clean and neat. _____ 3. Be on time. _____ 4. Be friendly and cheerful. _____ 5. Do not smoke or chew gum. _____ 6. Look at the interviewer and listen carefully. _____ 7. Try to answer questions fully, in a clear, strong voice. _____ 8. Let the interviewer know why you think you would be good for the job. _____ 9. Ask questions about any important things the interviewer did not talk about. _____ 10. Thank the interviewer for seeing you. _____ 11. _____ _____ 12. _____ *These points were included in the workbook, *Janus Job Interview Guide*, available from Janus Book Publishers, 3541 Investment Boulevard, Suite 5, Hayward, CA 94545. **INTERVIEW APPEARANCE** 8. Given instructions in appropriate physical appearance, _____ _____ will list eight of the following characteristics of grooming and dress required for a job interview. (Criterion: 100%)

continued

TABLE 11–7 Task Delineation for Job Seeking Skills (cont'd.)

Date of Skill Acquistion	Behavioral Objective

_____ a. Clean hair.

_____ b. Hair neatly combed.

_____ c. Clean body.

_____ d. Clean teeth.

_____ e. Clean shaven.

_____ f. Naturally applied makeup.

_____ g. Clean fingernails.

_____ h. Clean and neatly pressed clothes.

_____ i. Simple and conservative dress.

_____ j. _____

_____ k. _____

9. After meeting criterion on Objective #8, _____
_____ will attend the program on a specified date, dressed and groomed appropriately for a job interview. (Criterion: 100%)

10. Given class discussion and activities of appropriate social behaviors for an interview, _____ will list ten of the following social behaviors or demonstrate these in a role-play situation. (Criterion: 100%)

_____ a. Attend interview with pen, resume, and social security card.

_____ b. Arrive on time for interview.

_____ c. Arrive alone for interview.

_____ d. Walk and stand straight.

_____ e. Speak in a clear, strong voice.

_____ f. Look straight at the interviewer as much as possible.

_____ g. Listen carefully to what the interviewer says in the job interview.

_____ h. Wait until interviewer has stopped talking to ask or answer questions.

_____ i. Keep conversation on job related subjects.

_____ j. Thank the interviewer for seeing you.

_____ k. _____

_____ l. _____

_____ m. _____

continued

TABLE 11-7 Task Delineation for Job Seeking Skills (cont'd.)

Date of Skill Acquistion	Behavioral Objective
	_____ n. _____

INTERVIEW SKILLS

11. Given a video taped presentation of an interview and discussion of questions generally asked by an interviewer, _____ will respond personally to _____ of the following typical interview questions. (Criterion: 100%)

   _____ a. Describe your past work experience.

   _____ b. List the schools you have attended.

   _____ c. How long have you known your references?

   _____ d. What is your birth date?

   _____ e. What is your address?

   _____ f. _____

   _____ g. _____

   _____ h. _____

12. Given class discussion and activities concerning appropriate questions to ask in an interview, _____ will list _____ of the following questions. (Criterion: 90%)

   _____ a. What are the hours?

   _____ b. What is the salary per week?

   _____ c. Does your company provide insurance benefits?

   _____ d. What is the appropriate dress?

   _____ e. _____

   _____ f. _____

   _____ g. _____

13. Given a simulated interview situation, _____ will ask interviewer appropriate questions that were not covered by the interviewer using questions listed in Objective #12. (Criterion: 90%)

14. Given a simulated interview situation, _____ will arrive at the appropriate time dressed and groomed appropriately, will demonstrate appropriate social skills, and will ask and answer appropriate interview questions. (Criterion: _____)

continued

TABLE 11–7   Task Delineation for Job Seeking Skills (cont'd.)

Date of Skill Acquistion	Behavioral Objective
	15. Given completed simulated interview and suggested time for follow-up by interviewer, client will make appropriate contact by telephone or in person at designated time. (Criterion: 100%)
	16. Given completed simulated interview, and no time-line suggestions from interviewer, client will contact interviewer (by telephone or in person) to follow-up twice weekly. (Criterion: 100%)
	USING THE WANT ADS
	The following objectives require prerequisite skills in use of the newspaper which are detailed in the Community Living Skills Task Delineation.
	17. Given a list of abbreviations used in the help-wanted sections of the classified ads, _____ will match abbreviations with corresponding completed words. (Criterion: 90%)
	18. Given the newspaper, _____ will locate the help-wanted section of the classified ads. (Criterion: 100%)
	19. After locating the help-wanted section of the classified ads, _____ _____ will select _____ ads which are related to job clusters identified in long- or short-range occupational goals as identified in the Career Exploration Task Delineation. (Criterion: 100%)
	APPLICATION OF JOB-SEEKING SKILLS
	20. After demonstrating skills specified in Objectives 1–19, _____ _____ will make an appointment with a Vocational Rehabilitation Counselor, will arrange for transportation, will arrive on time for appointment, will demonstrate appropriate physical and social interview appearance, and will obtain specific information regarding placement services procided by Vocational Rehabilitation. (Criterion: 100%)
	21. After demonstrating skills specified in Objectives 1–19, _____ _____ will make an appointment at the State Employment Agency, will arrange transportation, will register for placement services, will arrive on time for interview dressed and groomed appropriately, and will exhibit previously demonstrated appropriate interview skills during the interview situation. (Criterion: 100%)
	22. Given the help-wanted section of the newspaper, _____ _____ will identify _____ of the jobs advertised, will arrange for an interview, arrange transportation, arrive on time dressed and groomed appropriately, and follow previously demonstrated interview skills during the interview situation. (Criterion: _____)

Source: Weyandt, B., & Dowdy, C. A. (Eds.) (1985). *Task delineations for employment skills*. Birmingham, Al.: University of Alabama at Birmingham., pp. 5–12. Reprinted with permission.

Program. An excellent resource for teaching job seeking skills is *Pathways: A Job Search Curriculum*. This material is available from Milt Wright and Associates, 17624 Romar Street, Northridge, California 91325.

Job Maintenance Skills   One of the biggest problems for individuals with disabilities is job retention and job advancement. Michaels (1989) suggests that specific areas to be taught in this field include:

1. accepting criticism—changing behavior to reflect input;

2. dealing with supervisors/managers—including discussing the disability and requesting appropriate accommodations;

3. evaluating your own performance-monitoring task completion and providing self-feedback;

4. goal setting—developing short- and long-term goals and monitoring progress;

5. developing a vocational plan—short- and long-term plans, including goals for career advancement and job up-grading;

6. developing social skills—appropriate behavior/interactions for the job setting.

In the Spark's Center Transitional Program (Weyandt & Dowdy, 1985), students were asked to provide reasons for the necessity of the following behaviors and to demonstrate the appropriate job behavior given simulated job situations requiring the behavioral responses.

1. Exhibit appropriate appearance

2. Demonstrate punctuality

3. Respond appropriately to constructive criticism

4. Exhibit appropriate interaction with coworkers

5. Exhibit appropriate interaction with employer

6. Contact employer when ill or late

7. Follow supervisor's direction

8. Complete all assigned tasks

9. Ask supervisor questions when unsure of procedures

Additional behaviors to target can be obtained from research in which employers are asked to describe desirable employees. Chamberlain (1988) conducted research in which employers were asked to rank the employee factors related to job success. The factors were grouped into categories, and the top four categories are presented in table 11–8.

It is important to note that approximately one half of the factors are in some way connected to social skills. The importance of social skills on the job are seldom refuted;

TABLE 11-8 Rank Order of Factors Related to Job Success

FACTORS

Work-Related (Category Rank=1)

working independently of direct supervision
following instruction
being able to adapt to new work situations
responding appropriately to supervisor correction
understanding the work routine

Personal (Category Rank=2)

efficiency
interest in the job
maintaining an appropriate personal appearance
neatness on the job
stamina/physical abilities

Communication (Category Rank=3)

initiating contact with supervisor when necessary
being able to read or write
being able to communicate basic needs
responding appropriately to questions/statements
reading and following community and/or safety signs

Social (Category Rank=4)

getting along well with others
pleasantness
refraining from exhibiting irritating behaviors
being sociable/initiating appropriate contacts
displaying a socially acceptable attitude

Source: Chamberlain, E. E. (1988). Employers perception of factors related to job success. *Career Development for Exceptional Individuals, 11* (2), p. 30. Reprinted with permission.

however, few high school teachers include social skill training as a part of the curriculum for students with mild disabilities. The original models also did not focus on the importance of social skills and relationships.

Transition Model

This chapter has addressed a variety of roles that are the responsibility of the high school special education teacher. These include areas that address the immediate needs of students with disabilities, such as preparing for the high school graduation exam and techniques for facilitating success in the regular classroom. The real focus has been on the responsibilities that prepare students for their future demands in independent living, post-secondary training, and employment. However, many of the models for transition that impact on high school programming have had a very narrow focus.

The model proposed by Madeline Will (1984) may be described as a unidimensional view of transition from school to work (Clark & Kolstoe, 1990), with the single outcome focus as employment. In this model, persons with disabilities are described as reaching employment with either no special services, time-limited services, or ongoing services. No special services include community agencies or programs such as community colleges available to all persons. An example of time-limited services would be those of a Vocational Rehabilitation Agency. The ongoing services have become known as supported employment. In supported employment an individual, usually with severe disabilities, requires a job coach to be able to obtain and maintain competitive employment. This transition model, which was articulated by the Office of Special Education and Rehabilitative Services (OSERS) (Will, 1984), is considered a narrow approach to a very complex problem (Halpern, 1985). Even the references to other desired outcomes of transition, such as social, personal, and leisure success, were noted to be desirable because they enhanced the opportunities to obtain employment and increased the enjoyment of the benefits of employment (Will, 1984).

A subsequent model proposed by Halpern (1985) revised the OSERS model and suggested that successfully living in the community should be the primary target of a transition program. The dimensions of successful community living include employment, but equal in importance is the individual's residential environment and the quality of their social network. Unlike Will (1984) who proposed that success in employment would likely result in success in the other areas, Halpern (1985) suggested that success in each area must be a curricular goal in an effective transition program.

Clark (1990) proposed that for high school students with disabilities to receive an individualized curriculum that addresses life-career development and transitions, a special curriculum should be in place. He further noted that students in primarily resource and regular classes should have career development curricula infused into both school settings. An example of an integrated curricula was provided earlier in the APL model (1981). Clark and Kolstoe (1990) also suggested that students primarily in self-contained classes should be provided community-based instruction. A version of this process is the work-study program often available in schools. In the work-study program, students spend a portion of their school day in the classroom setting working on subjects that will facilitate independent adult living—money management, social skills, transportation. The remainder of the school day is spent off campus on a job site.

Clark and Kolstoe (1990) also proposed a school-based career development and transition education model for adolescents with handicaps. This model is more broadly based than those of Will (1984) or Halpern (1985). The focus is on four content area components recommended for all students with disabilities; the components include values, attitudes, and habits; human relationships; occupational information; and acquisition of job and daily living skills. Clark proposed that learning experiences and instruction in these four content areas begin in preschool and continue throughout adult working and retirement years.

Regardless of the course of study options available in high school (such as work evaluation or work adjustment, cooperative education or work-study, vocational or technical or fine arts education, or college prep or general education), Clark and Kolstoe advocate for the inclusion of instruction in career development and transition knowledge and skills for all students with disabilities. Outcome data reported earlier in the chapter supports the need for these areas of instruction. Failure to make a life-career development model a legitimate curricular option for a standard diploma in every high school denies an appropriate education opportunity for many students with disabilities (Clark and Kolstoe, 1990).

SUMMARY

This chapter described the process of planning effective education plans for transitioning students with mild disabilities into independent living and work or post-secondary settings. The first section reviewed the developmental stage of adolescence, including the physical, psychological, personality, and cognitive changes normally experienced by adolescents. The characteristics specific to adolescents with mild disabilities were then reviewed to examine the difficulties added in the presence of a disability. Cognitive differences were found to impose limitations in situations requiring problem-solving, reasoning, and language skills. Difficulties with social and behavioral skills creates problems in developing peer relations and performing successfully in school and work settings. The common academic deficits impact daily living activities as well as the ability to pursue post-secondary training and advanced levels of employment.

The third section of the chapter reviewed the societal influences on adolescents. Cognitive and perceptual limitations make understanding the changing roles for males and females in contemporary society difficult. Poor self-esteem and the need for peer approval may lead to an increased risk for becoming sexually active and facing an unplanned pregnancy or the possibility of AIDS. Alcohol and drug abuse were also found to be more prevalent among populations characterized by low self-esteem, difficulties with social interactions, stress, and depression. Suicide was also explored as a major risk for persons with mild disabilities.

The high school curriculum was discussed as needing to address the current and future challenges of these students. Several common approaches were reviewed, including basic skills remediation, tutorial, learning strategies, functional curriculum, and the work-study model. The role of the special education teacher proposed in the chapter evolved from a focus on the individual strengths and needs of students rather than one approach adopted through an administrative decision. A thorough review was provided for each of the components in the role of the high school teacher. These include preparing students for content classes, the high school graduation exam, post-secondary training programs, independent living, employment, and counseling for today's crises. Specific recommendations were made regarding the scope of the curriculum and corresponding materials available.

Finally, several transition models were described beginning with the mandate from federal government in 1984. The most comprehensive included four content area components: 1. values, attitudes, and habits; 2. human relationships; 3. occupational information; and 4. acquisition of job and daily living skills.

REFERENCES

Adult Performance Level Project (APL) (1975). *Adult functional competency.* Austin, TX: University of Texas Office of Continuing Education.

Alley, G.R., & Deshler, D.D. (1979). *Teaching the learning disabled adolescent: Strategies and methods.* Denver: Love Publishing.

Anderson, T., & Magnusson, D. (1990). Biological maturation in adolescence and the development of drinking habits and alcohol abuse among young males: A prospective longitudinal study. *Journal of Youth and Adolescence, 19,* 33–44.

Brolin, D. (1989). *Life centered career education: A competency based approach.* Reston, VA: The Council for Exceptional Children.

Brown, D.S. (1989). Workforce composition in the year 2000: Implications for clients with learning disabilities. *Rehabilitation Counseling Bulletin, 33,* (1), 80–84.

Buttrill, J., Niizawa, J., Biermer, C., Takahashi, C., & Hearn, S. (1989). Serving the language disabled adolescent: A strategies based model. *Language, Speech, and Hearing Services in Schools, 20,* 170–184.

Chamberlain, E.E. (1988). Employers perception of factors related to job success. *Career Development for Exceptional Individuals, 11* (2), 30.

Chesler, B. (1982). ACLD committee survey on LD adults. *ACLD Newsbrief, 145,* 1, 5.

Clark, G.M., & Kolstoe, O.P. (1990). *Career development and transition education for adolescents with disabilities.* Boston: Allyn and Bacon.

Cruickshank, W.M. (1978). *Learning disabilities: Information please.* Quebec, Canada: Quebec Association for Learning Disabilities.

Cullinan, D., Epstein, M.H., & Lloyd, J.W. (1983). *Behavior disorders of children and adolescents.* Englewood Cliffs, NJ: Prentice-Hall.

Dowdy, C.A., Carter, J., & Smith, T.E.C. (1990). Differences in transitional needs of high school students with and without learning disabilities. *Journal of Learning Disabilities, 23,* (6), 343–348.

Dowdy, C.A., Smith, T.E.C., & Nowell, C. (In Press). Accessing vocational rehabilitation services for persons with learning disabilities. *Journal of Learning Disabilities.*

Deshler, D.D., & Schumaker, J.B. (1986). Learning strategies: An instructional alternative for low-achieving adolescents. *Exceptional Children, 52,* 583–589.

Dossetor, D.R., & Nicol, A.R. (1989). Dilemmas of adolescents with developmental retardation: A review. *Journal of Adolescence, 12,* 167–185.

Drew, C. J., Logan, D.R., & Hardman, M.L. (1988). *Mental retardation—A life cycle approach,* 4th Ed. Columbus, OH: Merrill.

Edgar, E. (1987). Secondary programs in Special Education: Are many of them justifiable? *Exceptional Children, 53,* 555–561.

Edgar, E. (1988). Employment as an outcome for mildly handicapped students: Current status and future directions. *Focus on Exceptional Children, 2* (1), 1–8.

Epstein, M.H., Polloway, E.A., Patton, J.R., & Foley, R. (1989). Mild retardation: Student characteristics and services. *Education and Training in Mental Retardation, 24,* 7–16.

Goldstein, A., Sprafkin, R., Gershal, N., & Klein, P. (1980). *Skillstreaming the adolescent: A structured learning approach to teaching prosocial skills.* Champaign, IL: Research Press.

Guetzloe, E. (1988). Suicide and depression: Special education's responsibility. *Teaching Exceptional Children, 20,* 25–28.

Halpern, A.S. (1985). Transition: A look at the foundations. *Exceptional Children, 51,* 479–486.

Halpern, A.S., Close, D. W., & Nelson, D. J. (1986). *On my own: The impact of semi-independent living programs for adults with mental retardation.* Baltimore: Paul H. Brookes.

Hammer, T., & Vaglum, P. (1990). Use of alcohol and drugs in the transitional phase from adolescence to young adulthood. *Journal of Adolescence, 13,* 129–142.

Havighurst, R. J. (1953). *Human development and education.* New York: Longman's, Green.

Hudson Institute (1987). *Workforce 2000, work and workers for the 21st century.* Indianapolis, IN: Author.

Johnson, J.L. (1988). The challenge of substance abuse. *Teaching Exceptional Children, 20,* 29–31.

Kauffman, J.M. (1989). *Characteristics of behavior disorders of children and youth,* 4th Ed. Columbus, OH: Merrill.

Kennedy, J.H. (1990). Determinants of peer social status: Contributions of physical appearance, reputation, and behavior. *Journal of Youth and Adolescence, 19,* 233–244.

Kerr, M.M., Nelson, C.M., & Lambert, D.L. (1987). *Helping adolescents with learning and behavior problems.* Columbus, OH: Merrill Publishing.

Knowles, M. (1984). *The adult learner: A neglected species,* 3rd Ed. Houston: Gulf Publishing Co.

Kokaska, C.J., & Brolin, D.E. (1985). *Career education for handicapped individuals,* 2nd Ed. Columbus, OH: Merrill.

McDowell, R.L. (1981). Adolescence. In G. Brown, R. McDowell, & J. Smith. *Educating adolescents with behavior disorders.* Columbus, OH: Merrill.

Larson, R., Kubey, R., & Colletti, J. Changing channels: Early adolescent media choices and shifting investments in family and friends. *Journal of Youth and Adolescence, 18,* 583–599.

Mercer, C.D. (1987). *Students with learning disabilities,* 3rd Ed. Columbus, OH: Merrill.

Mercer, C.D., & Mercer A.R. (1985). *Teaching students with learning problems,* 2nd Ed. Columbus, OH: Merrill.

Michaels, C.A. (1989). Employment: The final frontier—Issues and practices for persons with learning disabilities. *Rehabilitation Counseling Bulletin, 33,* (1), 67–73.

Mithaug, D.D., Martin, J.E., & Agran, M. (1987). Adaptability instruction: The goal of transitional programming. *Exceptional Children, 51,* 397–404.

Mehring, T.A., & Colson, S.E. (1990). Motivation and mildly handicapped learners. *Focus on Exceptional Children, 22,* 1–7.

Mori, L.F., & Masters, A.A. (1986). *Teaching secondary students with mild learning and behavior problems.* Rockville, Maryland: Aspen Publications.

Neel, R.S., Meadows, N., Levine, P., & Edgar, E.B. (1988). What happens after special education: A statewide follow-up study of secondary students who have behavioral disorders. *Behavioral Disorders, 13,* 209–216.

Nelson, C.M. (1988). Social skills training for handicapped students. *Teaching Exceptional Children, 20,* 19–23.

Ness, J., & Price, L.A. (1990). Meeting the psychosocial needs of adolescents and adults with LD. *Intervention, 26,* 16–21.

Patton, J.R., Cronin, M.E., Polloway, E.A., Hutchison, D., & Robinson, G.A. (1989). Curricular considerations: A life skills orientation. In G.A. Robinson, J.R. Patton, E.A. Polloway, & L.R. Sargent. (1989). *Best Practices in Mild Mental Disabilities.* Reston, VA: The Division on Mental Retardation of the Council for Exceptional Children.

Payne, J.S., & Patton, J.R. (1981). *Mental retardation.* Columbus, OH: Merrill.

Polloway, E.A., Epstein, M.H., Patton, J.R., Cullinan, D., & Luebke, J. (1986). Demographic, social, and behavioral characteristics of students with educable mental retardation. *Education and Training of the Mentally Retarded, 21,* 27–34.

Polloway, E.A., Patton, J.R., Epstein, M.H., & Smith, T.E.C. (1989). Comprehensive curriculum for students with mild handicaps. *Focus on Exceptional Children, 21,* 1–12.

Polloway, E.A., Patton, J.R., Payne, J.S., & Payne, R.A. (1989). *Strategies for reaching mildly handicapped learners.* Columbus, OH: Merrill.

Polloway, E.A., & Smith, T.E.C. (1992). *Language instruction for students with disabilities.*

Ritter, D.R. (1990). Adolescent suicide: Social competence and problem behavior of youth at high risk and low risk for suicide. *School Psychology Review, 19,* 83–95.

Rusch, F.R., & Phelps, L.A. (1987). Secondary special education and transition from school to work: A national priority. *Exceptional Children, 53,* 487–492.

Sabornie, E.J., & Beard, G.H. (1990). Teaching social skills to students with mild handicaps. *Teaching Exceptional Children, 23,* 35–38.

Scarr, S., Weinberg, R.A., & Levine, A. (1986). *Understanding development.* New York: Harcourt Brace Jovanovich.

Schaeffer, A.L., Zigmond, N., Kerr, M.M., & Heidi, E.F. (1990). Helping teenagers develop school survival skills. *Teaching Exceptional Children, 23,* 6–9.

Shea, T.M., & Bauer, A.M. (1991). *Parents and teachers of children with exceptionalities,* 2nd Ed. Boston: Allyn & Bacon.

Smith, T.E.C., & Dowdy, C.A. (1989). The role of study skills in the secondary curriculum. *Academic Therapy, 24,* 479–490.

Smith, T.E.C., Price, B.J., & Marsh, G.E. (1986). *Mildly handicapped children and adults.* St. Paul, MN: West.

Spirito, A., Hart, K., Overholser, J., & Halverson, J. (1990). Social skills and depression in adolescent suicide attempters. *Adolescence, 25,* 543–552.

U.S. Department of Labor (1977). *Dictionary of occupational titles,* 4th Ed. Washington, D.C.: U. S. Government Printing Office.

Vogel, S.A. (1990). Postsecondary counseling for adults with learning disabilities in Dowdy, C.A., Perry, B.D. (Eds.). *Bridge to success for adults with learning disabilities: A training series.* pp. 7–8. Birmingham, AL: University of Alabama at Birmingham.

Wehman, P., Kregel, J.K. & Barcus, J.M. (1985). From school to work: A vocational transition model for handicapped students. *Exceptional Children, 52,* 25–37.

Weyandt, B., & Dowdy, C.A. (Eds.) (1985). *Task delineations for employment skills.* pp. 5–12. Birmingham, Al.: University of Alabama at Birmingham.

Will, M.C. (1984). *OSERS programming for the transition of youth with disabilities: Bridges from school to working life.* Washington, DC: Office of Special Education and Rehabilitative Services (OSERS), U.S. Department of Education.

Woodward, D.M. (1981). *Mainstreaming the learning disabled adolescent,* Rockville, Maryland: Aspen Publications.

Woodward, D.M. (1983). *The learning disabled adolescent.* Austin, TX: Pro-Ed.

Young, G.A., Rathge, R., Mullis, R., & Mullis, A. (1990). Adolescent stress and self-esteem. *Adolescence, 25,* 333–341.

Zigmond, N., & Thornton, H. (1985). Follow-up of post secondary age learning disabled graduates and drop-outs. *Learning Disabilities Research, 1* (1), 50–55.

Computers and Students with Mild Disabilities

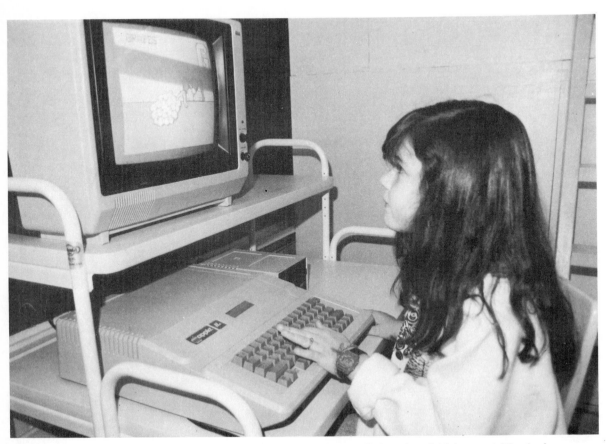

Chapter 12 was written by: Ernest Singletary, University of Alabama at Birmingham

Outline

OBJECTIVES

After reading this chapter, you will be able to:

- define technology;

- describe the role of technology in schools;

- describe the role of computers in schools;

- discuss the effects of computers on instruction;

- describe recent trends in the use of technology in schools;

- define computer-assisted instruction;

- describe how computer-assisted instruction can be used in schools;

- describe the role of computers and special education;

- discuss how schools should plan for computers in classrooms;

- describe specific applications of computer technology in schools;

- define assistive devices;

- discuss some of the resources necessary for computer usage;

- discuss how computers will likely be used in the future in schools.

Introduction

We live in an ever-changing, highly technological world. Automatic teller machines (ATMs), FAX machines, computers with voice output, and computerized telephone operators with speech capabilities that have high quality output are just a few of the examples. More and more schools are exploring the use of computers and other technologies to enhance educational opportunities for students (David, 1991). While technology has been heralded for several years as the salvation for education, new and unique ways to use technology in education have been slow to develop. There has been a phenomenal increase in the number of computers in schools and the availability of software, but many teachers are still struggling with how to efficiently implement the technology.

One area that is receiving a great deal of attention is the use of computer technology in special education programs. In order to meet the needs of students with disabilities, schools need to develop new and more efficient ways to provide appropriate services to this group of students. Computer technology is one way to provide such services. Through computer technology, teachers are better able to individualize instruction, motivate students, and provide the immediate feedback and reinforcement that are so vital to students with disabilities.

This chapter will investigate the role of technology and instruction relative to students with mild disabilities. The role of technology in the schools will be explored, and the status of technology will be reviewed. Ways to use technology, especially computers, with special education populations will be presented, with tips on how to implement technology in your school programs. Finally, the future of computer technology will be presented and discussed.

Technology in the Schools

Technology has been available and used in public school programs for many years. Film projectors, slide projectors, tape recorders, and opaque projectors are examples of the technology that has been used by teachers for several decades. Think about your years in elementary and secondary schools. It is likely that even in the most rural and poor districts, some technology was used for instructional purposes, at least occasionally.

DEFINING TECHNOLOGY

Technology can be defined in many different ways. Heinich, Molenda, and Russell (1985) state that technology is:

1. A process—the systematic application of scientific or other organized knowledge to practical tasks, the process of devising reliable and repeatable solutions to tools.

2. A product—the hardware and software that result from the application of technological processes.

3. A mix of process and product—used in instances where: (a) the context refers to the combination of technological processes and resultant products; (b) process is inseparable from product (p. 402).

Technology "embraces every possible means by which information can be presented. It is concerned with the 'gadgetry' of education and training, such as television, language laboratories and the various projected media, or, as someone once said, 'everything from computers to dinner ticket dispensers'" (Percival & Ellington, 1988, p. 13).

There is also a technology of instruction that focuses the many forms of technology on the instructional process. The technology of instruction can be described as a teaching and learning interchange that results in the application of technology to teaching and learning. It should be a reliable and effective method of instruction that utilizes technology and the scientific principles of human learning (Heinich *et al.*, 1985). Examples of technology that can be applied to instruction include instructional television, audiovisual kits, such as filmstrips, videocassette technology, closed-circuit television, and computers (Smith, 1990).

The technology discussed in this chapter will be computer technology—microcomputer hardware and software utilized by students with mild disabilities in grades K through twelve. We acknowledge that there is a great deal of technology available other than that which is computer related; however, our focus will be on the use of the microcomputer, since this is the most powerful form of technology currently available for educational purposes.

THE ROLE OF TECHNOLOGY IN SCHOOLS

The primary role of technology in schools is to enhance the teaching-learning-management process. Technology in education has never intended to replace the teacher, but to facilitate teaching (Gagne, 1987). When computers were first being discussed as an educational tool, many teachers were actually fearful of losing their jobs to machines. However, there is a general consensus that there will always be the need for the human involvement in teaching. Computers are only used to help teachers provide appropriate programs to students.

While technology has become an integral part of our educational processes, there are some concerns about our overuse or inappropriate use of technology (Collins, 1991). Critics are concerned that our educational system will become dehumanized if we rely too heavily on technology in the classroom. Human qualities, such as loving, knowing, and decision making, must be included in our instructional activities to maintain the "human" element of teaching and learning (Hatch, 1984).

COMPUTERS IN SCHOOLS

The 1980s have seen microcomputers become a fixture on the American education scene. Their expansion has been so complete that it is difficult to go into a school and not find at least one microcomputer. Although each classroom may not have its own computer, students generally have the opportunity to use computers at least on a rotating basis (Wallace, Cohen, & Polloway, 1988). Much of the computer technology available in schools was generated by teachers who wanted to get one step ahead in educating children. It has been the interest of teachers, not administrators, that has pushed our educational system as far as it has gone toward technological competence. A few teachers have been interested and motivated to maximize the use of computer technology in their classrooms (Smith, 1990).

THE ROLE OF COMPUTERS IN SCHOOLS

Computers play a vital role in schools today. They are involved with instruction, administration, and a combination of both. Although computers have been present in educational settings for only a few years, it is already difficult to imagine schools without microcomputers, at least in the principal's office and library. The future will only see the future consolidation of computers and schools. In fact, it is likely that computers will become such an obvious part of our education that they will go unnoticed in classrooms, where they would have attracted significant attention just a few years ago.

THE STATUS OF COMPUTERS IN SCHOOLS

The growth in the number of computers in schools has been truly amazing (Rich, 1991). From a very few computers just a few years ago, the number has increased to hundreds of thousands. The increase continues at such a rapid pace that it is difficult to accurately document how many computers are in schools.

According to Goodspeed (1988), during the 1986–1987 school year, the number of computers in schools increased to more than 2 million. This represented a twenty-five percent increase from the 1985–1986 year. Of the computers in schools, fifty-nine percent are made by Apple Computers, sixteen percent by Tandy, eleven percent by IBM, and nine percent by Commodore. The Apple Computer company appears to be winning the numbers game in schools. The latest report from Quality Education Data reports that Apple computers can be found in more than eighty percent of the schools that have computers (McCarthy, 1989).

The domination of Apple computers in schools has recently increased with the addition of new MacIntosh models. These new generation MacIntosh computers are affordable for schools and target educational purposes. The MacIntosh will likely replace the domination of the Apple IIE in schools. Its user-friendly approach, with a "mouse" and "windows" make its adaption in public schools very likely.

THE EFFECTS OF COMPUTERS ON INSTRUCTION

Most of the research investigating computers and instruction has resulted in positive conclusions (Majsterek, 1989; Higgins & Boone, 1990). For example, it has been found that computers help students learn material in less time than conventional instructional procedures, facilitate attention and motivation, and increase time on task (Lindsey, 1987). In a recent study, comparisons were made between students with disabilities and their nondisabled peers regarding computer usage. One of the conclusions was that the level of engagement with the learning task using the computer was eighty to eighty-five percent for both groups. This engagement level is significantly higher than for other types of instruction (Cosden, Gerber, Semmel, Goldman, & Semmel, 1987).

While there is concern among critics that computers will be used to keep students busy rather than involved in creative activities (Majsterek, 1989), most professional educators are optimistic about the role computers will play in education in the future. They foresee computers as being used for a wide set of activities, ranging from drill and practice, to creative written expression.

Advantages of Computers

There are numerous advantages to using computers in the classroom. While these advantages apply to all students, they are especially related to students who are experiencing mild learning and behavior problems. Advantages include:

- students can learn at their own pace;
- high speed feedback to the learner provides excellent reinforcement;
- slow learners find the computer very patient;
- color graphics, animated graphics, and music can add realism and motivation to activities;
- record keeping ability of computers facilitates individualized instruction;
- the memory capacity of computers keeps students progress up to date and allows them to pick up where they left off;
- computers expand teachers' span of control;
- motivation is improved simply by the novelty of using a computer;
- instruction through computer technology is reliable from learner to learner, regardless of teacher attitudes, time of day, or other variables that can affect instruction;
- computers can make instruction more effective (students learn more) and more efficient (students learn in less time) (Kearsley, 1983).

Disadvantages of Computer Technology

There always seems to be a "downside" to innovations, and using computers in educational settings is no exception. There actually are disadvantages in using technology in the classroom. These include expense, limited teacher expertise in implementation, and quality of software. Table 12–1 (on page 466) summarizes some of the disadvantages of using computers in the classroom.

TRENDS IN TECHNOLOGY IN SCHOOLS

The numbers of computers in schools have continued to increase dramatically over the past decade (Smith, 1990). As technologies have become cheaper to purchase and easier to use and as computer software has become more available, the number of computers has grown rapidly. A key finding in the ninth annual survey of states regarding the use of computer technology in schools was that the key issue related to continued expansion of computers in classrooms is funding. During the most recent reporting year, more than ninety percent of the states responding to the survey indicated a leveling of spending for hardware,

TABLE 12-1 Limitations of Computers

■ Computer instruction is relatively expensive even with significant recent cost reductions.

■ Computer designed specifically for instruction/learning have lagged behind those for business purposes.

■ There is limited availability of high-quality, direct-instruction materials.

■ Software developed for one computer system cannot be used with other systems.

■ Design of learning materials for computers is difficult and time consuming.

■ Computerized instruction may limit creativity.

■ Learners may resist highly structured format of instruction.

■ Novelty of learning on the computer may be diminishing.

■ Teachers may not be skilled in appropriate use of computers.

■ Some students may develop anxiety over computer use.

■ A few students may monopolize computers in classrooms.

■ There are too few computers to go around in most schools.

Source: Heinich et al., 1985; Smith, 1990.

software, and training. States where funding has increased somewhat are shifting their emphasis from securing equipment and materials to training (Bruder, 1989). More and more school personnel are realizing that equipment alone does not ensure a valid computer program; trained personnel must be present also.

With respect to training as a priority, Bruder (1989) reported:

■ 23 states require computer courses to earn a degree (with varying hours);

■ 18 states require a course on integrating technology into the curriculum;

■ 94 percent of respondents do not require inservice training in computer technology, but 93 percent provide such training to teachers who request it;

■ 67 percent related that states fund training;

■ inflation has raised the cost of training in 26 states from $32.8 million to $36.3 million;

■ 32 states provide some form of credit for training in technology (pp. 26–27).

Bruder's report indicates that even when a lack of trained personnel was cited as the greatest problem in advancing computers in classrooms, funding was still the base problem. Of programs that receive special support for computer usage, special education had the most support, followed by programs for at-risk students and students classified as gifted.

Computer Usage in Schools

"Microcomputers in schools" has been the most prevalent buzz phrase of the 1980s; the 1990s will likely witness the widespread acceptance and management of computers through a more thorough planning system at the school, district, and state levels. Computers have primarily been used for administrative and instructional purposes. The administrative uses focus on facilitating the day to day paper flow that exists in schools, and developing useful data bases on students, personnel, and materials. Instructional uses of computers include computer assisted instruction (CAI) and computer managed instruction (CMI).

ADMINISTRATIVE USES OF COMPUTERS

There are numerous ways to use computers to assist administrators in schools. These include 1. grade tracking, 2. attendance records, 3. generating individual education programs, 4. testing students, 5. developing and keeping track of budgets, 6. class scheduling, and 7. reporting performances of students (Kinzer *et al.*, 1986). Some schools use computers for these purposes extensively, while others continue to rely on manual management processes. Larger districts that have a much greater administrative burden are more likely than small districts to have a comprehensive administrative computer system.

One of the most laborious and time consuming administrative tasks for teachers of students with mild disabilities is the development of IEPs. New computer software programs are available to assist teachers and administrators with this activity. The result of a computerized IEP program is an IEP printout that details goals and objectives; a method of tracking these goals and objectives is included in the computer program. Computerized IEP programs have their advocates as well as critics. Advantages of a computerized IEP system include :

- compliance with Public Law 94-142 is easier;
- assessment and curriculum staff can collaborate easier through their collective input;
- it is not necessary to regenerate new goals and objectives for each student;
- quality of the IEP is enhanced;
- regular classroom teachers can become more involved;
- curriculum objectives can be consistent across IEPs;
- computerized printouts provide an organized set of goals/objectives and activities; and
- information is readily accessible for reporting and planning (Budoff *et al.*, 1985).

Computerized IEP programs enable school officials to generate thousands of goals and objectives for many different topics (Lint, 1984). If this process can be developed to a point where the end products are truly individualized, much valuable teacher time could be saved and redirected to instructional activities (Gearheart, Weishahn, & Gearheart, 1988).

While some districts have chosen to use computerized IEPs, there is a great deal of controversy over the use of these machine-generated intervention programs. The primary concern over the use of computerized IEPs is whether or not a computer-generated program can truly be individualized (Gearheart *et al.*, 1988). Many argue that without dialogue and debate among members developing an IEP, a truly individualized program cannot be developed. This is an area that needs to be investigated in order to determine whether or not the continued development of computerized IEP programs is justified.

INSTRUCTIONAL USES OF COMPUTERS

There are numerous uses of computers in the instructional process. These include computer-managed instruction and computer-assisted instruction. Some districts use computers solely to track student progress, while others incorporate computers into many instructional activities with students.

Computer-Managed Instruction

One useful area for computers is computer-managed instruction (CMI). CMI can be defined as a management system that enables teachers and administrators to develop and implement programs for students and keep track of student's progress. Comprehensive CMI programs enable the teacher to do the following.

- assess entry skills of a pupil,

- prescribe appropriate learning experiences (both print and nonprint),

- reassess progress,

- assign additional learning exercises if warranted or to "promote" a student to the next module, and

- keep complete dated records on each pupil including a record of particular areas of difficulty. (Bartel, 1990, p. 513)

Records on up to 10,000 students can be maintained with CMI. These records can include the child's diagnosis, prescribed intervention program, data collected throughout the school year, and a mechanism for reporting the information. This system works extremely well with competency based educational programs through its comprehensive record keeping abilities. Keeping track of students' daily progress helps teachers organize instruction and facilitates accountability (Reid, 1988). Just centralizing the records of students in special education through CMI can result in numerous benefits (Chandler, 1987).

Authoring Languages   One method of implementing CMI is through authoring languages. Authoring languages can be defined as "software designed to allow non-programmers to create computer-based learning materials by responding to prompts or completing simple forms" (Lockard *et al.*, 1990, p. 430). They enable teachers to design their own computer-managed instructional programs when commercial programs are not available. When using an authoring language, teachers are able to insert text, aids, and even test questions onto a "template" without having progamming skills (Bartel, 1990). The result is that teachers, most of whom are not trained in programming, are able to interact with the computer and develop a program for their students.

Ther are numerous authoring systems on the market. These include Pilot and SuperPilot. A recent, very powerful system is the Multi-Sensory Authoring Computer System (MACS), which was developed at John Hopkins University. The system uses sound, color, vocabulary, numbers, and graphics in its programs. Students using the MACS receive immediate feedback and are able to interact with the program. The program includes options for distractions, specified amount of time for viewing cues and prompts, and different ways to indicate correct responses (Panyan, 1988). Table 12–2 lists examples of authoring systems available on the market.

TABLE 12–2 Examples of Authoring Programs for Students with Mild Disabilities

MACS (A multi-sensory authoring computer system)
Johns Hopkins University
Center for Technology in Human Disabilities
2301 Argonne Drive
Baltimore, MD 21218

Early Learning I, II, and Mix n Match
(Preschool and elementary level programs used with keyboard, PowerPad, single switch, or Touch Window.)
Marblesoft
21805 Zumbrota NE
Cedar, MN 55011

Following Directions: One and Two Level Commands
(For training commands and spatial concepts. Uses Touch Window or joy stick.)
Laurezte Learning
110 East Spring Street
Winnooski, VT 05404

Writer Rabbit
(For early writing and reading, grades 2-4.)
Learning Company
6493 Kaiser Drive
Fremont, CA 94555

Word Attack
(Vocabulary building program with data disks for grades 2-9, SAT, roots, and prefixes.)
Davidson & Associates
3135 Kashiwa St.
Torrance, CA 90505

Mystery Sentences
(Clues are given to build sentences.)
Scholastics
4460 Black Avenue, Ste. J
Pleasanton, CA 94566

Source: Tanenhaus, J. (1989). What's new in special education software? Part two. *Closing the Gap, 9,* 12-15.

While some CMI programs are only used to keep records, others are much more comprehensive in their scope. Some prepare report cards, evaluations for special programs, individual educational programs, and other reports. The continued expansion of CMI means that the role of computers in this area will likely continue to grow well into the 1990s (Reid 1988).

One use of computers is the evaluation of students with disabilities. Assessing students with disabilities using traditional means takes time from regular and special education teachers. Therefore, a mechanism for assessing students with less teacher-time would be beneficial. Salend and Salend (1985) discussed some implications of using microcomputers in classroom testing; they noted numerous advantages, including:

1. speed of the test item presentation can be regulated and matched to student;

2. physical organization of the test can facilitate performance;

3. computer graphics and colors can be used to highlight important parts;

4. students can respond to test items in several ways different to those available without computers;

5. the need for handwriting is minimized, which is very beneficial to students whose handwriting is a major deficit area;

6. instant feedback and reinforcement are motivating factors;

7. tests can be administered in a game-like format which increases motivation.

In addition to these advantages of using microcomputers in testing, there are several disadvantages. Chief among disadvantages to using computers in evaluation is the fact that some students do not know how to operate the computer and may not have keyboard skills. Another major limitation could be the amount of time it takes teachers to program the test. Teachers may spend considerably more time developing a test for use on a computer than they would for a more traditional, paper-pencil test, especially as they begin to use computers for testing purposes. As more and more tests become commercially available on computers, and as teachers develop a file of tests on computer disks, this limitation will resolve itself.

Someone in the schools must be responsible for evaluating the CMI programs being used. Often this will fall to an administrator or an individual who has been designated as the "computer specialist" for the school. Since much of the computer application in a school may occur in the special education programs, special education teachers or supervisors may be involved. Table 12–3 represents a list of questions that could be used to evaluate CMI programs. These questions could be modified to fit any CMI program.

Another rapidly developing use of computer technology and assessment is computer-analysis of test scores. Examples include the Woodcock-Johnson compuscore, and similar computer applications of raw scores obtained from the Peabody Individual Achievement Test-Revised (PIAT-R) and Kaufman Test of Educational Achievement (K-TEA). These programs enable evaluators to feed raw scores into the computer for analysis. The computer programs complete the analysis of the raw scores and provide a variety of comparisons and analyses for the evaluator to use in determining appropriate intervention techniques. These computer-assisted test interpretations save analysis time and provide a

TABLE 12–3 Evaluating CMI Programs

Is the program sensitive to the learning styles of different children?

Does the program reflect a sound understanding and clear conception of the curriculum?

Does the program have a research base? How recent is it?

Does the program reflect excellent test construction?

Are the directions clear and concise?

Is the program more than generally diagnostic?

Are parallel tests available for retakes?

Do the tests demand more than simple recall of information?

Is the record keeping accurate for both individuals and groups?

Does the program print hard copies of progress for both individuals and groups?

Source: D.K. Reid (1988). *Teaching the learning disabled.* Boston: Allyn & Bacon, p. 419. Reprinted with permission.

more error-free computation of scores. As they continue to be developed, they will likely include prescriptions based on certain intratest score comparisons.

COMPUTER-ASSISTED INSTRUCTION

A popular method of using computers in school programs is computer-assisted instruction (CAI). CAI can be defined as a two-way interaction between the learner and computer (Smith, 1990). It is an active, not a passive instructional system (Lockard, Abrams, & Many, 1987). CAI is the way most schools use computers in instruction. Nelson and Waack (1985) found that out of a sample of 202 schools, the use of CAI ranged from a low of 56.5 percent of kindergarten classes to a high of 81.5 percent in third grade classes. At the high school level, CAI was used most often in math and science instruction, 92 percent and 85 percent respectively.

CAI can be extremely beneficial in the classroom. "Properly designed CAI acts as an electronic blackboard where the programmer's instructions, in the form of software, act as a master teacher with a finely tuned sensitivity to student needs" (Sloane *et al.*, 1989, p. 2). CAI guides students in a structured instructional program, and provides feedback to students regarding performance.

There are several advantages to using CAI.

- It is interactive, not passive.

- It provides instant feedback, not delayed feedback.

- It often motivates students and maintains their attention.

- It can help individualize instruction (Sloane *et al.*, 1989).

McCormick and Haring (1990) categorized CAI into five groups: 1. drill and practice, 2. tutorial, 3. simulations, 4. problem solving, and 5. word processing. Additional ways include microcomputer-based laboratories to measure physical phenomena, cognitive development programs, and computer programming that can be used to help students develop logical thinking skills (Majsterek, 1989).

Although there are a wide variety of applications for CAI, the most prevalent application in schools is through drill and practice (Cosden *et al.*, 1987; Lindsey, 1987). Teachers may not take advantage of the many ways CAI can be used to improve instruction. They simply may have students sitting at the computer involved in drill and practice exercises because they have limited skills on maximizing the use of computers in the classroom. While CAI, when properly utilized, can be a wonderful asset in the classroom, it can also be detrimental to students if CAI is used as a teacher substitute (Gearheart, Weishahn, & Gearheart, 1988). The purpose of CAI, as with any technology, is to enhance instruction, not be used as a replacement of teachers and teaching. CAI is doomed to failure if it is used as a substitute teacher.

Drill and Practice

As stated, the most common way computers are used in the classroom is drill and practice. The primary purpose of drill and practice is to reinforce skills that have previously been learned and to develop a functioning level that becomes automated (Hasselbring & Goin, 1989). Drill and practice means just that, drill and practice certain activities. Doll (1987) states that drill and practice programs "provide students repetitious exercise on materials or facts already presented by a teacher or school library media specialist" (p. 69). Students should not be involved in computer-assisted drill and practice activities if they have not previously learned the skill or material. Practicing something that you do not know how to do will not lead to improvement. In fact, it could lead to frustration and a lessening of motivation.

While drill and practice is the most popular form of CAI, it is also the most criticized. Critics contend that drill and practice overuse has resulted in the computer being little more than an electronic flashcard. Drill and practice should not be used to replace needed instructional time. Students who need to be tutored in a subject area do not need to spend a great deal of time in drill and practice activities in that subject (Kinzer et al., 1986). Drill and practice alone will not teach new skills (Hasselbring & Goin, 1989).

When used appropriately, drill and practice on the computer can be very beneficial, especially to students with mild disabilities. An example provided by Kinzer *et al.* (1986) shows a way drill and practice could benefit students with mild disabilities. In the example, students would be provided drill and practice activities in subtraction before they begin a lesson in long division. The purpose of the drill and practice would be to increase the fluency level of the student in subtraction, which would be an important skill for long division.

For students with mild disabilities, drill and practice activities can be extremely beneficial. Many students with mild mental retardation, learning disabilities, and emotional problems, have memory problems and require longer periods to learn material. For these students, practicing a skill already learned can facilitate their retention and fluency in the skill.

Teachers can use drill and practice activities in a variety of ways. The most logical is for individual students to practice on skills in which they are experiencing problems. For example, a student with learning disabilities who has problems decoding unfamiliar words might use a drill and practice program to work on phonetic analysis. A student who has math problems might devote twenty minutes daily to an individual program that practices calculation skills. Drill and practice programs can also be used with groups of students. Students can be organized into small teams, usually no more than three or four students, and compete with other teams in successfully completing drill and practice programs. Regardless of how drill and practice programs are used, teachers must ensure that they are used in a positive manner to enhance and develop skills rather than a vehicle to keep students occupied for a period of time.

Tutorials

Unlike drill and practice, tutorials are designed to introduce new materials to students (McCormick & Haring, 1990). Tutorials are actual instructional activities designed to teach students new skills, not simply practice previously learned skills. An example of a tutorial program for students with mild mental retardation was given by Hasselbring and Goin (1989). They described a program to teach students to recall facts that combined drill and practice with recall. After facts are acquired, the drill and practice activities help students develop recall skills.

Using the tutorial program in conjunction with drill and practice appears to be an excellent method of teaching new skills to students with disabilities, as well as improving their fluency and competence. One important aspect of tutorials is the branching that occurs. Students acquire competence in certain skills and are "branched" into other activities. Another important component of tutorials is the documentation of the performance of the student.

Simulations

Problem-solving skills are taught in a realistic context in simulations (McCormick & Haring, 1990). Computer simulations can be used to replicate almost any kind of environment. For example, a simulation of a job interview would be an excellent way to help prepare a secondary student with mild disabilities for a real job interview. A major advantage in computer simulations is that the person receiving training can experience complicated, real-life situations without any risk for failure (Yin & Moore, 1987). In the job interview example, the student is in no danger of actually losing the job because the entire episode is a simulation.

Numerous topics that are important for students with mild disabilities can be adapted to simulation programs. For example, these students frequently experience deficits in social skills. While problems in social skills are bad enough, the real problem is when deficient social skills negatively impact on a wide variety of activities, including getting along with friends, getting along on a job, and working with adults, such as teacher and parents. Simulations can be used to train students with disabilities how to deal with certain social situations. By using real-life scenarios in a training format, students can experience situations and decide what actions they should take.

Hasselbring and Goin (1988) suggest the following guidelines when determining when simulations would be appropriate as an instructional activity.

1. When the learning objectives are complex and students are unlikely to be able to develop the needed skills in a real-life environment (for example, work skills).

2. When the time scale of the real-life event is too long or too short to allow efficient learning (for example, money management).

3. When the real-life experience involves danger or high cost (such as driver training).

4. When the real-life event cannot be carried out in a normal teaching environment (for instance, voting) (p. 406).

Students generally enjoy computer simulations. Therefore, allowing students to use computers in simulation activities can be a positive reinforcer for appropriate behaviors or successful completion of certain tasks. Simulations can therefore be the primary method of instruction for a particular skill, or a reinforcer to encourage students to achieve specific skills.

Problem-Solving Programs

This component of CAI teaches students a systematic way to solve problems (McCormick & Haring, 1990). Through the use of problem-solving programs, students are encouraged to develop logical thinking skills, problem-solving skills, and strategy development. Teaching problem-solving skills using the computer goes well beyond the drill-and-practice activities that are the focus of many CAI programs (Turkel & Podell, 1984). The problem-solving activities involve a process that can use any subject content, thus facilitating instruction while enhancing problem-solving abilities (Reid, 1988).

Problem-solving activities can be combined with simulations for "real life" situations. For example, students can be involved in a simulated situation that requires problem-solving skills. In one of the most popular simulations and problem-solving programs, *Oregon Trail,* students simulate participation on a trail drive. They have to make several decisions such as what to take with them, what routes to take, and whether to ford a river or go extra miles to get to a crossing. These kinds of problem-solving activities used with simulations provide motivation to students and enable them to develop problem-solving abilities. Teachers need to ensure that during these kinds of activities students do not simply use trial-and-error methods, but think through various solutions to problems (Hasselbring & Goin, 1989).

Zimmerman (1988) compared students with learning disabilities and students without learning disabilities in their problem-solving abilities using computers. Results revealed no significant differences between the groups. In stating these results, it was noted that "The computer may have supplied a necessary link for students with LD to self-generate strategies for feedback purposes. Further, the computer may have dealt with motivational, attributional, and other affective factors that influenced the outcomes of this study but that were not explored or controlled" (p. 640). The results seem to suggest that using the computer in problem-solving activities may be very beneficial for students with learning disabilities.

Word Processing Programs

Word processing programs provide a mechanism for students to write (McCormick & Haring, 1990). They are now used successfully with students as early as first grade. Several programs, specifically designed for young students, include Bank Street Writer,

Paper Clip, and Writing Assistant. These are very user-friendly programs and relatively simple to use (Reid, 1988).

Since many students with mild disabilities exhibit problems in written expression, the word processing component of CAI can greatly facilitate writing skills. Using word processing programs has several advantages for students with mild disabilities who are mainstreamed into regular classes (Salend, 1990).

- It minimizes spelling errors through "spell-check" capabilities.

- It helps overcome handwriting problems by enabling students to present a neat, legible copy that looks polished.

- It provides motivation to write through using the computer.

- It facilitates text revisions through editing modes that enable the writer to insert words, delete words or sentences, and move entire sections.

- It improves selection of words used through a thesaurus component.

- It eliminates the time-consuming and often error-plagued process of copying and recopying papers.

One potential difficulty for students using word processing programs is the requirement to have keyboard skills. Students can often learn the commands required of the programs, but with limited keyboard skills, their progress with word processing programs will be limited (Salend, 1990). Therefore, one area where instruction may be needed is keyboard training. There are actually numerous computer programs available for keyboard training. By using these keyboard training software packages, students become familiar with the computer, often lose their initial fears about using the computer, and develop the necessary skills required to use word processing programs.

Word processing programs can be used in a variety of ways in teaching writing. Teachers can do most of the keyboard activities and have students give them handwritten drafts of stories, or teachers can have students doing the actual writing using the word processing program. This latter method is better when teaching students to take advantage of the computer in writing activities. Table 12–4 (on page 476) describes several different ways for this use.

To ensure proper usage of CAI with students who are disabled, teachers should ask two main questions.

1. Does the courseware engage the student in "successful" learning?

2. Will the CAI augment teacher-directed instruction? (Majsterek, 1989)

By posing and answering these questions, teachers are more likely to use CAI programs with students who have disabilities in an effective manner. Using CAI to simply occupy the time of these students is a waste of valuable resources.

COMPUTERS AND SPECIAL EDUCATION

Computers have been used in special education programs for many years. Teachers of students with disabilities are always trying to find new ways to enhance the success of this

TABLE 12–4 Uses of Word Processing Programs in Teaching Writing

The following suggestions include those developed at Bank Street College, which began using word processing with students in 1979.

1. Give the students a time limit for their writing, such as:
   a. writing until the screen is full,
   b. writing for fifteen minutes,
   c. writing until there is nothing left to say.
2. Type several sentences out of order. Have the students rearrange them sequentially.
3. Give the students the beginning and ending of a story and ask them to supply the middle.
4. Have the student retell a folk tale in an original style.
5. Develop a classroom newspaper. Have different journalists contribute various articles and have the students edit the paper.
6. Type a passage with exposition or action words in one verb tense. Have the student change the tense of the passage.
7. Type a long passage and merge the paragraphs into one. Have the students break the passage into appropriate paragraphs.
8. Type a passage with a few words capitalized. Have the students replace each capitalized word with a lower-case synonym.
9. Type the instructions and skeleton of a business letter. Have the students use this form letter to request information about their projects.
10. Have students send letters developed on their word processing program to electronic "pen pals" in different parts of the country.
11. Type a passage with repetitious words and sentences. Have the students edit the writing.
12. Team pairs of students to work on a project and edit one another's work.

Source: D.K. Reid (1988). *Teaching the learning disabled.* Boston: Allyn & Bacon, p. 422. Reprinted with permission.

population. As a result, they were one of the first groups to try computers with their students. Lindsey (1987) believes that computers are directly and indirectly having an impact on the delivery of special education and related services to children and adults with disabilities in a variety of educational settings. In the area of special education, computer technology is primarily being used 1. as a compensatory tool, 2. in instructional management, and 3. in the delivery of instruction.

The application of computer technology to special education populations is relatively new, but growing rapidly (Majsterek, 1989). As a result, a great deal of research has not been completed regarding the usage of computers and special education. However, the data that have been collected generally support the benefits of using computers with students who are mildly disabled. For example, studies have shown that students with disabilities, like their nondisabled peers, may actually achieve at a higher level as a result of using computers. In addition, there has been a substantial increase in the number of students with disabilities who receive computer-assisted instruction (Lindsey, 1987). After comparing students with disabilities and their nondisabled peers on problem-solving tasks using the computer, Zimmerman (1988) even raised the question "Can the microcomputer equalize deficits and aid the student who has problems with traditional teaching and testing environments?" (p. 640).

Professionals in special education must begin to use technology more effectively with students who are disabled. Advantages that can be used to facilitate performances of students with disabilities must be exploited. Special education must "thoughtfully and carefully begin to reshape its instructional approaches in order to prepare the exceptional individual to use current and future technologies as vocational, educational, recreational, and prosthetic tools" (Cain, 1984, p. 239).

Planning for Computer Usage

Before the full-scale implementation of microcomputer technology into instructional programs, schools must have plans and policies in place. For example, schools need to know where microcomputers are needed, what kinds of software will be required for certain groups of children, what the priorities are for the school, and who will be in charge of making decisions regarding computer technology in classrooms.

When computer technology started becoming available to schools, teachers who were interested in trying computers with their students simply did so. There was limited planning by the teacher, and virtually none at the school or district level. Planning for the use of computer technology at the state level was not even considered. In addition to limited planning, most schools did not even have goals for their computer programs (Woolfolk, 1990). As more and more teachers started using computers and ordering computer software for their students, school administrators initiated planning efforts. To this point, however, most schools have had very few policies regarding the use of computer technology in the classroom (Geisert & Futrell, 1990).

DEVELOPING POLICIES FOR COMPUTER USE IN SCHOOLS

In order for schools to have an efficient computer program for instructional and administrative purposes, they must develop and implement a plan and policies. At the state level, policies for hardware and software selection are just being developed. Bruder (1989) reported that only five states have policies regarding hardware adoption while seven states reported policies on adopting software. While these numbers are extremely low, data collected by Bruder revealed that several additional states are considering adopting such policies.

In addition to policy development at the state level, local education agencies need policies for computer programs. There are numerous questions that should be considered when developing a plan for computer usage in schools. Examples of questions include:

- At the elementary level:
  1. Will we teach our sequence in Logo competencies all together at one grade level, or teach them across grade levels?
  2. How will new transfer students learn the expected level of word processing to benefit from regular instruction?

■ At the secondary level:

1. Will the school offer a separate computer course, mini-course, or unit, for example, or will the mandated skills be integrated into existing courses?

2. How will the school confront the equity questions with a unit, or by the efforts of every teacher who has computers in the classroom?

3. If a high school student does not know keyboarding, how and when will it be taught? (Geisert & Futrell, 1990, p. 216)

Many additional questions should be considered during the plan and policy development. While there is no way that a school can consider all of the questions necessary, initial questions at least result in a starting place for developing a plan and policies.

The entire school district should develop a plan for computers in classrooms. This necessitates that the planning effort should be community-wide. Table 12–5 describes the steps that should be taken in such a planning effort.

TABLE 12-5 Steps in Community-Wide Planning Effort for Computers in Schools

STEP	ACTION
1	Form a community-wide committee of teachers, parents, administrators, and community members.
2	Survey community and school personnel to determine overall computer needs of schools.
3	Set priorities based on needs.
4	Determine how technology, including computers and software, might reduce high priority needs.
5	Determine which computer software is needed to to meet needs.
6	Determine what hardware is necessary to run software.
7	Develop plans for training school personnel.
8	Set goals for school year; include getting hardware and software.
9	Secure equipment and materials; implement plan.
10	Evaluate accomplishments.

Source: Geisert & Futrell, 1990.

SELECTING HARDWARE AND SOFTWARE

Selecting Hardware

Schools that are expanding their computer capabilities often purchase additional computers. There are Apples, IBMs, Commodores, Radio Shacks, and others, plus clones of many of these brand-name computers. Not only do schools have to determine which company to buy from, but what models to purchase. For example, Apple computers come in the old line IIE version and the newer MacIntosh models. Some computers have color monitors, while others do not. Some computers even have voice output capabilities, while others do not. What should schools buy? What do they need?

The main computer line that has dominated the educational scene has been the Apple IIE series. Recently, Apple Computers, Inc., announced that the IIE series would be replaced by the MacIntosh LC. The newer MacIntosh will be capable of using Apple IIE software, as well as software specifically designed for the MacIntosh systems. The main market that the MacIntosh LC targets is schools.

Although the Apple systems have been dominant in education, school personnel may want to consider other brands of computers. For this reason, effort needs to go into planning for the computer hardware needs of the school. If there is no one on the school staff with the expertise to make decisions regarding hardware selection, school administrators should consider working with personnel from other schools, personnel from the state department of education, or paid consultants to help make appropriate decisions. Spending a little money when developing a computer education program could result in buying the right equipment, thus saving time and money in the long run.

Selecting Software

A key component in the success of computer programs for students with disabilities is the software that is available (Shanahan & Ryan, 1984). Appropriate software goes a long way in enhancing the quality of computer-based programs (Chandler, 1987). There are literally thousands of companies that currently produce software, and many of these companies concentrate their efforts on school-based markets. Therefore, school personnel must be cognizant of their software needs and which particular programs represent their best buys.

To date, there is not a great deal of good software available for educational purposes. Although more and more educational software has been developed during the past several years, there is still not any software that is appropriate for all students in all subjects. The limited budgets that schools have had for educational software also restricts the number of programs that schools can purchase in a given academic period (Woolfolk, 1990).

The limited amount of good educational software and the limited budgets to purchase software make it imperative that schools buy the best programs that are available. This requires attention to the way software is purchased. There are several problems in selecting appropriate software: many teachers are not aware of the software that is available (Wallace & Rose, 1984), companies may not be willing to loan software for evaluation purposes for fear of it being copied and not purchased (Smith, 1990), and there is limited knowledge about what to look for when evaluating software (Jolicoeur & Bergen, 1988). Regardless of the problems, software should be thoroughly evaluated before it is purchased. Buying the wrong software can doom the computer education program.

One way to approach software selection is through a selection committee similar to committees that choose textbooks. The committee should include people who are 1. knowledgeable about courses where the materials will be used, 2. knowledgeable about computer technology and education, and 3. experienced in software selection.

One way to review educational software is to use a comprehensive checklist. This ensures that you collect similar information about different software programs for comparison purposes. Figure 12–1 provides an example of a software evaluation checklist. The purpose of such a checklist is simply to have an organized way to record information about particular programs.

Specific Applications of Technology

There are numerous programs that have been developed to teach specific academic skills. For special education teachers, using these specific skills packages might be the most beneficial use of the computer. It would allow individualized instruction and enable the teacher to work with other students while one student works on the computer. The programs can be used to teach initial skills as well as reinforce those already learned.

COMPUTER TECHNOLOGY AND READING

Computer technology can be used to teach reading in a number of different ways. These include the typical computer-assisted instruction activities: 1. drill and practice, 2. tutorials, 3. simulations, and 4. problem solving (Wallace, Cohen, & Polloway, 1989). As a result of the demand for programs, software companies have developed reading programs that can:

- reinforce sight words,

- expand vocabularies,

- provide drill in phonics,

- analyze words according to structural analysis, and

- test comprehension (Mercer, 1987, p. 401).

Research in reading points out that most students with disabilities have problems at the word level in decoding and word recognition skills. Drill-and-practice activities work well to help students improve decoding skills. Current research is insufficient on which to draw any general conclusions about the use of computer programs and reading deficiencies (Hasselbring & Goin, 1989); however, it has been concluded that drill-and-practice activities do enhance decoding skills. Therefore, special education teachers should continue to work with their students on these skills. The main caution is not to rely too much on computers in reading instruction.

Schipper (1991) describes a way to help students with reading problems with a word processing program. Teachers create large signs of compound words from a story that is

FIGURE 12–1 Computer Software Evaluation Form

Computer Software Evaluation Form

Reviewer's Name: _____ Date of Review: _____
Address/Phone #: _____ ( ) _____
Program Title: _____
Size: 5" _____ 3.5" _____
Package Title: _____
Copyright Date: _____
Microcomputer (brand, model, memory): _____
Hardware and/or Peripherals: _____
Necessary Software: _____
Producer: _____ Author(s): _____
Back-up Copy Policy: _____ Cost: _____

PART 1 – Program Overview and Description
1. Subject area and specific: _____
2. Prerequisite skills necessary: _____
3. Target audience: _____ Regular _____ Special needs _____ Category
4. Appropriate grade level (circle): N K 1 2 3 4 5 6 7 8 9 10 11 12
   college
5. Type of program (check one or more):
   _____ Simulation   _____ Testing
   _____ Educational Game   _____ Classroom Management
   _____ Drill and Practice   _____ Remediation
   _____ Tutorial   _____ Enrichment
   _____ Problem Solving   _____ Other (specify)
   _____ Authoring System
6. Appropriate group instructional size: __ individual __ small group __ class
7. Is this program an appropriate instructional use of the computer? _____
8. Briefly list the program's objectives. Are they clearly stated in the
   program or in the documentation?
   Are they educationally valuable?   Are they achieved?
9. Briefly describe the program. Mention any special strengths or
   weaknesses. _____
   _____

continued

FIGURE 12-1   Computer Software Evaluation Form (cont'd.)

PART 2 – Evaluation Checklist
Please answer Yes, No, or Not Applicable for each question below.
To add information, or to clarify an answer, use "Comments" at the end of
each section.

EDUCATIONAL CONTENT
1. Is the program content accurate? _____
2. Is the program content appropriate for intended users? _____
3. Is the difficulty level consistent for material, interest, and vocabulary? __
4. Is the program content free of racial or sexual bias? _____
   Comments: _____
   _____

PRESENTATION
1. Is the program free of technical problems? _____
2. Are the instructions clear? _____
3. Is the curriculum material logically presented and well organized? _____
4. Do graphics, sound, and color enhance the presentation? _____
5. Is the frame display clear and easy to read? _____
   Comments: _____
   _____

INTERACTION
1. Is the feedback effective and appropriate? _____
2. Do cues help students answer questions correctly? _____
3. Can students access the program "menu" for help? _____
4. Can students control the pace and sequence of the program? _____
5. Are there safeguards against students "bombing" the program? _____
   Comments: _____
   _____

TEACHER USE
1. Is the recordkeeping possible within the program? _____
2. Does the teacher have to monitor student use? _____
3. Can the teacher modify the program? _____
4. Is the documentation clear and comprehensive? _____
   Comments: _____
   _____

FIGURE 12-1   Computer Software Evaluation Form (cont'd.)

PART 3 – OVERALL SUMMARY
Check one.
_____ Excellent Program. Recommend without hesitation.
_____ Pretty good program. Consider purchase.
_____ Fair. But might want to wait for something better.
_____ Not useful. Do not recommend purchase.

Note: Adapted from Media Lab, UAB.

   Some demographic data is required regarding the person conducting the rating. The title of the program and the nature of the disk should be documented.

being read in the class with a word processing program. Students then use the words to provide a visual representation of the word to facilitate vocabulary development. Another way to use computers to help students with poor reading skills is to take advantage of speech output of computer technology. Students can then "read" the story on the computer while listening to the story (Schipper, 1991).

COMPUTER TECHNOLOGY AND WRITTEN EXPRESSION

Word processing packages, as previously noted, provide an excellent vehicle for teaching written expression skills. These programs make writing much easier than using the traditional paper and pencil approach. Students can make changes and even check for specific types of errors. Each new draft does not require the student to start over again and rewrite the entire story. Teachers can point out certain changes that need to be made and those changes can be made on the spot. Telling students they have to rewrite an entire four page paper to change a few sentences and make some paragraph indentions is very discouraging. Word processing packages enable students to make these changes very easily and rapidly.

Several word processing programs have been developed specifically for young students and students with disabilities. One of the most popular, the Bank Street Writer, enables students to use word processing with simple, easy to understand commands. This program includes 1. write, 2. edit, and 3. transfer modes (Wallace & McLoughlin, 1988). With this program, as well as with other word processing programs, students are able to edit their work, add or delete sections, and even spell-check their work prior to printing (Wallace *et al.*, 1989). Other programs that are used frequently in schools include the Grammar Problems for Practice by Milliken; Verb Viper, Word Invasion, and Word Master by DLM; and The Writing Adventure by DLM (Mercer, 1987).

Although it is obvious that word processing programs make writing easier, especially to obtain a "clean" and "neat" final copy, how word processing packages help students learn to write has not been fully investigated. Hasselbring and Goin (1989) reviewed the research on this topic and concluded that teaching task-specific writing skills was much more beneficial than teaching generic writing skills. Their basic conclusion was that "more research is needed before a clear understanding of the relationship between the writing process and the computer can be drawn" (p. 405). Still, they recommend that teaching keyboard and word processing skills should be a part of the curriculum for students with mild disabilities.

Schipper (1991) suggests several ways computers can be used to enhance written expression skills. These include having students use computers to sequence story events, changing stories, and keeping logs and journals. The use of computers in written expression exercises can be easily implemented with teachers using a minimum of creativity.

COMPUTER TECHNOLOGY AND SPELLING

Teaching spelling skills to students with disabilities has long been recognized as a problem. These students simply have problems remembering spelling rules and remembering how specific words are spelled. Microcomputer usage has made spelling instruction much more successful. By using this technology, teachers are able to individualize spelling instruction

TABLE 12-6 Examples of Software for Spelling Instruction

NAME OF PROGRAM	PRODUCER	DESCRIPTION
The Spelling System	Milliken	■ for use with Apple II ■ teaches major principles and patterns in spelling English ■ teaches many irregularities ■ teachers can add words ■ contains 4 diskettes & workbook
Spelling Wiz	DLM Teaching Resources	■ for Apple II, IBM, Commodore, Tandy, & Atari ■ focuses on 300 commonly misspelled words in grades 1–6 ■ uses game format
Spelltronics	Educational Activities	■ for Apple II, TRS-80, Commodore, Atari ■ uses letter cloze technique ■ teaches 240 words ■ correct answers are rewarded ■ words are grouped according to concept

Source: C.D. Mercer (1987). *Students with learning disabilities,* 3rd Ed. Columbus, OH: Merrill.

in a way that can accommodate the wide variety of spelling problems presented by some students. Research to date suggests that students with spelling problems benefit a great deal from interventions with computers (Wallace *et al.,* 1989).

Spelling software programs use a variety of techniques to teach spelling skills. These include games, such as hangman and crossword puzzles; the cloze technique to teach generalization skills; and built-in spell-check programs. In addition to spelling instruction, computer software enables spelling assessment (Wallace & McLoughlin, 1988). Table 12–6 describes some of the spelling programs that are available.

Regardless of which computer program is used in spelling instruction, the programs should result in skills deemed desirable by teachers. Hasselbring and Goin (1989) recommend that spelling instructional programs:

■ require the use of long-term memory,

■ be limited in the size of the practice set of words,

■ require practice spread over several different times, and

■ emphasize speed as well as accuracy.

COMPUTER TECHNOLOGY AND MATH

For many students, math is their worst subject. Students with disabilities are even more likely to experience problems in math than their nondisabled peers. Recently there has been a rapid increase in the number and types of math software programs available for students who are experiencing math problems. While most of these programs focus on drill and practice and skill instruction (Wallace & McLoughlin, 1988), they enable teachers to individualize math instruction and focus on specific math skill deficits. Software programs that focus on math instruction use a variety of different formats for motivational purposes. These include games, animation, and sound effects. The self-correcting and immediate feedback capabilities of software programs enable students to find out immediately how they have done. As Mercer (1987) points out, this keeps the students from simply practicing errors.

Hasselbring and Goin (1989) note that for students with some math skills, drill and practice activities work well to help develop fluency, or automaticity. However, for students who cannot remember certain math facts, drill and practice alone will not be beneficial. For these students it is recommended that teachers use a combination of drill and practice and tutorial. The tutoring activities will teach new skills, and the drill and practice will help develop fluency in that skill.

There are several different math programs available that can be used in special education programs. The following provides an example of some of these programs (Mercer, 1987). Keep in mind that these are only examples of programs. Also, with the rapid changes in computer technology, new programs are developed and old programs are changed constantly. Therefore, before purchasing a specific program for any subject area, you should get as much information as possible about different programs that are available to meet specific needs of your students.

Academic Skill Builders in Math This program, produced by DLM Teaching Resources, can be used on Apple, IBM, Commodore, Tandy, and Atari computers. It includes six individual programs in each of the four basic math operations and combinations of operations. Games provide the basic format for the instructional activities.

Basic Skills in Math Love Publishing Company produces this math software package that is designed to work on the Apple II series computers. This program assesses a student's skills in the basic math functions and then branches into an individual program based on the student's performance. Visual and auditory reinforcement are given for correct responses, and after a student achieves mastery at a certain level, a game reinforcer is provided.

Math Sequences This program is produced by Milliken for the Apple and Atari computers. It includes twelve diskettes that focus on drill-and-practice activities for students in grades one through eight. The materials can also be used for older students who are in need of remediation. When students miss a problem more than once, the program presents a step-by-step explanation of how to correctly solve the problem. Records for each student are maintained in the management component of the program.

Math Skills—Elementary Level and *Math Skills—Junior High Level* These programs are produced by Encyclopedia Britannica Educational Corporation. The programs are designed for the Apple computers. Drill-and-practice activities are presented at each different level. Immediate feedback is provided students and instructional activities are presented if students miss problems.

COMPUTER TECHNOLOGY AND OTHER SKILLS

In addition to the basic skills, computer technology can be used to enhance development in other areas. For example, computer programs can help students develop better listening skills. Students can be given directions to follow or questions to answer, and the responses can be recorded immediately through a computer program; immediate feedback is given to the student (Wallace *et al.*, 1989). This program improves listening skills by helping students focus on important auditory cues. The immediate feedback provided facilitates the development of listening.

Assistive Devices

Assistive devices can be defined as "a wide variety of aids, tools, and equipment used by handicapped people to function more effectively in the classroom, the home, and the workplace. These are devices that compensate for sensory, communication, mobility, and manipulation deficits" (Elting, 1987, p. 70). When used properly, assistive devices can help students overcome a wide variety of physical and sensory problems.

Many different assistive devices are available for persons with disabilities. These range from simple, mechanical aids, such as canes and page turners, to very sophisticated computer aids. Examples of these sophisticated computer aids are speech synthesizers, text-to-braille software programs, and computers that "read" materials. Microcomputers represent the most promising development in the area of assistive devices for the future (Elting, 1987). Examples of the use of microcomputers to facilitate communication include voice output components, and sophisticated language boards.

A problem for some persons with physical disabilities is their inability to physically manipulate equipment. For example, a child with cerebral palsy, which significantly restricts arm movements, might be very intelligent but unable to communicate due to speech problems and limited arm and hand use. In order for this person to access and use a computer, various adaptive devices must be used. Microswitches and other adaptive equipment can facilitate access to computers. An example is a mercury switch. The mercury switch operates by turning something on when the device is held upright, and turning it off when the device is horizontal. Even individuals with severe physical problems are capable of operating mercury switches with head movements and other similar physical actions (Parette, Strother, & Hourcade, 1986). Table 12–7 (on page 488) describes some alternative methods of inputting information into computers that will enable many persons with physical problems to use computer technology.

One area where assistive technology is used extensively with students who have disabilities is speech input-output. Speech input-output devices enable students who have reading problems that result from sensory deficits or learning disabilities to obtain information that would be impossible without the devices. These mechanisms also help students who have oral expression problems. Students with cerebral palsy, severe speech impairment, or those with expressive aphasia may be able to communicate with speech output

TABLE 12-7 Alternative Methods of Inputting Information into Computers

1. *Voice recognition.* The computer recognizes speech of user and converts speech into action.

2. *Key guard.* A device that modifies the traditional keyboard to change the size and spacing of the keys.

3. *Graphics tablet.* A small slate that may be covered by templates of words, pictures, numerals, and letters that are input when touched by a special stylus.

4. *Adapted switches.* The student activates the system by using an adapted switch, which is controlled by pressure or body movements. Switches can be activated by foot, head, cheek, chin, and eye movements.

5. *Scanning systems.* An array of letters, phrases, and numerals are displayed on the screen at a rate that is adjusted to the student's need. The student selects the message from the scanner by use of the keyboard or a switch.

6. *Touch screens/light pens.* Devices that allow the student to activate the computer by touching the screen.

7. *Joysticks.* The student controls the movement of the cursor by moving a stick in different directions.

8. *Mouthsticks.* A tool that is placed in the mouth and used to press buttons and activate switches.

9. *Headbands.* The student wears a headband that allows control of the computer through head or eye movements.

10. *Sip and puff systems.* The student sucks on a long command tube attached to a computer or wheelchair.

11. *Skateboard.* A block of wood on rollers attached to the student's arm is moved in different directions to control cursor movements.

Source: S.J. Salend (1990). *Effective mainstreaming.* New York: MacMillan, p. 279. Reprinted with permission.

devices in a much more efficient manner than without them. Wetzel (1991) believes that the availability of such technology will increase in the future and therefore make learning easier for students who require such devices for optimal learning.

Selecting appropriate assistive devices for students with disabilities is a very important function. With technology moving so rapidly, it is virtually impossible for school personnel to keep up with all of the advances that are being made in the area of technology and disabilities. There may be specific devices available that would greatly enhance the success of a particular student, but local school personnel and parents might be unaware of the equipment.

One way to avoid the problem of not knowing what is available is to utilize assistive device services. Elting (1987) reported that several states have already developed state-supported assistive device programs, including Pennsylvania, Missouri, Florida, Ohio, New Jersey, California, and Massachusetts. These information centers provide a centralized support system that keeps up to date with the latest developments in assistive devices for persons with disabilities. Schools and parents can access current information simply by contacting these programs.

Resources for Computer Usage

As a result of the computer technology explosion, computer software and hardware entrepreneurs have multiplied rapidly. Many of these software and hardware companies specialize in educationally oriented wares. For many teachers and administrators who are not trained proficiently in computer technology, knowing what to buy and where to buy it can be a problem. Therefore, personnel from schools responsible for purchasing materials and implementing programs need to rely on information from sources that are knowledgeable about computer technology and education.

There are numerous sources of information that will help school personnel make decisions about hardware and software purchases. Wallace *et al.* (1988) list sources for computer-assisted programming and computer software and equipment in tables 12–8 and 12–9. Table 12–10 provides a listing of guides to special education resources for computers.

TABLE 12–8 Sources of Computer-Assisted Programming

Bulletin on Science and Technology
  for the Handicapped
AAAS
1515 Massachusetts Avenue, NW
Washington, DC 20005

Closing the Gap
P.O. Box 68
Henderson, MN 56044

Communication Enhancement
  Clinic
The Childrens Hospital
300 Longwood Avenue
Boston, MA 02115

Communication Outlook
Artificial Language Laboratory
Computer Science Department
Michigan State University
East Lansing, MI 48824

Department of Speech Pathology
  and Audiology
University of South Alabama
Mobile, AL 36688

Journal of Special Education Technology
Exceptional Child Center
Utah State University
Logan, UT 84322

LINC Resources, Inc.
1875 Morse Road, Suite 225
Columbus, OH 43299

Software Registry
CUSH
James Fitch, Editor
Department of Speech Pathology and
  Audiology
University of South Alabama
Mobile, AL 36688

The Handicapped Source
101 Route 46 East
Pine Brook, NJ 07058

Trace Center International Software and
  Hardware Registry
University of Wisconsin-Madison
314 Waisman Center
1500 Highland Avenue
Madison, WI 53706

Source: S. Edwards (1987). Preschool handicapped children. In G. Wallace, S.B. Cohen, & E.A. Polloway, (Eds.). *Language arts*, Austin, TX: Pro-Ed., p. 362. Reprinted with permission.

Table 12-9 Sources of Computer Software and Equipment

Aspen Systems Corporation P.O. Box 6018 Gaithersburg, MD 20877	Institute on Technology P.O. Box 1155 Brookline, MA 02146	Prentke Romich Company 8769 Township Road 513 Shreve, OH 44676-9421
Crestwood Company P.O. Box 0406 Milwaukee, WI 53204	Intellectual Software 798 North Avenue Bridgeport, CT 06606	Quest Publishers and Distributors, Inc. P.O. Box 7952 Richmond, VA 23221
Don Johnston Developmental Equipment 981 Winnetka Terrace Lake Zurich, Il 60047	Koala Technologies Corp. 3100 Patrick Henry Drive Santa Clara, CA 95950	Softkey Systems, Inc. 4737 Hibiscus Avenue Edina, MN 55435
EKEG Electronics Co., Ltd. P.O. Box 46199 Station G Vancouver, BC V6R 4G5	Laureate Learning Systems, Inc. One Mill Street Burlington, VT 05401	Street Electronics Corp. 1140 Mark Avenue Carpinteria, CA 93013
Graphic Learning Corporation P.O. Box 4649 Richmond, VA 23229	Parrot Software 190 Sandy Ridge Road State College, PA 16803	Unicorn Engineering Co. 6201 Harwood Avenue Oakland, CA 94618

Source: S. Edwards (1987). Preschool handicapped children. In G. Wallace, S.B. Cohen, & E.A. Polloway, (Eds.). *Language arts,* Austin, TX: Pro-Ed., p. 360. Reprinted with permission.

Table 12-10 Guide to Special Education Resources

1. Apple Computer Resources in Special Education and Rehabilitation
   (Details hardware and software, and product catalogs)
   Office of Special Education
   Programs/MS 43 F
   Apple Computer Inc.
   20525 Mariani Avenue
   Cupertino, CA 95014

2. Catalyst
   (A quarterly newspaper highlighting reviews, and resource guide)
   Western Center for Microcomputers in Special Education
   1259 El Camino Real, Suite 275
   Menlo Park, CA 94025

3. Closing the Gap
   (Bi-monthly publication on technology for the handicapped with a special February edition
   documenting resources which are highly recommended).
   Closing the Gap
   P.O. Box 68
   Henderson, MN 56044

4. Computer Disability News
   (A quarterly paper reviewing articles and books plus a column listing public domain software)
   Computer Disability News
   The Easter Seal Society
   70 East Lake St.
   Chicago, IL 60601

5. IBM National Support
   Center for Persons with Disabilities Resource Guides
   (5 different guides for mobility, hearing, speech, language, learning, and vision)
   IBM National Support Center for Persons with Disabilities
   P.O. Box 2150
   Atlanta, GA 30055

Source: Morgan, B. (1990). A guide to special education resources. *Electronic Learning,* February, 26–27.

Software for students with disabilities has flooded the markets over the past several years. It ranges from materials on teaching reading to materials that focus on social skills. To show the wide variety of available software, examples are described below:

Syllable Square Grades three through twelve. This syllable-oriented word game challenges students to put syllables together to form over 1,500 words. The object of the game is to put two- and three-syllable words together to clear the board. It can be used with one or two players and is game oriented. Helps students develop hand-eye coordination, sequencing, reading, and spelling skills. (Cambridge Development Laboratory, 1991 catalog)

The Children's Writing and Publishing Center Grades two through eight. This desktop publishing in an easy-to-use format helps students improve their skills in the area of written expression and makes writing fun and rewarding. (Cambridge Development Laboratory, 1991 catalog)

Memory Match Grades one through four. This is a concentration game that allows students to play the computer or other students. The program requires students to use observation and thinking skills. (Cambridge Development Laboratory, 1991 catalog)

Where in Europe is Carmen San Diego? Grades four through twelve. This program helps students develop deductive reasoning, reference and research skills, and teaches history, economics, government, and culture. It is part of a series that targets different geographic areas. (Cambridge Development Laboratory, 1991 catalog)

Math and Me Grades K through two. This colorful and motivating program teaches basic math skills. Students are given opportunities for determining the correct answer, even after a failure. (Cambridge Development Laboratory, 1991 catalog)

IBM Spelling Series Grades four through twelve. Using a combination of practice, tests, and games, this program helps students develop spelling skills with most familiar words used at various ages. (BrainTrain, 1991–1992 catalog)

That's My Story Grades two through eight. This program encourages students to write using a motivational structure. Uses twelve short story starters to help get students started. (BrainTrain, 1991–1992 catalog)

Muppetville Grades Preschool through one. Using the Muppet characters, it helps students learn memory, matching, discrimination, addition, visual-association, and self-testing skills. (BrainTrain, 1991–1992 catalog)

Stickybear Reading Grades K through two. Using animated characters, it helps students develop vocabulary and reading comprehension skills. Students match words and pictures. (BrainTrain, 1991–1992 catalog)

These examples of computer software are briefly described to convey the wide range of different materials available for educational use. Teachers and school personnel must evaluate software to determine if it meets their needs and the needs of their students. Purchasing software because it looks good, is inexpensive, and because other people like it are not sufficient reasons.

The Future and Computers in Special Education

Although the future is difficult to predict, all signs point to a very positive outlook regarding the use of computer technology with special education populations. As computers become easier to operate, as teachers become more skilled in adapting curricula to computer uses, and as research identifies the best ways to teach students using computers, the application of this technology to special education should become more successful.

Several current trends in technology are predicted to continue in the future. For example, the miniaturization of hardware will likely continue (Heinich et al., 1985). It was not but a very few years ago that computers capable of performing any major task were huge, actually taking up space in several rooms. Now, microcomputers the size of notebooks can perform more activities in a much quicker time than many of the old "mainframe" computers.

It is likely that in the future, students in our schools will use computers just as they use calculators today. All students will have access to computers through a variety of input devices, many of which are not even presently developed. Computers will be an integral part of schools, classrooms, and student's equipment and materials (Lockard *et al.*, 1987). Technology to alter states of human consciousness and provide bionic extensions of the brain will even become available as we move into the twenty-first century (Heinich, 1985).

Specific predictions concerning computers and education were made by Nickerson and Zodhiates (1988).

1. The speed of the devices used for computing and for storing information will continue to increase, while their size, power requirements, and cost will continue to decrease. These trends have characterized computer technology for several decades and will probably continue to do so for the foreseeable future.
2. Computer systems that realize orders of magnitude increase in computing power by exploiting parallel multi-processor architectures will become increasingly common.
3. Remote wireless terminals will provide access to computer networks and thereby to central repositories of information of nearly every conceivable type.
4. Microprocessor-based computing power will be everywhere—in household appliances, in hand tools, in games and toys, in clothing.
5. Software will be available for an increasingly extensive array of applications and much of it will have potential for serving educational purposes.
6. Software also will be developed that will permit the supplementation of conventional text with dynamic graphics, including process simulations, that should enhance the effectiveness of expository material.
7. Multimedia communication facilities, allowing the mixing of text, images, and speech will become widely available.
8. User-oriented languages and "front ends" to applications software will become increasingly easy for people without technical training to use. How soon truly natural-language capabilities will be available is difficult to say; however, systems with useful aspects of natural language and limited speech input and output capabilities will proliferate.
9. Computer-based information services addressed to a diversity of objectives—job posting, want ads, selective news, information searches—will also proliferate.
10. Increasingly powerful tools to facilitate interacting with very large data bases—both for directed searching and for browsing—will be developed (p. 2).

The role of teachers in the future of technology is critical. Teachers will be the ones who help develop a vision about how computer technology can be used (Lockard *et al.*, 1987). This vision will then be used by scientists and technicians to develop the actual hardware and software to turn classrooms in the next century into computerized learning centers.

For special education, rehabilitation, and other programs that provide services to persons with disabilities, the future of technology is unimaginable. Even in the 1990s we are seeing computer technology used to enable very incapacitated persons with quadriplegia to function in a "normalized" environment; machines actually read to persons who are blind. Computer technology is helping persons with paralysis move their immobile arms and legs. And, certain assistive devices permit individuals with physical disabilities to access a multitude of aids.

With all of these benefits already existing for persons with disabilities as a result of technology, the future can only be very bright. Computers will undoubtedly continue to make persons with disabilities more capable of achieving at their maximum levels, regardless of what those levels may be. Since this is a major goal of special educational services, computer technology will continue to be a major part of intervention programs provided by special education teachers.

The use of computers in conjunction with video discs will likely increase in the future. Video disc technology uses discs, similar to records, for audio-visual productions. They can be used either alone, or in conjunction with computers. When video discs are used with computers, students have the capability of interacting with the program. They can use the computer keyboard or a special touch sensitive monitor to interact. As video disc technology expands, its use with computers will likely be increased, making this new technology

SUMMARY

This chapter has focused on technology and students with mild disabilities. Although technology was defined as including a variety of different machines and approaches, computer technology was the main topic in this chapter. It was initially pointed out that our world is in a technological revolution. What is new in technology today is already out of date tomorrow. Technology seems to be moving faster and faster; the future will likely see even more rapid gains made than in the past.

The next section of the chapter focused on how computers are used in schools. It was noted that the number of microcomputers in schools currently exceeds two million, with the number continuing to increase each year. The effects of computers on instruction was discussed. It was generally concluded that the use of computers in education resulted in positive outcomes by students. Computers have been found to be motivating, capable of maintaining attention, and providing timely reinforcement and feedback to students.

Computers are used in schools two primary ways: for administrative purposes and for instruction. Administratively, computers assist in tracking students, keeping records, and developing individual education programs. For instructional purposes, computers are used either in computer-managed instruction or computer-assisted instruction. In computer-managed instruction, computers assess students' skills, develop appropriate programs, and track students' progress through an education program. The record keeping capabilities of computer-managed instruction make life for teachers and administrators much easier, and the quality of services likely improve.

Computer-assisted instruction (CAI) is the most popular way computers are used in schools. CAI can be implemented with 1. drill and practice, 2. tutorials, 3. simulations, 4. problem solving, and 5. word processing. Drill and practice is the most likely used component of CAI. Using this strategy, students practice basic skills that they have learned. Drill and practice should be used only if the student has learned a skill. Having a student engage in drill-and-practice activities on computers in skills in which they are not competent is of little use to the student.

Tutorials are used to teach new skills to students and is often used in conjunction with drill and practice. Simulations offer an opportunity to "simulate" real-life situations for learning purposes. Problem-solving components of CAI teach students to analyze situations and apply problem-solving steps to resolve the problem. Problem solving and simulations are often used together to have students solve problems in a simulated situation. Finally, word processing allows students to write using computers and software. Word processing programs enable students to add text, change text, delete text, and often even spell-check text. These components make the writing process much easier for students, especially students with mild disabilities.

One section of the chapter focused on the need to initiate planning when implementing computer programs. District plans and policies regarding computer instruction should be developed before widespread activities begin. Also, select activities should occur before purchasing hardware and software for the district. Without adequate equipment and materials, the best school program will not be successful.

The final section of the chapter dealt with the future of computer technology in schools. Our world is continuing in a technology frenzy that is not likely to slow down. As our "chips" get smaller and more powerful, our computer technology changes in its scope. Better applications of technology to educational settings will likely develop from research and practice. The use of microcomputer technology in special education, especially with mildly disabled populations, will only increase substantially.

REFERENCES

Bruder, S. (1989). Ninth annual survey of the states. *Electronic Learning, 9*, 22–28.

Bruder, S. (1990). Computer coordinator survey. *Electronic Learning, 9*, 24–29.

Budoff, M., Thorman, J., & Gras, A. (1985). *Microcomputers in special education.* Cambridge: Brookline Books.

Cain, E.J. (1984). The challenge of technology; Educating the exceptional child for the world of tomorrow. *Teaching Exceptional Children, 16*, 239–241.

Chandler, H.N. (1987). Database. *Journal of Learning Disabilities, 20*, 58–59.

Collins, A. (1991). The role of computer technology in restructuring schools. *Phi Delta Kappan, 73*, 28–35.

Cosden, M.A., Gerber, M.M., Semmel, D.S., Goldman, S.R., & Semmel, M.I. (1987). Microcomputer use within micro-educational environments. *Exceptional Children, 53*, 399–409.

Cosden, M., & Semmel, M. (1987). Developmental changes in micro-educational environments for learning handicapped and non-learning handicapped elementary school students. *Journal of Special Education Technology, 8*, 1–13.

David, J.L. (1991). Restructuring and technology: Partners in change. *Phi Delta Kappan, 73*, 37–40.

Doll, C. (1987). *Evaluating educational software.* Chicago: American Library Association.

Elting, S. (1987). Special education assistive device services. *Teaching Exceptional Children, 19*, 70–71.

Gagne, R.M. (1987). *Instructional technology: Foundations.* Hillsdale, NJ: Lawrence Erlbaum Associates.

Gearheart, B.R., Weishahn, M.W., & Gearheart, C.J. (1988). *The exceptional student in the regular classroom,* 4th Ed. Columbus, OH: Merrill.

Geisert, P., & Futrell, M. (1990). *Teachers, computers, and curriculum.* Boston: Allyn and Bacon.

Goodspeed, J. (1988). Two million microcomputers now used in U.S. schools. *Electronic Learning, 7*, 16.

Hammill, D.D., & Bartel, N.R. (1990). *Teaching students with learning and behavior problems*, 5th Ed. Boston: Allyn & Bacon.

Haring, N.G. Introduction. In N.G. Haring & L. McCormick (Eds.). *Exceptional Children and Youth*, 5th Ed. Columbus, OH: Merrill.

Hasselbring, T.S., & Goin, L.I. (1989). Use of Computers. In G.A. Robinson, J.R. Patton, E.A. Polloway, & L.R. Sargent (Eds.). *Best Practices in Mild Mental Disabilities*. Reston, VA: Division on Mental Retardation, Council for Exceptional Children.

Hatch, J.A. (1984). Technology and devaluation of human processes. *Educational Forum, 48*, 243–251.

Heinich, R., Molenda, M., Russel, J. (1985). *Instructional media*, 2nd Ed. New York: Macmillan.

Higgins, K., & Boone, R. (1990). Hypertext: A new vehicle for computer use in reading instruction. *Intervention, 26*, 26–31.

Hofmeister, A.M. (1989). Teaching with videodiscs. *Teaching Exceptional Children, 21*, 52–54.

Jolicoeur, K., & Berger, D.E. (1988). Implementing educational software and evaluating its academic effectiveness: Part I. *Educational Technology, 28*, 7–13.

Kinzer, C., Sherwood, R., & Bransford, J. (1986). *Computer strategies for education: Foundations and content-area applications*. Columbus, OH: Merrill.

Lindsey, J. (1987). *Computers and exceptional individuals*. Columbus, OH: Merrill.

Lint, G. (1984). *PennStar IEP and planned course system*. Harrisburg, PA: Pennsylvania Department of Education.

Lockard, J., Abrams, P., & Many, W. (1990). *Microcomputers for educators*, 2nd Ed. Glenview, IL: Scott, Foresman.

Majsterek, D.J. (1989). Computer-assisted instruction for elementary schoolchildren with learning disabilities. *LD Forum, 15*, 31–33.

McCarthy, B. (1989). The K-12 hardware industry. A heated race that shows no sign of letting up. *Electronic Learning, 8*, 5–9.

Mercer, C.D. (1987). *Students with Learning Disabilities*, 3rd Ed. Columbus, OH: Merrill.

Nelson, P., & Waack, W. (1985). The status of computer literacy/computer-assisted instruction awareness as a factor in classroom instruction and teacher selection. *Educational Technology, 25*, 23–26.

Nickerson, R., & Zodhiates, P. (1988). *Technology in education: Looking toward 2020*. Hillsdale, NJ: Lawrence Erlbaum Assoc.

Panyan, M. (1988). MACS Training, Project RETOOL. Prescott, AZ.

Parette, H.P, Strother, P.O., & Hourcade, J.J. (1986). Microswitches and adaptive equipment for severely impaired students. *Teaching Exceptional Children, 19*,15–18.

Percival, F., & Ellington, H. (1988). *A handbook of educational technology*. London: Kogan Page.

Reid, D.K. (1988). *Teaching the learning disabled*. Boston: Allyn & Bacon.

Rich, T. (1991). Computer technology and education: Past performance and future promise. *Educational and Training Technology International, 28*, 147–152.

Salend, S.J. (1990). *Effective mainstreaming*. New York: Macmillan.

Salend, S.J., & Salend, S.M. (1985). Implications of using microcomputers in classroom testing. *Journal of Learning Disabilities, 18*, 51–53.

Schipper, D. (1991). Practical ideas: Literature, computers, and students with special needs. *The Computing Teacher, 19*, 33–37.

Shanahan, D., & Ryan, A.W. (1984). A tool for evaluating educational software. *Teaching Exceptional Children, 16*, 242–247.

Sloane, H., Gordon, H., Gunn, C., & Mickelsen, V. (1989). *Evaluating educational software: A guide for teachers*. Englewood Cliffs, NJ: Prentice-Hall.

Smith, T.E.C. (1990). *Introduction to education*, 2nd Ed. St. Paul: West Publishing.

Tannenhaus, J. (1989). What's new in special education software? Part Two. *Closing the Gap, 9,* 12–15.

Tannenhaus, J. (1990). Public domain software: A hidden resource. *Closing the Gap, 10,* 16–17.

Turkel, S.B., & Podell, D.M. (1984). Computer-assisted learning for mildly handicapped students. *Teaching Exceptional Children, 16,* 258–262.

Wallace, G. and McLoughlin, J.A. (1988). *Learning Disabilities: Concepts and Characteristics,* 3rd Ed. Columbus, OH: Merrill.

Wallace, G., Cohen, S.B., & Polloway, E.A. (1988). *Language arts: Teaching exceptional students.* Austin, TX: Pro-Ed.

Wallace, J., & Rose, R.M. (1984). A hard look at software: What to examine and evaluate (with an evaluation form). *Educational Technology, 24,* 35–39.

Wetzel, K. (1991). Speech technology II: Future software and hardware predictions. *The Computing Teacher, 19,* 19–21.

Woolfolk, A.E. (1990). *Educational psychology.* Englewood Cliffs, New Jersey: Prentice-Hall.

Yin, R.K., & Moore, G.B. (1987). The use of advanced technologies in special education: Prospects from robotics, artificial intelligence, and computer simulation. *Journal of Learning Disabilities, 20,* 60–63.

Zimmerman, S.O. (1988). Problem-solving tasks on the microcomputer: A look at the performance of students with learning disabilities. *Journal of Learning Disabilities, 21,* 637–641.

TABLE AND FIGURE CREDITS

Table 2–3	From "Needs of learning disabled adults" by F. J. Hoffman, K. L. Sheldon, E. H. Minskoff, S. W. Sautter, E. F. Steidel, M. B. Bailey, & L. D. Echols (1987). *Journal of Learning Disabilities, 20,* 43–52. Copyright 1987 by the Donald D. Hammill Foundation. Reprinted by permission.
Figure 2–1	Reprinted with the permission of Merrill, an imprint of Macmillan Publishing Company from *Characteristics of Behavior Disorders of Children and Youth,* Fourth Edition by James M. Kaufman. Copyright © 1989, 1985, 1981 by Merrill Publishing Company.
Figure 3–1	From Special education as development capital, *Exceptional Children, 37,* p. 236. Copyright 1970 by The Council of Exceptional Children. Reprinted with permission.
Figure 3–2	Adapted figure from *Exceptional Children in the Schools, Special Education in Transition,* Second Edition by Lloyd M. Dunn, copyright © 1973 by Holt Rinehart and Winston, Inc., reprinted by permission of the publisher.
Figure 4–4	Reprinted with permission of Merrill, an imprint of Macmillan Publishing Company from *Developing and Implementing Individual Education Programs,* Third Edition by Bonnie B. Strickland and Ann P. Turnbull. Copyright © 1990, 1982, 1978 by Merrill Publishing Company.
Table 5–1	From *Informal Assessment in Education* by Gilbert R. Guerin and Arlee S. Maier by permission of Mayfield Publishing Company. Copyright © 1983 by Mayfield Publishing Company.
Tables 5–3 and 5–4	Reprinted with the permission of Merrill, an imprint of Macmillan Publishing Company from *Direct Instructional Reading,* Second Edition by Douglas Carnine, Jerry Silbert, Edward J. Kameenui. Copyright © 1990 by Macmillan Publishing Company. Copyright © 1979 by Macmillan Publishing Company.
Table 5–7	Reprinted with the permission of Merrill, and imprint of Macmillan Publishing Company from *Students with Learning Disabilities,* Third Edition by Cecil D. Mercer. Copyright © 1987, 1983, 1979 by Merrill Publishing Company.
Table 5–9	"The Dolch Word List Reexamined" by Dale D. Johnson, *The Reading Teacher,* February 1971, pp. 455–456. Reprinted with permission of Dale D. Johnson and the International Reading Association.
Table 6–1	Reprinted with permission from the *Journal of School Psychology, 24,* S. Graham, A review of handwriting scales and factors. Copyright © 1986, Pergamon Press plc.
Table 6–5	Reprinted with the permission of Merrill, an imprint of Macmillan Publishing Company from *Teaching Students with Leaning Problems,* Third Edition by Cecil D. Mercer and Ann R. Mercer. Copyright © 1989 by Macmillan Publishing Company. Copyright © 1985 by Macmillan Publishing Company.
Table 6–9	Reprinted with the permission of Merrill, an imprint of Macmillan Publishing Company from *Language Assessment and Intervention for the Learning Disabled,* Second Edition by Elizabeth Hemmersam Wiig and Eleanor Semel. Copyright © 1984, 1980 by Bell & Howell Company.
Figure 6–2	From "Write right—or left: A practical approach to handwriting" by R. A. Hagin (1983), *Journal of Learning Disabilities, 16,* 266–271. Copyright 1983 by the Donald D. Hammill Foundation. Reprinted by permission.

INDEX